TACTICAL EMERGENCY CARE

CARE

Military and Operational Out-of-Hospital Medicine

Robert A. De Lorenzo, MD, FACEP

MAJOR, MEDICAL CORPS, U.S. ARMY

Robert Porter, MA, EMT-P, Flight Paramedic

AIRONE, ONONDAGA COUNTY SHERIFF DEPARTMENT

Brady
Prentice Hall
Upper Saddle River, New Jersey 07458

Library of Congress Cataloging-in-Publication Data
De Lorenzo, Robert A.
 Tactical emergency care : military and operational out-of-hospital medicine /
Robert De Lorenzo and Robert S. Porter.
    p.   cm.
 Includes bibliographical references and index.
 ISBN 0-8359-5325-4 (alk. paper)
 1. Medicine, Military. 2. Emergency medicine. 3. Disaster medicine. I.
Porter, Robert S., 1950–   . II. Title.
RC971.D4 1998
616.9'8023--dc21   98-52453
                                                                          CIP

Publisher: Julie Alexander
Acquisitions Editor: Sherene Miller
Editorial Assistant: Jean Auman
Marketing Manager: Tiffany Price
Marketing Coordinator: Cindy Frederick
Director of Production and Manufacturing: Bruce Johnson
Managing Production Editor: Patrick Walsh
Senior Production Manager: Ilene Sanford
Production Editor: Larry Hayden IV
Creative Director: Marianne Frasco
Photography: Skip Surre, Joshua Vayer
Cover design: Marianne Frasco
Composition: Lido Graphics
Presswork and Binding: R.R. Donnelley, Harrisonburg, Virginia

 ©1999 by Prentice-Hall, Inc.
Upper Saddle River, New Jersey 07458

Printed in the United States of America

10 9 8 7 6 5 4

ISBN 0-8359-5325-4

Prentice-Hall International (UK) Limited, *London*
Prentice-Hall of Australia Pty., Limited, *Sydney*
Prentice-Hall Canada Inc., *Toronto*
Prentice-Hall Hispanoamericana, S.A., *Mexico*
Prentice-Hall of India Private Limited, *New Delhi*
Prentice-Hall of Japan, Inc., *Tokyo*
Editoria Prentice-Hall do Brasil, Ltda., *Rio de Janeiro*

Contents

Preface

This textbook was borne out of a need for a professionally written emergency care text dealing with tactical medicine issues. It is designed to complement existing and successful emergency care teaching textbooks. This text builds on the strong foundation of recognized emergency care principles and practices. It is not intended to replace these principles but rather build on them. As such, the goal of this book is to present the principles of tactical emergency care against the backdrop of the nationally recognized curriculums and standards for emergency care and prehospital education. In that vein, we have strived to present as much new or reworked material as possible, drawing from the very best medical and military sources available.

The intended audience is students and practitioners of emergency care in the tactical environment, including Army combat medics, Navy and Coast Guard corpsmen, Air Force medical technicians, and civilian EMTs and paramedics supporting tactical law enforcement and SWAT teams and paramilitary forces. Special operations medics, independent-duty corpsman and technicians, physicians, physician assistants, and nurses will also appreciate the state-of-the-art tactical medical approach. Disaster medical workers will find the principles of this text valuable in their work, particularly in light of the austere conditions faced in many disasters. EMS providers, including first responders, EMTs, and paramedics wishing to expand their knowledge or with an interest in preparing for situations not covered in traditional EMS textbooks, will find this volume particularly helpful. Hazardous materials experts will especially appreciate the detailed coverage of self-protection and decontamination of nuclear, biologic, and chemical agents.

Because this textbook appeals to a wide variety of prehospital providers, both in and out of the military, police, and tactical units, we have adopted the generic term *medic* to describe the tactical field provider. The time-honored title of medic is borrowed from military usage and dates back at least to World War II, when it referred to enlisted (and sometimes officer) medical personnel. For this textbook, the medic may be trained at various levels, including basic or advanced life support. Nonetheless, to maintain unity, we will usually use the term *medic* to describe all the various tactical providers, unless specifically stated otherwise. Certainly, all providers are expected to operate at their level of training and within their system of medical control.

Where possible, this book focuses on the primary standard of care found in the tactical environment. As such, this textbook encompasses a broad mix of basic and advanced life support techniques and strategies, and even introduces some new (to the traditional out-of-hospital arena) approaches. The textbook assumes the reader is well grounded in the principles of basic emergency medical technology practice. Airway, breathing, and bleeding control are emphasized along with rapid removal from the hostile environment. Penetrating trauma is a big part of tactical medicine and receives emphasis.

Trauma is by no means the only component of tactical field care, however. Care of nuclear, biologic, and chemical casualties is now a great concern, as is preventive care and environmental medicine. A new concept in civilian EMS (but a tradition in the military) is the out-of-hospital practice of providing ambulatory care for minor field problems, such as headache and sore throat. A chapter is devoted to this new concept, using the successful military model as a springboard. A chapter is also devoted to the emerging field of tactical law enforcement medical support, or tactical EMS.

The emerging threat of terrorist attack using weapons of mass destruction, including biologic agents, nuclear weapons, incendiary devices, chemical agents, and explosives (the so-called BNICE threats) is covered in detail. All domestic providers from civilian rescuers to National Guard service members need to be familiar with this material. Finally, several appendices outline specific and useful information on field drugs, tactical airway management and fluid administration, manual carries, and protection against nuclear, chemical and biologic threats.

It is our goal to provide the first textbook on tactical emergency care. We have relied on the best sources of information from all three military services, law enforcement medical support organizations, and others with an interest in tactical care. A thorough review of the literature supports the recommendations and guidelines in the text. Readers desiring this information are directed to the reading list at the end of each chapter. In some cases, our advice goes beyond what any one military service or agency uses as established doctrine. This was necessary to provide a single recommendation that was usable in most, if not all, services and circumstances. In all cases, however, the tactical medical recommendation is based on sound medical principles and represents the very best in patient care. Readers wishing to offer suggestions for improvement are invited to contact the authors through the publisher. Lastly, we wish to thank our friends and colleagues for supporting us in this project, and especially to my (R.A.D.) wife Karen for her patience and loving support.

R.A.D. & R.S.P.

NOTICES

Drugs and Drug Dosages

Every effort has been made to ensure that the drug dosages presented in this textbook are in accordance with nationally accepted standards. When applicable, the dosages and routes are taken from the American Heart Association's Advanced Cardiac Life Support Guidelines. The American Medical Association's publication *Drug Evaluations*, and the material published in the *Physician's Desk Reference*, are followed with regard to drug dosages not covered by the American Heart Association's guidelines. It is the responsibility of the reader to be familiar with the drugs used in his or her system, as well as the dosages specified by the medical director. The drugs presented in this book should only be administered by direct order, either verbally or through accepted standing orders, of a licensed physician.

Gender Usage

The English language has historically given preference to the male gender. Among many words, the pronouns "he" and "his" are commonly used to describe both genders. Society evolves faster than language and the male pronouns still predominate in our speech. The authors have made great effort to treat the two genders equally, recognizing that a significant percentage of paramedics are female. However, in some instances, male pronouns may be used to describe both male and female paramedics solely for the purpose of brevity. This is not intended to offend any readers of the female gender.

Photographs

Please note that many of the photographs contained in this book are taken of actual emergency situations. As such, it is possible that they may not accurately depict current, appropriate, or advisable practices of emergency medical care. They have been included for the sole purpose of giving general insight into real-life emergency settings.

Body Substance Isolation Precautions and Personal Protective Equipment

Emergency response personnel should practice Body Substance Isolation (BSI), a strategy that considers ALL body substances potentially infectious. To achieve this, all emergency personnel should utilize personal protective equipment (PPE). Appropriate PPE should be available on every emergency vehicle. The minimum recommended PPE includes the following.

- **Gloves.** Disposable gloves should be donned by all emergency response personnel BEFORE initiating any emergency care. When an emergency incident involves more than one patient, you should attempt to change gloves between patients. When gloves have been contaminated, they should be removed as soon as possible. To properly remove contaminated gloves, grasp one glove approximately one inch from the wrist. Without touching the inside of the glove, pull the glove half-way off and stop. With that half gloved hand, pull the glove on the opposite hand completely off. Place the removed glove in the palm of the other glove, with the inside of the removed glove exposed. Pull the second glove completely off with the ungloved hand, only touching the inside of the glove. Always wash hands after gloves are removed, even when the gloves appear intact.

- **Masks and Protective Eyewear.** Masks and protective equipment should be present on all emergency vehicles and used in accordance with the level of exposure encountered. Masks and protective eyewear should be worn together whenever blood spatter is likely to occur, such as arterial bleeding, childbirth, endotracheal intubation, invasive procedures, oral suctioning, and clean-up of equipment that requires heavy scrubbing or brushing. Both you and the patient should wear masks whenever the potential for airborne transmission of disease exists.

- **HEPA Respirators.** Due to the resurgence of tuberculosis (TB), prehospital personnel should protect themselves from TB infection through use of a high-efficiency particulate air (HEPA) respirator, a design approved by the National Institute of Occupational Safety and Health (NIOSH). It should fit snugly and be capable of filtering out the tuberculosis bacillus. The HEPA respirator should be worn when caring for patients with confirmed or suspected TB. This is especially true when performing "high hazard" procedures such as administration of nebulized medications, endotracheal intubation, or suctioning on such a patient.

- **Gowns.** Gowns protect clothing from blood splashes. If large splashes of blood are expected, such as with childbirth, wear impervious gowns.
- **Resuscitation Equipment.** Disposable resuscitation equipment should be the primary means of artificial ventilation in emergency care. Such items should be used once, then disposed of.

Remember, the proper use of personal protective equipment ensures effective infection control and minimizes risk. Use ALL protective equipment recommended for any particular situation to ensure maximum protection. Consider ALL body substances potentially infectious and ALWAYS practice body substance isolation.

Department of Defense

The opinions or assertions in this text are solely the authors' and do not necessarily represent the official views of the Department of Defense.

AUTHOR BIOS

Robert A. De Lorenzo, MD, FACEP
Major, Medical Corps, Flight Surgeon, US Army
Ft. Sam Houston, Texas
Clinical Associate Professor of Military and Emergency Medicine
Uniformed Services University of the Health Sciences
Bethesda, Maryland

Robert De Lorenzo is a major in the US Army on active duty. He has over 18 years experience in traditional EMS settings, including basic EMT, paramedic, training officer, and medical director. He is also expert in military medicine and specializes in tactical emergency medicine. He is author of numerous EMS and military articles in the medical peer-review and EMS literature.

Robert S. Porter, MA, EMT-P
Senior Advanced Life Support Educator, Madison County EMS
Hamilton, NY
Flight Paramedic, AirOne, Onondaga County Sheriff Department
Syracuse, NY

Bob Porter is the Senior Advanced Life Support Educator for Madison County, New York, and a flight paramedic with AirOne, of the Onondaga County Sheriff's Department. He is coauthor of the successful Brady series of EMS textbooks including Paramedic Emergency Care and Intermediate Emergency Care. He has over 25 years of EMS education and administrative experience and is considered a national leader in EMS education.

Contributing Author

Joshua S. Vayer, BA, CSA
Director, Casualty Care Research Center &
Research Assistant Professor of Military and Emergency Medicine
Uniformed Services University of the Health Sciences
Bethesda, Maryland

GENERAL REVIEWERS

The authors are grateful to the following individuals who shared their time and expertise in helping integrate the wealth of material in this book. Their efforts were instrumental in shaping the final form of the book. Their appearance here does not constitute endorsement by their respective agencies.

Guillermo J. Pierluisi, M.D
Dept. of Emergency Medicine
University of Pittsburg

Mary Ann Harrison
Joint Special Operations
Medical Training Center
Ft. Bragg, NC

LCdr. Richard Wolfe
Naval School of Health
Sciences, Bethesda, MD

TECHNICAL REVIEWERS

The authors are grateful to the following reviewers for sharing their technical expertise. Their voluntary contributions were an enormous help in achieving the best book possible. Their appearance here does not constitute endorsement by their respective agencies.

Col. James A. Pfaff, MD, FACEP
Brooke Army Medical Center, Ft. Sam Houston, TX

Sgt. 1st Class Robert Malloy, EMT-P
US Army Medical Department
Center and School, Ft. Sam Houston, TX

Cmdr. Jerry Mothershead, MD, FACEP
Naval Medical Center
Portsmouth Naval Base, VA

Sgt. 1st Class David A. Scott, LPN, EMT

US Army Medical Department Center and School, Ft. Sam Houston, TX

Cmdr. Garry B. Criddle, RN
US Coast Guard/Public Health Service, Washington, DC

Capt. Steven W. Salyer, PhD, PA-C
Brooke Army Medical Center, Ft. Sam Houston, TX

Jon R. Krohmer, MD, FACEP
Kent County EMS
Grand Rapids, MI

Col. Craig H. Llewellyn, MD, MPH, US Army (Ret.)
Uniformed Services University of the Health Sciences, Bethesda, MD

Jeff T. Dyar, NREMT-P
National Fire Academy, Federal Emergency Management Agency, Emmitsburg, MD

Maj. Brian Zachariah, MD, FACEP, USAR
University of Texas
Southwestern Medical Center, Dallas, TX

Sgt. 1st Class Roger Hillhouse, RRT, CVT, EMT
US Army Medical Department Center and School, Ft. Sam Houston, TX

Henry J. Siegelson, MD, FACEP
Emory University, Atlanta, GA

LTC Cliff Cloonan, MD, FACE
Joint Special Operations
Medical Training Center
Ft. Bragg, NC

Jonathan F. Politis, NREMT-P
Emergency Medical Services
Colonie, NY

Maj. Peter Forsberg, MA, PA-C, US Army (Ret)
University of Texas Health Science Center, San Antonio, TX

Mstr. Chief Louis P. Brockett, NREMT, IDC
Naval Hospital, Patuxent River, MD

Sgt. Maj. Bradley Ennis
US Army Medical Command, Ft. Sam Houston, TX

Capt. Eric M. Johnson, RN, NREMT
US Army Medical Department Center and School, Ft. Sam Houston, TX

CMSgt Robert Loftus, EMT, USAF
Command Medical Service Manager, Langley Air Force Base, VA

Eric Poach, EMT-P
EMS Outreach Specialist
Mercy Hospital of Pittsburg, PA

MSgt Richard Ellis, NREMT-P, USAF
USAF EMT Program Manager, Wichita Falls, TX

James Jones, Director of Emergency Preparedness
Niagara Mohawk Corp. Nuclear Power Plant, Oswego, NY

Ptl. James S. Holman, EMT-P
Alleghany County Bureau of Police, SWAT, Pittsburgh, PA

Andrew Dorman, Supervisory Special Agent
Federal Bureau of Investigation, Bomb Data Center, Washington, DC

Chris Thompson, EMT-P, USN (Ret)
Rural Metro Ambulance Service
Syracuse, NY

Staff Sgt. Everett Taylor, CVT
Brooke Army Medical Center
Ft. Sam Houston, TX

Sgt. 1st Class Steven Newsome, EMT, CVT
US Army Medical Department Center and School
Ft. Sam Houston, TX

1

THE TACTICAL ENVIRONMENT OF CARE

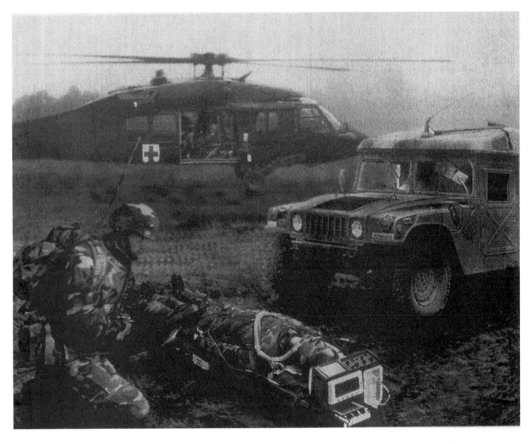

The medic's equipment and tactical ambulances are depicted in this artist's conception of the not-too-distant future.

OBJECTIVES

After reading this chapter, you will be able to:

1. Describe the tactical environment and the impact it has on emergency care.
2. Understand the overriding importance of the mission in all military and many other tactical operations.
3. Know the principles of medical control in all aspects of tactical emergency care.
4. Describe the three stages of care in the tactical setting.
5. Know the primary elements and priorities of each of the three stages of care.
6. Understand the role of scene size-up, patient movement, and bleeding control in care under fire.
7. Know the role of the initial and focused assessment, ABCs, spinal immobilization, relief of tension pneumothorax, intravenous fluid resuscitation, and cardiac arrest treatment in tactical field care.
8. Understand the role of the ongoing assessment, oxygen therapy, continued intravenous fluid therapy, and patient monitoring in casualty evacuation.

CASE

You are the combat medic assigned to Charlie Company, 1-10th Light Infantry Battalion. While on patrol with the lead platoon, you contact the enemy and shots are fired. The platoon leader immediately halts the platoon to return fire while the platoon sergeant directs the machine gun crews to ready their weapons. Everyone, including you, hits the ground and finds cover and concealment. Shots ring out from all sides, and a thick haze soon covers the battlefield.

As an armed member of the team, you instinctively find a good defensive position, and return fire as directed by your sergeant. The long hours of combat training and drilling now pays off as you clutch your rifle, looking for a good target. The fighting continues for what seems like an eternity (but in reality lasts less than 2 minutes) and then abruptly stops. The enemy has withdrawn, and the platoon leader calls a cease fire.

Soon, the cries of "medic! medic!" are heard. You grab your aid bag and go to work. Someone directs you to Jones, who was "point man." He was out in front of the patrol when the shooting started. Now he is located in a small clearing, near where the enemy had just been. Quickly, you high crawl through the mud and weeds to reach him. He is able to speak and says he is shot in the thigh. You position him between the enemy and yourself, and after donning latex gloves, conduct a rapid search for severe bleeding, finding only oozing blood on his legs. Fearing the return of the enemy, you grab his web gear and quickly drag him behind a large rock.

Now in the relative safety of good cover, you begin the initial and focused assessments, and discover Jones is alert and oriented, with normal vital signs. A serious gunshot wound to the thigh is confirmed. Bleeding is easily controlled with direct pressure. To conduct the detailed assessment, you remove his garments, replacing his protective flak vest and helmet after checking the body surfaces for injuries. Since evacuation is at least 2 to 3 hours away, an IV is started, and morphine 2 mg is injected for pain relief, followed by cefazolin 2 gm for infection prophylaxis. By now, several platoon members have assembled a makeshift litter from a poncho, and the casualty is removed from the firefight zone to the predetermined casualty evacuation point 2 kilometers to the rear.

INTRODUCTION

The **tactical medic** frequently operates in an environment very different from traditional emergency medical services (EMS). Direct fire, hostile enemy attacks, chemical weapons threats, harsh and austere conditions all characterize many tactical operations. This changes many of the priorities, and shifts the emphasis of emergency care. This chapter discusses the unique aspects of the tactical environment and the impact it has on emergency medical care. In this text, the term *medic* refers to all tactical field personnel, including Army medics, Navy corpsmen, Air Force medical technicians, special operations medical personnel, and civilian EMTs and paramedics.

ENVIRONMENT

Wars and other tactical operations occur in all corners of the globe and in all possible conditions. Extremes of weather are common, as is prolonged exposure to the elements. Darkness is common, and light discipline precludes the use of flashlights or lanterns. Additionally, continuous operations can run 24, 48, or 72 hours or longer, with no opportunity for sleep. Civilian law enforcement operations may involve prolonged operations under similar conditions. These severe conditions challenge the medic in his or her responsibility to support the mission.

Tactical operations may occur across the globe and in many different environmental conditions. In addition to the heat, cold, moisture, and wind of the temperate climate, you may face the temperature and physical extremes of mountain, jungle, desert, and arctic environments. Special concerns associated with each of these environments may affect your activities and focus during operations and combat.

Mountain

Because of the rugged terrain of mountainous areas, you will frequently encounter fractures and sprains. Bitter cold and wind may induce cold and hypothermic injuries, while personnel may also suffer from severe sunburn and snow blindness. Increased altitude may cause altitude sickness until personnel become acclimated, and the lower atmospheric pressure reduces respiratory system effectiveness, especially in seriously injured patients.

Jungle

Here you must anticipate and protect against the extreme heat and humidity leading to heat exposure and exhaustion while you balance fluid loss with electrolyte replacement. The jungle heat and humidity also encourages bacterial growth, making it hard to assure the water supply without diligent purification and aggressive sanitation that is essential for disease control. The prevalence of disease also complicates wound healing, so it is imperative to observe body fluid isolation techniques and keep wounds as clean as possible. The jungle environment is also hard on equipment, inducing mechanical and electrical equipment corrosion and shortening medical supply shelf life.

Desert

Heat and lack of water characterize most desert environments. However, note that deserts frequently experience great changes in temperature from daytime to nighttime, as much as 70 degrees. The lack of water and excessive heat contribute to dehydration, heat exposure, and exhaustion, and the sun may cause severe sunburn and eye injuries to the unprotected. Shelter from the sun and heat during the day and warm clothing and blankets for the nights may be essential. Sand may induce excessive equipment wear and tear and premature failure, while blowing sand may reduce visibility. Excessive heat may also significantly reduce the shelf life of medical supplies.

Arctic

The arctic or any severely cold environment can have harsh and devastating effects on tactical forces. Cold, especially when it combines with wind, quickly cools the body's surface, resulting in frostbite, freezing, or hypothermia. Damp clothing or fluids (like water or auto, home, or stove fuel) on the skin greatly increase the rate and severity of heat loss. Even temperatures above freezing can seriously injure wet, cold limbs, especially feet, over time. Increased darkness associated with arctic winter and the unpredictability of weather patterns add to the risk, yet in sunlight, snow blindness becomes common without protective eye wear. Wind or helicopter-blown snow may create white-out conditions, and snow may cover ground obstacles, leading to poor footing and an increase in leg and foot injuries. Severe cold reduces battery power and charge life and may result in the freezing of supplies. During combat, thermal detection of troops becomes easier in the very cold environment.

 Whenever your unit is to deploy in adverse environment conditions, whether mountainous, jungle, desert, or arctic, plan accordingly. Bring the necessary supplies and water. Also consider sheltering against the sun, heat, wind, cold, contamination, or precipitation. Use available land contours or existing structures to provide casualties and the fighting force with shelter or construct ones to protect them from the adverse environment.

MOBILITY

High Mobility

Because tactical units, ships, and aircraft are mobile, the medic must be prepared to pack light. For example, an infantry medic may be limited to one small shoulder pack (in addition to a rifle and other equipment) that he or she has to carry 10 or 12 miles each day. Civilian tactical operations are not usually as arduous, but missions can require entry into forests, deserts, mountains, or other remote areas. Common tools of emergency care, such

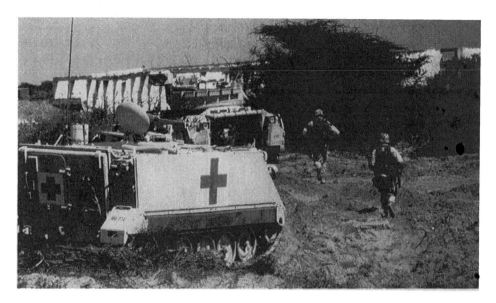

Figure 1-1 Tactical ambulances are designed for rough terrain and harsh conditions.

as oxygen bottles, wheeled stretchers, and intravenous fluids are prohibitively heavy and cannot easily be man-packed in this situation. However, not all medics walk to work. Some are assigned to a ship, aircraft, or vehicle and have the benefit of carrying additional equipment, including some heavy or bulky items.

Tactical Equipment

Much of the equipment used by the medic is similar or identical to the equipment used by traditional civilian EMS providers. Other equipment is tailored to suit the conditions of the tactical environment and is especially rugged, and has a nonreflective finish (to maximize camouflage and concealment). Equipment for waterborne operations should float, if possible, and aircraft equipment must be especially lightweight.

Tactical Ambulance

Tactical ambulances serve the same purpose as their civilian counterparts: to transport patients. Tactical ambulances, however, are frequently more austere and are designed for more rugged conditions than are traditional civilian ambulances (Figure 1-1). Tactical ambulances such as the military **Humvee** can also carry four **litter (nonambulatory) patients** at a time over very rough terrain. Consequently, patient care is much more challenging for the medic in the back of a tactical ambulance.

Helicopters

The military pioneered the use of helicopters to transport casualties, and it remains critical to effective patient evacuation (Figure 1-2). Like their ground counterparts, military helicopter ambulances can carry more patients but have less medical equipment than

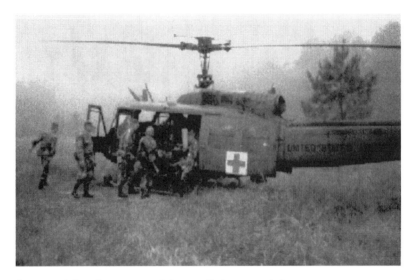

Figure 1-2 The military pioneered the use of helicopter ambulances.

their civilian counterparts. Chapter 8, Tactical Evacuation, discusses evacuation principles in greater depth.

TACTICAL MISSION

Depending on whether the tactical medic supports a military unit or civilian law enforcement operation, he or she will have slightly different duties and responsibilities. The civilian tactical medic will often be a sworn peace officer with an obligation to uphold the law and keep the peace. The first priority, after personal safety, is the safety of the public. The military medic, on the other hand, has a duty to protect the constitution, defend the nation, and obey all lawful orders. Implied in this duty is the obligation to carry out the mission to the best of his or her abilities, regardless of the challenges or obstacles in the way. *Thus, the military medic gives first priority to the mission, and places his or her own welfare after it.* History is full of examples where medics in the face of overwhelming odds risked their lives to accomplish their sworn duty. This honorable tradition carries through to the present and is part of what makes military emergency care special.

Personal Safety

Placing the mission above personal safety has important implications for the practice of the military medic. For example, to reach a wounded soldier, the medic may have to expose himself or herself to enemy gunfire while crawling to the casualty (Figure 1-3). This is in direct contrast to a civilian EMS provider, who is under no obligation to take excessive risks to rescue another person. Nonetheless, both military and civilian tactical medics have a strong tradition of selfless service and courageous duty.

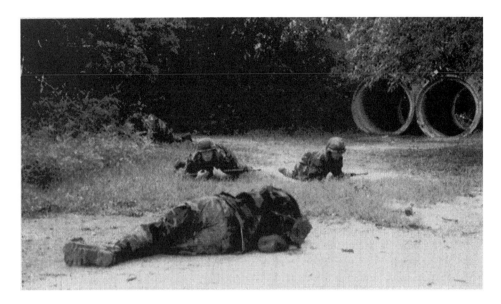

Figure 1-3 Approach the casualty keeping a low profile.

Mission First

Although the slight differences in mission priority will occasionally force military and civilian tactical medics to choose different courses of action under similar circumstances, these situations will be infrequent. Instead, the similarities between military and civilian tactical operations are strong, and the principles of tactical medicine apply to both. This is seen with the tactical operational maxim of "mission first." In the tactical setting, medical care may be only a small, and possibly dispensable, part of the overall mission. If the tactical situation is such that performing the medical mission threatens the overall unit mission, then the medic may have to stop or modify his or her medical care. An example might be delaying a casualty's evacuation until a hostile threat is neutralized.

Who's in Charge?

This subordination of the medical mission to the overall tactical mission brings up the point of who is in charge. In all units, the chain of command dictates the actions of the unit and all its members. This does not change if the unit sustains casualties. The unit's leaders remain in charge and continue the focus on the overall mission. *Certainly, the medic provides input to the leader on medical matters, but it is the unit leader, not the medic, who decides the timing and resources for care and evacuation.* This is quite different from what occurs in the traditional civilian situation. When injury or illness occurs, the top priority is the health and welfare of the patient.

Medical Direction

All tactical care provided by the medic is an extension of the physician's professional services. The general principles of **medical direction** do not change when in the tactical environment. The extreme conditions sometimes encountered during tactical operations, however, require flexibility and adaptability on the part of medic and physician director to make medical direction work. It is critical for the medic to establish a good working relationship with the medical director. In law enforcement units, the medical director may be the local EMS medical director. In an Army or Marine Corps medical platoon, the medical director is the battalion or brigade surgeon. On board ship, the vessel's medical officer is the medical director. In aviation units, a flight surgeon may fill the role of medical director. *In all cases, the physician must be regularly involved in training, evaluation, and utilization of medics and medical activities and missions.*

For their part, physicians must be motivated to provide supervision, training, and guidance to the medic and to their leaders and commanders. It is also highly desirable for the physician to be knowledgeable and skilled in EMS and prehospital care. In some cases, a physician assistant (PA) is available to assist the physician with medical direction. A PA can extend the physician's influence and expand the positive impact of medical control. The PA must always have a close working relationship with the medical director, who is ultimately responsible. PAs should strive for the same degree of knowledge and excellence in EMS and prehospital care as would physician medical directors. When used in this text, the term *physician* also refers to the physician assistant (except where specifically noted).

ROLE OF THE MEDIC

The medic in a tactical unit or on board a ship or aircraft performs many duties in addition to providing emergency care. When circumstances dictate, the medic may give priority to other missions. Fortunately this is rare. Most of the time, the medic will be able to accomplish all of his or her tasks, including ambulatory care (sick call), preventive medicine, field sanitation, and psychological (combat) stress control. All these roles are discussed later in the textbook.

PRINCIPLES OF CARE

In a hostile situation, medical care takes on a new dimension. Not only must the patient be cared for, but the medic must take an active role in protecting (and possibly defending himself or herself, the patient, and the team). This need for protection and defense can greatly alter the amount and type of care that can be provided to the patient. The remaining sections discuss the principles of care in the hostile environment.

TABLE 1-1

STAGES OF CARE

- Care under fire
  Casualty under effective hostile fire
- Tactical field care
  Casualty no longer under effective hostile fire
- Combat casualty evacuation care
  Care rendered once casualty is being transported by ground vehicle, aircraft, or boat

Stages of Care

The care provided in a hostile environment can be divided into three stages: (1) care under fire, (2) tactical field care, and (3) casualty evacuation care. Care under fire is the medical care provided to the casualty while still under effective hostile fire. Tactical field care occurs once the casualty is no longer under effective hostile fire. Combat casualty evacuation care is rendered once the casualty is being transported by a ground vehicle, aircraft, or boat (Table 1-1).

CARE UNDER FIRE

Care under fire encompasses all care provided by the medic while the patient (and medic) are still under effective hostile fire. The overriding concern in this situation is protection and defense against hostile fire. Obviously, medical care is very restricted and geared toward removing the patient and medical team from hazards. Table 1-2 outlines the management principles of **care under fire**.

TABLE 1-2

MANAGEMENT PRINCIPLES OF CARE UNDER FIRE

- Defend self and casualty (return fire)
- Use cover and concealment—avoid direct fire
- Protect casualty from hostile fires
- Remove casualty from imminent hazard
- Stop life-threatening hemorrhage with a tourniquet

Adapted, in part from Butler KF, Hagmann J, Butler EG; Tactical Combat Casuallty Care in Special Operations. Milit Med 1996; 161 (s): 3-16.

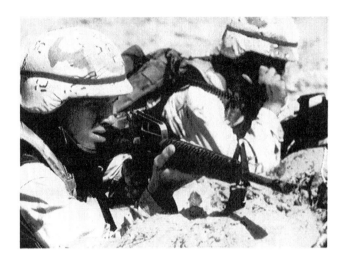

Figure 1-4 A key difference between civilian prehospital providers and tactical medics is the ever-present need for self-defense.

Scene Size-Up

The focus of tactical scene size-up involves defending and protecting yourself, your team, and your patient from hostile fire. If armed (and authorized to do so), return fire. Military medics are routinely armed with an automatic rifle or semiautomatic pistol and should not hesitate to use it if clearly warranted (Figure 1-4). In fact, under the **Laws of War (Geneva Conventions)**, medics have an obligation to defend patients in their care. Of course, once the threat has subsided, military medics may not engage in offensive tactics (such as pursuing a fleeing enemy). Such action contradicts their noncombatant status under the Laws of War. Sworn law enforcement officers, of course, must follow their police department's rules on engaging and apprehending suspects when faced with this situation.

Rules of Engagement

The medic supporting tactical law enforcement must follow his or her unit's standard procedures when faced with fire. If armed, there are probably strict **rules of engagement** that must be followed. If unarmed, then the key action is to take immediate cover. The decision to arm the medic (or not) in a tactical law enforcement team is a matter of local control. There is no "correct" approach; however, all individuals carrying firearms must be fully qualified and trained to use them.

Cover and Concealment

Cover provides protection against small arms fire (for example, large tree, ditch, or boulder), whereas **concealment** merely hides your presence from the enemy (Figure 1-5). Cover is preferable if available; however, in a pinch, concealment (for example, bushes, plaster drywall, or tall grass) will suffice. The key is to find it quickly and get your patient and yourself behind it immediately.

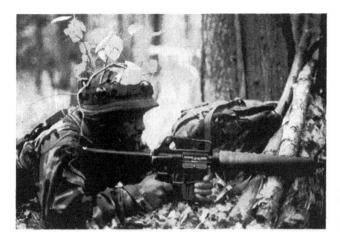

Figure 1-5 Cover and concealment are used to avoid hostile fire.

Moving the Casualty

Getting the patient to cover (or concealment) may entail moving the casualty a few meters (yards). Tell the casualty to move as quickly as possible to cover while maintaining a low profile. If the casualty is unable to move, the medic may need to drag him or her using one of the techniques described in chapter 8, Tactical Evacuation. Although there is a small risk in moving a casualty (of worsening injuries), the benefits of protection far outweigh any potential risk. *When under hostile fire, the medic should never hesitate immediately to move a patient who is exposed to hostile fire.* There is simply no time to evaluate and immobilize suspected cervical spine or skeletal injuries before movement takes place.

Movement Principles

Ideally, choose a technique that is least likely to worsen the casualty's injuries. If a spine or long bone (for example, femur, tibia, radius, or humerus) fracture is suspected, try to move the casualty along the long axis of the body. If the patient has an open abdominal wound, try to avoid placing excess pressure on the abdomen. However, the medic must use whatever technique accomplishes the goal in the most expedient fashion: immediate removal of the casualty from imminent danger.

Initial Assessment and Care

Once the casualty is out of imminent danger, the medic can provide very limited medical care. Care in this situation is restricted because of the continued risk of hostile fire and the limitations of the tactical environment. Limited sight (often complete darkness or thick smoke) is common on operations, and any artificial light may expose your position to the enemy. Night vision equipment can assist in this regard but is not always available. The medic must also maintain a low profile to avoid exposure to hostile arms. This makes rendering care difficult because visualization of the whole patient at once is

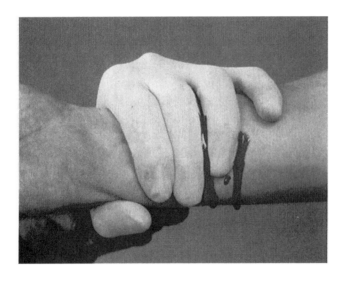

Figure 1-6 Direct pressure, with a gloved hand alone, if necessary, is almost always successful in controlling bleeding.

impossible. If possible, place the casualty between the enemy and yourself. This provides a small margin of concealment for your movements as you begin treatment.

Hemorrhage Control

The primary thrust of tactical initial assessment is the detection and control of life-threatening hemorrhage. Severe exsanguinating bleeding must be controlled in the care-under-fire stage. Direct pressure, with a gloved hand alone, if necessary, is almost always successful (Figure 1-6). Only life-threatening bleeding is addressed at this stage. Actively flowing or spurting blood qualifies for this purpose, whereas oozing or mostly clotted blood does not.

Apply a Tourniquet

If the medic cannot maintain direct pressure, or if the casualty must be moved under fire, apply a tourniquet (Figure 1-7). If the wound is on the head or trunk, apply a pressure dressing (Figure 1-8). Tourniquets are acceptable under these circumstances to save a life and prevent unacceptable delays in removing the patient from under fire.

ABCs

Airway and breathing management is deferred in this stage because this management requires too much time and places the medic at unacceptable risk of hostile fire exposure. The only exception, perhaps, is a simple readjustment of the casualty's head and neck to relieve upper airway obstruction by the tongue and palate. Artificial ventilation is likewise not performed at this stage. Removal of the casualty's body armor (for example, ballistic vest, kevlar helmet and protective armor system [PASGT]) is contraindicated unless it is necessary to access a potential bleeding site.

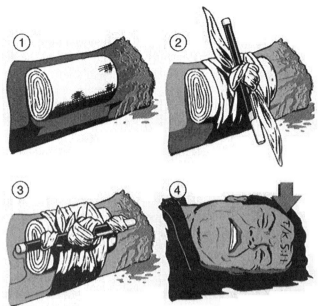

Figure 1-7 A tourniquet is applied to stop life-threatening bleeding when other measures have failed or are not possible.

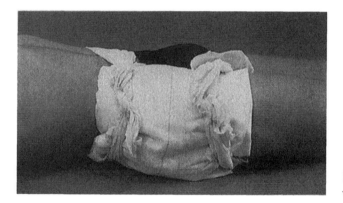

Figure 1-8 A pressure dressing will stop most bleeding.

Evacuation

Once the casualty is reached and rapidly assessed for life- threatening bleeding, it is necessary to remove the casualty to relative safety. Movement from this point may require a manual carry or the use of a field litter. However, until relative safety has been reached, the priority of expedient movement applies.

TACTICAL FIELD CARE

Tactical field care is the care rendered after the casualty is removed from the immediate threat of hostile fire. It encompasses all the emergency care provided in the field and is the type of medicine traditionally within the realm of the combat medic, corpsman, or emergency medical technician. Unlike care under fire, the medic and patient are not at imminent risk of being shot. This affords benefits of providing more intensive emergency treatment. *Tactical field care focuses on management of the airway and breathing, dressing of wounds, and splinting of fractures.* This is not to suggest that tactical field care is the same as civilian-style prehospital care. They both share the same principles and goals, but tactical field care focuses on the types of problems likely to be encountered in the tactical environment. Furthermore, there remains some risk of fire or threat, and care is adjusted accordingly. Table 1-3 outlines the general approach to patient management in the tactical field care stage. Specific circumstances may require variation of this approach, and the medic in the field should be authorized to adjust care as indicated.

TABLE 1-3

GENERAL APPROACH TO PATIENT MANAGEMENT IN TACTICAL FIELD CARE
INITIAL ASSESSMENT AND MANAGEMENT

- Airway
  Manual methods
  Naso or oropharyngeal airways
  Endotracheal intubation
  Cricothyrotomy or cricothyrostomy
- Breathing
  Bag-valve-mask ventilation
  Needle decompression of tension pneumothorax
- Circulation
  Control bleeding with direct pressure or tourniquet
  Start large-bore (18-14 gauge) IV
  Fluid resuscitation with saline
- Focused and Detailed Assessment and Management
- Disability and drugs
  Rapid head-to-toe assessment for wounds, fractures
  Splint and dress as indicated
  Analgesia
  Antibiotics
  Evacuation

Adapted, in part from Butler KF, Hagmann J, Butler EG; Tactical Combat Casuallty Care in Special Operations. Milit Med 1996; 161 (sl): 3-16.

Initial Assessment and Management

The initial assessment in tactical field care is focused on the airway. All standard prehospital airway techniques come into play: manual airway maneuvers (Figure 1-9), oral and nasopharyngeal airways, orotracheal intubation, and in cases of complete upper airway obstruction (unrelieved), surgical airways. Table 1-4 outlines an approach to determining which technique to use. Of course, the specific tactical and medical situation may dictate variations, and provider training will limit certain options.

No special requirements are needed to manage the airway in the tactical field care stage. However, the medic should observe the following points: intubation and surgical airways, though potentially life-saving, also require extensive training and meticulous attention to detail to accomplish. Only trained and authorized medics should attempt these procedures. The light on the laryngoscope is a high-intensity white light, and care must be exercised if light discipline is a tactical concern. Digital endotracheal intubation may be an option in this circumstance (see Appendix D, Advanced Airway Procedures).

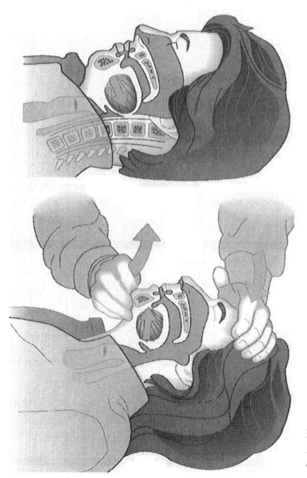

Figure 1-9 The head-tilt, chin-lift maneuver is the best method for initially opening the airway.

TABLE 1-4

AIRWAY MANAGEMENT IN TACTICAL FIELD CARE

- Awake, alert, and talking—no intervention indicated
- Unconscious or significant altered mental status
  Chin lift or jaw thrust maneuver, then
  Naso or oropharyngeal airway, if tolerated
- Unconscious casualty: advanced management
  No airway obstruction: orotracheal intubation
  Complete unrelieved upper airway obstruction: needle cricothyrostomy or cricothyrotomy
  Light restricted environment: digital intubation (patient must be completely unresponsive)

In a similar fashion, cricothyrotomy (as opposed to needle cricothyrostomy) requires adequate lighting. The red color of blood and tissue can make the performance of this technique under red lens light almost impossible. Of less concern is the possibility of contamination by dirt, mud, and debris. Since this procedure is performed only in acute life-threatening airway obstruction, the benefits far outweigh any risks of contamination (see Appendix D, Advanced Airway Procedures).

Spinal Immobilization

The issue of spinal immobilization frequently raises concern when treating casualties. On the one hand, medics are traditionally taught to protect the cervical spine in the rare but devastating chance a neck fracture is present. On the other hand, it is known from research and experience that this type of injury is very unlikely in the tactical environment. Table 1-5 provides a balanced approach to deciding when to immobi-

TABLE 1-5

CERVICAL IMMOBILIZATION IN TACTICAL FIELD CARE

- Cervical spine immobilization not indicated for:
  Penetrating head or neck trauma
  Falls from standing or off low (1-2 meters) objects
- Cervical spine immobilization indicated (if feasible) for unconscious casualties or conscious casualties with neck pain and
  High speed (>30 mph or 50 km/h) vehicle crash
  Falls from great height or direct blunt neck trauma
  Blast injury
  Any casualty where neurological signs are indicative of cervical spine injury

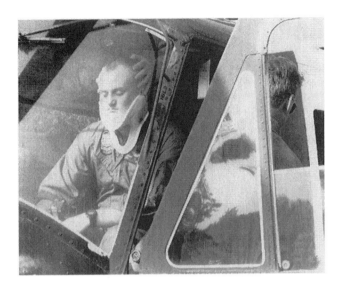

Figure 1-10 High-speed vehicle crash is one mechanism where cervical spine immobilization in the tactical environment is important.

lize the cervical spine in the tactical environment. *In general, penetrating (gunshot, shrapnel, knife) wounds to the neck or short falls (such as when a standing person falls) do not require cervical immobilization. In contrast, high-speed motor vehicle crashes or high falls are examples of situations where cervical immobilization is ordinarily indicated in the tactical environment* (Figure 1-10).

Breathing

Breathing or ventilation of the patient is straightforward and follows the same principles of basic and advanced life support. The best choice for field use is the bag-valve-mask (Figure 1-11). This device is compact and lightweight, and can be used in intubated and unintubated patients. A disadvantage is the high degree of attention required by the medic to maintain an adequate airway and ventilation. An intubated patient requires at least two hands, one to hold the endotracheal tube and the other to compress the bag. A casualty without an endotracheal tube may require two rescuers, one to manually maintain the airway and mask seal, the other to compress the bag.

Immediate Versus Expectant?

The high intensity of services needed to resuscitate and sustain a casualty with apnea or ineffective respirations may adversely affect the ability of the medic to carry out other care or perform other missions. Depending on the tactical situation, this type of casualty may be considered immediate (warranting aggressive and immediate care) or expectant (not expected to survive). See the discussion on cardiopulmonary resuscitation (CPR) later in this chapter for more information.

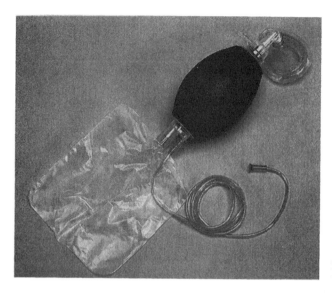

Figure 1-11 The bag-valve-mask is the best method of providing positive pressure ventilation.

Suspected Tension Pneumothorax

Casualties suffering penetrating torso (chest or back) trauma should always be evaluated for tension pneumothorax. *Signs and symptoms of tension pneumothorax include difficulty breathing, tachycardia, decreased breath sounds, and hyper-resonance to percussion on the affected side (the affected side is nearly always the side with the penetrating wound). Deviated trachea, jugular vein distension, hypotension, and altered mental status are late signs* (Figure 1-12). Tension pneumothorax is an imminent lifethreat and easily corrected in the field; therefore, an aggressive search for this problem is mandatory in penetrating torso trauma.

Relief of Tension Pneumothorax

Casualties with penetrating torso trauma and signs of tension pneumothorax should be immediately decompressed. Needle thoracostomy is performed on the affected side by placing a long (> 2") 14-gauge or larger diameter angiocatheter in the 2d or 3d intercostal space (midclavicular line; Figure 1-13). Place the needle over the superior edge of the rib to avoid the inferior neurovascular bundle. Skin preparation with betadine, alcohol, or in a pinch, a clean rag is adequate prior to inserting the needle. Successful placement is confirmed by a rush of air and/or blood though this is not always encountered. Casualties will sometimes improve dramatically but not always. Instead, expect less worsening of the casualty's condition. Leaving the catheter in place (removing the needle) and open to the air is satisfactory. If necessary, loosely cover the catheter opening with a nonocclusive dressing.

Sucking Chest Wounds

Traditional medic training places a lot of emphasis on aggressively treating sucking chest wounds. In the past, training manuals emphasized the early placement of occlusive (air-tight) dressings over such chest wounds. Current emergency care dictates a different

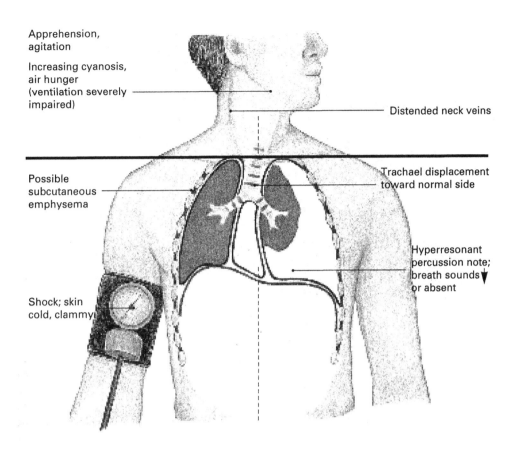

Apprehension, agitation

Increasing cyanosis, air hunger (ventilation severely impaired)

Distended neck veins

Possible subcutaneous emphysema

Trachael displacement toward normal side

Hyperresonant percussion note; breath sounds ▾ or absent

Shock; skin cold, clammy

Figure 1-12 Signs and symptoms in tension pneumothorax.

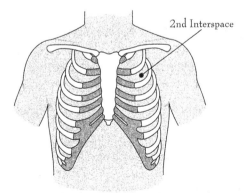

2nd Interspace

Figure 1-13 Relief of tension pneumothorax is accomplished by placing a large bore needle over the rib at the 2nd or 3rd intercostal space.

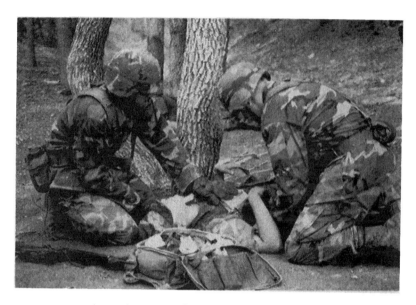

Figure 1-14 Applying a dressing to a chest wound.

approach: placement of a nonocclusive dressing (such as gauze) over the wound, followed by a careful search and relief of tension pneumothorax (Figure 1-14). If necessary, provide positive pressure ventilation using bag-valve-mask. This approach is not only simpler and quicker than applying an occlusive dressing, but also addresses the key lifethreats in penetrating torso trauma.

Circulation

Management of circulation in the tactical field care stage focuses on the control of bleeding, obtaining intravenous access, and initiating fluid resuscitation. Rarely in the field will chest compressions and cardiopulmonary resuscitation be performed, however. Instead, in most cases of a casualty without a pulse, resuscitation is not attempted.

Bleeding Control

Any serious bleeding not already controlled is managed at this point. Direct pressure, elevation of the extremity, and pressure dressings are the preferred methods of control. In this stage of care, a tourniquet should hardly ever be necessary. Any tourniquets previously applied in the care-under-fire stage should be rechecked but not removed.

Intravenous (IV) Access

IV access through a peripheral vein is indicated in all casualties sustaining serious injury or illness. For adult casualties, access is best obtained with an 18-gauge or larger catheter (Figure 1-15). Critically injured casualties should have two IV lines initiated. Upper extremity peripheral veins are preferred, however, in young healthy casualties (≤60 years

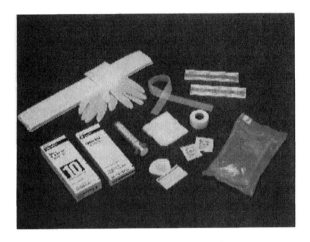

Figure 1-15 Supplies needed to initiate an intravenous infusion.

old), a lower extremity vein may be used. The external jugular vein may also be used in any patient in whom it is visible or palpable. Standard technique is used to start IV lines in the field, and no special preparation or requirements are needed.

Intravenous Fluids

The fluid of choice for all casualties is normal saline (0.9% saline). This fluid can be safely used in all situations, including trauma, burns, head injury, respiratory, and cardiac illness, as well as in pediatric patients. It has the advantage of being inexpensive, readily available, and compatible with all field medications. Ringers Lactate is an acceptable alternative. Other solutions such as hypertonic saline, albumin, or Hespan may have slight advantages in selected cases, but none has the universal application of normal saline, and therefore will not be discussed in this text.

Fluid Resuscitation

Not all casualties require fluid resuscitation. It is important for the medic to distinguish which casualties will benefit from intravenous fluids. Table 1-6 outlines a basic approach to deciding which casualties should get IV fluids. Casualties not exhibiting early or late signs of

TABLE 1-6

FLUID RESUSCITATION IN TACTICAL FIELD CARE

- Controlled hemorrhage without shock: no fluids necessary
- Controlled hemorrhage with shock: normal saline 1000 ml; may repeat if significant shock persists up to 3000 ml
- Uncontrolled intra-abdominal or thoracic hemorrhage with shock: normal saline 1000 ml total

shock (tachycardia, tachypnea, altered mental status, prolonged capillary refill, hypotension) do not require fluids and should have their IV site saline locked.

Maintaining Access

In the tactical setting, it is desirable to initiate an IV on any casualty who may potentially go into shock or require intravenous medications. Once an IV is established, the optimal method of maintaining access is through a saline lock device. A saline lock will keep the IV catheter patent for several hours or more, and it is safe to use on all patients.

The alternative method, a "keep vein open" drip rate, is undesirable for several reasons. First, it requires constant observation. Manual rate controllers (thumbwheel stopcock and similar types) are notorious for changing drip rates during transport. The tactical medic, more than most prehospital providers, can ill-afford to keep a constant watch on IV drip rates. Second, a constant drip uses precious IV fluid, a heavy and bulky commodity in short supply in the tactical environment. Last, a constant drip requires the use of an IV pole or pressure bag, which is cumbersome and difficult to use in tactical ambulances.

Bolus Administration

The method of fluid administration recommended is the bolus method. This method is the easiest to remember, requires no complex rate-time calculations, and is quickest to accomplish. In the tactical environment, there is little advantage to the patient or medic to administer fluids at a proscribed rate. Intermittent boluses, given as needed, accomplish the same thing.

To administer a bolus, simply open the stopcock as wide as possible until the desired volume is infused (Figure 1-16). Then discontinue the infusion and reestablish the saline lock, if necessary. If available, a pressure infuser will speed up the bolus infusion. Use a burette or similar device in children to assure accurate bolus administration and reduce the risk of fluid overload.

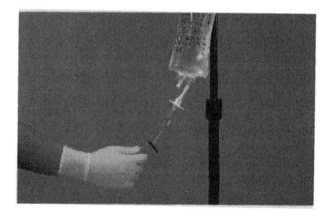

Figure 1-16 To administer a fluid bolus, turn the stopcock wide open until the desired amount of fluid has infused.

Fluid Resuscitation in Shock

Casualties with controlled external hemorrhage but exhibiting one or more signs of shock require an initial bolus of 1000 ml of normal saline (pediatric dosage is 20 ml/kg). This may be repeated up to a total of 3000 ml if necessary. The goal is modest improvement (not elimination) of the signs of shock. Restoration of blood pressure (BP) to "normal" values is counterproductive and not indicated. If a casualty has controlled hemorrhage and normal mental status, additional fluid is not warranted, even if the BP is relatively low. In this case, a systolic BP ≥ 80 is acceptable for an adult casualty. These fluid guidelines are also indicated for severe burns.

Intra-Abdominal and Thoracic Bleeding

Uncontrolled and continued bleeding inside the abdomen or thoracic cavity is a particularly difficult situation. Experience has shown that these types of injuries do not benefit from an extensive fluid resuscitation in the field. In fact, the casualty may do better if fluid is restricted to an initial 1000 ml saline bolus (20 ml/kg for children), even if signs of shock are present. Medical antishock trousers (MAST) or pneumatic antishock garments are contraindicated in these cases and, in fact, may do more harm than good.

Detailed Assessment and Treatment

After successfully addressing the casualty's ABCs, the medic should turn attention to the casualty's other injuries (Figure 1-17). Disrobe the casualty as much as practical, keeping or replacing critical environmental clothing (for example, winter parka) and protective

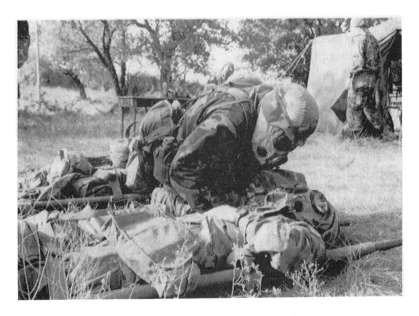

Figure 1-17 Detailed assessment can be challenging in the tactical environment.

garments (personal armor, kevlar helmet, NBC mask). Bandage or splint any significant injuries that are detected. Chapters 3 and 4 describe in further detail the care of specific injuries encountered on the conventional battlefield. Refer to any standard prehospital textbook for the general care of trauma casualties.

Medications

Drug therapy plays a small but important role in the field care of casualties. All medics should be trained and qualified to provide a limited range of parenteral (IV, IM, or SQ) and aerosolized medications to casualties. Table 1-7 lists several important categories of medications for use by medics in tactical field care. Appendix A, Medications for the Tactical Environment, provides additional details on the use of these and other medications used in the tactical environment.

Cardiopulmonary Resuscitation

The treatment of cardiac arrest in the tactical environment is somewhat different from the conventional prehospital approach. *All casualties in the field suffering cardiac arrest as a result of penetrating or blunt trauma are considered unresuscitatable and, therefore, dead.* No attempt should be made to resuscitate these patients.

Nontraumatic Cardiac Arrest

Most victims of nontraumatic (for example, sudden death due to myocardial infarction) cardiac arrest are usually not resuscitatable, given the austerity of care available in the tactical environment. Additionally, the tremendous distances and difficulties in evacuation preclude adequate care for most victims of cardiac arrest. Resuscitation in these circumstances should not be attempted unless the medic and team leader are ready to commit large amounts of time, energy, personnel, and equipment necessary to attempt a resuscitation in the tactical environment.

TABLE 1-7

TYPICAL PARENTERAL (IV, IM, SQ) MEDICATIONS FOR CASUALTY CARE

DRUG TYPE	TYPICAL EXAMPLE
Antibiotic, prophylactic	Cefazolin
Analgesic, narcotic	Morphine
Adrenergic agonist	Epinephrine
Anticholinergic	Atropine
Oxime	Pralidoxime
Anticonvulsant	Diazepam

Evaluating Cardiac Arrest

The medic should perform all the usual measures in the initial assessment. First, open the airway and assess breathing. Be certain to look and listen carefully for any air movement or chest rise. If breathing is absent, immediately check for a carotid pulse. Use gentle pressure to feel the pulse; otherwise, the medic's own pulse may be felt instead. If the casualty is breathless and pulseless, he or she is considered dead, and no further signs of death need to be sought. Resuscitation is not indicated unless one of the few exceptions described in the next paragraph are present.

Tactical CPR Exceptions

There are a few, specific circumstances where CPR may be performed in tactical field care (Table 1-8). These are all injuries or illnesses where CPR has some potential for success. Certainly, CPR should be initiated only if the mission allows and resuscitative efforts can be continued throughout evacuation (see chapter 8, Tactical Evacuation). Adequate CPR and continued resuscitation dedicate at least two or three medics to the effort, plus another two to four litterbearers if a vehicle is unavailable. The mission leaders must be involved in the decision to commit these resources. Given the low probability for survival (probably less than 10%) in cardiac arrest, it may not be prudent to try cardiac arrest resuscitations in critical mission scenarios.

TABLE 1-8

SPECIFIC CIRCUMSTANCES WHEN CPR IS INDICATED IN TACTICAL FIELD CARE

SITUATION	CONSIDER CPR?
Penetrating or blunt traumatic arrest	No
Most nontraumatic arrest	No
Near-drowning	Yes
Hypothermia	Yes
Lightning/electrical injury	Yes
Chemical/biological agent	Maybe

CASUALTY EVACUATION CARE

At some point in the operation, the casualty will be moved toward the rear for additional care. The usual means of evacuation are by ground or air ambulance, but any means at hand, including man-carry and watercraft can be used. Chapter 8, Tactical Evacuation, discusses various techniques in detail. This discussion will be limited to outlining the principles of emergency care in this, the final stage of tactical care. (See chapter 9, Evacuation Care, for a detailed discussion of ongoing assessment and treatment in prolonged evacuation.)

Evacuation Care

Casualty evacuation care is an extension of stage 2, tactical field care, except the patient and medic are on the move. Table 1-9 shows this similarity and adds guidance on continued care. *Since evacuations can stretch into hours in the tactical environment, it is crucial for the medic to perform an ongoing assessment during transport.* Ideally, critical patients should have their mental status and vital signs reassessed every 5 minutes or less. Reassessment of endotracheal tube, breath sounds, hemorrhage, and other important clinical findings should occur every 15 minutes or less. Less seriously ill or injured patients can be rechecked less frequently. Certainly, any significant change in the patient's vital signs or status should prompt a thorough reassessment.

Oxygen Therapy

Supplemental oxygen should be available on all dedicated ground and air ambulances. *All critically ill or injured patients and any patient with dyspnea or shortness of breath should have supplemental oxygen provided.* Additionally, patients with an oxygen saturation less than 95% as measured by pulse oximetry (if available) should receive oxygen. Oxygen, however, can be in short supply in the tactical environment, and judicious use is advised (see chapter 9, Evacuation Care).

TABLE 1-9

CASUALTY EVACUATION CARE OUTLINE

- Airway
  Same as tactical field care (Table 1-3)
- Breathing
  Same as tactical field care, plus
  Oxygen therapy
- Circulation
  Same as tactical field care, except
  Controlled or absent hemorrhage without shock: saline lock
  Controlled hemorrhage with shock: normal saline 1000 cc bolus initially, may repeat
  Uncontrolled intra-abdominal or thoracic hemorrhage with shock: normal saline 1000 cc bolus total
  Isolated head wound with shock: normal saline 1000 cc bolus total
- Focused and detailed assessment and management
  Same as tactical field care
- Ongoing assessment
  Vital signs and mental status checked every 5 minutes for critical casualties, every 15 minutes for others
  Electronic noninvasive monitoring of heart rate, blood pressure, and oxygen saturation (if available)

Oxygen Administration

All critical patients should initially receive high-flow oxygen by nonrebreather mask. Patients with less serious signs or symptoms will tolerate the nasal cannula better. If pulse oximetry is available, it can be used to titrate the oxygen flow. Reduce the oxygen rate to keep the saturation ≥ 95%. This technique can reduce oxygen consumption while maintaining adequate oxygenation. Oxygen supply can be limited in the field, and reduced consumption can conserve a scarce supply.

Intravenous Fluid Therapy

Fluid therapy in the evacuation stage of care parallels the principles outlined for tactical field care (Table 1-6). However, since evacuation from remote or hostile locations can take many hours, IV fluids must be maintained. Table 1-9 outlines a basic approach to providing IV fluids to adult casualties. When not administering fluids, the IV site should preferably be locked with saline or, alternatively, maintained at a keep vein-open-rate.

Reassessment

Reassess the patient for any undiscovered injuries, and retake the vital signs. Recheck the placement of all tubes, IV lines, and monitor leads. Recheck the distal circulation of all splinted extremities, and adjust the splint as necessary. Keep the patient warm with a blanket, if appropriate.

Patient Monitoring

The noise and motion of the evacuation itself will dictate certain modifications to care. In particular, it becomes difficult to assess accurately pulses, respirations, and breath sounds. Therefore, the medic must use extra effort to assess these parameters accurately. Capillary refill is easy to measure during transport and is a reasonable indicator of impending shock. Refill should be less than 3 seconds when checked on the neck or trunk (avoid the hands and feet since cool or warm distal extremities can give false impressions). Chest expansion is usually easier to assess than breath sounds in a noisy environment. Observe for equal expansion (be sure to disrobe the casualty's thorax). Palpate the expansion by placing both hands on the chest, just inferior to the axilla.
If available, electronic monitors, including pulse oximetry, electrocardiograph, and end-tidal CO_2 (capnometry) monitoring can prove very helpful. Readers are referred to standard EMT and paramedic textbooks on the proper use of these aids.

Redosing of Medication

If not already given and indicated by wound severity or location, administer intravenous antibiotics (see Appendix A, Medications for the Tactical Environment). Except in very prolonged evacuations (> 8 hours), redosing is not needed. Narcotic analgesia should be administered and redosed in accordance with the treatment outlines described in chapter 3, Care of Ballistic and Missile Casualties, and Appendix A, Medications for the Tactical Environment. Assess degrees of pain, level of consciousness, blood pressure, and respiratory rate before and 5 minutes after administration of any narcotic analgesic.

Transfer of Care

Once the medical facility is reached, transfer the care of the patient to the receiving team. Give a brief verbal summary of the patient's condition and any changes that may have occurred en route. Provide a written summary of care on either a field medical card or other prehospital care report. When the mission is concluded, refuel, restock, and clean up.

SUMMARY

The tactical environment poses significant challenges to accomplishing medical care. Mission requirements, limited equipment, harsh weather, darkness, and hostile fire all require the medic to be familiar with his or her role and to adapt his or her medical approach to the tactical environment.

Tactical emergency care is divided into three phases: care under fire, tactical field care, and casualty evacuation. Each phase focuses on the priorities at hand and reflects the immediate tactical situation. In all phases, emergency care focuses on the most immediately life-threatening and potentially correctable medical problems.

FOR FURTHER READING

BUTLER FK, Hagmann J, Butler EJ: Tactical Combat Casualty Care in Special Operations. Military Medicine, 1996; 161, Suppl: 3-15.

DE LORENZO RA: Improving Combat Casualty Care and Field Medicine: Focus on the Military Medic. Military Medicine, 1997.

DE LORENZO RA: Military and Civilian Emergency Aeromedical Services: Achieving Common Goals with Different Approaches. Aviation, Space and Environmental Medicine, 1997; 68(1): 56-60.

BOWEN TE, Bellamy RF: Emergency War Surgery, 2nd Ed, U.S. Government Printing Office, Washington, DC, 1988.

WEINER SL, et al.: Trauma Management for Civilian and Military Physicians. WB Saunders, Philadelphia, 1986.

BELLAMY RF: Combat Trauma Overview, in Zajtchuk R, Bellamy RF (eds): Anesthesia and Perioperative Care of the Combat Casualty. Department of the Army, Washington, DC, 1995.

ZAJTCHUK R (ed): Conventional Warfare: Ballistic, Blast and Burn Injuries. Department of the Army, Washington, DC, 1991.

2

INJURY MECHANISMS FROM CONVENTIONAL WEAPONS

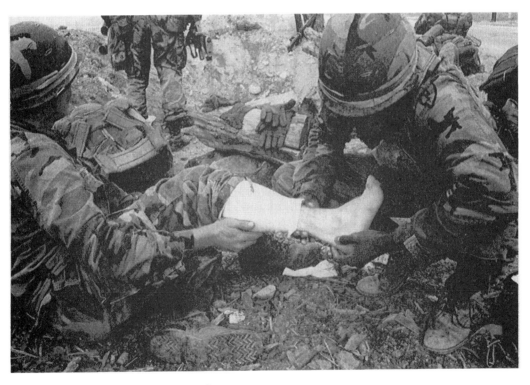

Medic dressing a penetrating extremity wound.

OBJECTIVES

After reading this chapter, you will be able to:

1. Apply the kinetic energy formula to determine the damage potential of a projectile.

2. Explain the energy exchange process between a projectile and an object it strikes.

3. Determine the effects profile, yaw, tumble, expansion, and fragmentation have on projectile energy transfer.

4. Describe the ballistic injury process, including direct injury, cavitation, temporary cavity, permanent cavity, and zone of injury.

5. Identify the relative effects a projectile has when striking various body regions and tissues.

6. Anticipate the injury types and extent of damage associated with handgun, assault rife, shotgun, artillery and cannon, and explosive fragmentation projectiles.

CASE

Your detachment is deployed to a United Nations peacekeeping assignment. Three days out, your outpost comes under artillery fire from an unknown origin. You are first on the scene, find a crater a few feet deep as cover, and size-up the scene. One shell has landed directly on a sentry post, destroying the small building with at least three soldiers lying in the debris. Artillery shells land about every 2 minutes in your proximity. You don your flack jacket, grab your aid bag, and rush to the closest casualty, keeping low and moving quickly. The first casualty has a large penetrating wound to the chest, does not respond to your questioning, does not appear to be breathing, and does not have a radial or carotid pulse. Moving to the second casualty, you find a soldier who is conscious but writhing with pain. His left leg has been blown off just below the knee. The wound is very jagged, and he is losing a lot of blood. You grab the casualty's belt, apply it as a tourniquet just above the knee, and tighten it until blood stops flowing from the wound. Further assessment notes that although the casualty is conscious, he isn't able to understand your questions. You drag him to the shelter of a shallow shell crater, and move quickly to the third casualty. This casualty has suffered a severe wound to the face with moderate bleeding and gurgling associated with attempts to breathe. You position the airway and note fluid and damaged tissue are interfering with his breathing. You turn the casualty's head to the side and drain, then wipe, the fluids from the airway. The patient still doesn't move air well so you lay out your intubation equipment. While the patient minimally fights the attempt, you insert the laryngoscope and locate the vocal cords (it's daytime so light discipline need not be observed). You place the endotracheal tube and note that some blood, then only condensation, moves through the tube with each patient breath. You auscultate good and bilaterally equal breath sounds and note the casualty is moving a good volume of air with each breath. Further patient assessment notes no other signs of injury, and you tie the casualty's hands to his belt to keep him from dislodging the endotracheal tube. After dragging him quickly back to your crater, you recheck the second casualty, administer morphine to relieve some of his pain, and return to monitor this patient. The artillery stops, and an evacuation team arrives with a field surgeon to transport your patients. Your commander later receives word that the two casualties are expected to recover, though with some disability, after a few weeks of care.

INTRODUCTION

Modern society has developed the process of injuring someone, either on the battlefield or city street, into a science. Weapons are designed to cause maximum damage either through the use of the easily carried and concealed handgun, the assault rifle capable of spraying a small to moderate area with high-energy projectiles, the hunting rifle with its bullet designed for maximum tissue damage or through the use of explosive detonation with associated projectiles. The result is a spectrum of missiles with the potential to do great damage to the human body. Understanding the principles of projectile travel and energy exchange will help you anticipate, then recognize, the potential for injury, whether to the marine, soldier, sailor, or airman during combat or to the civilian or tactical squad member in the urban setting.

THE PENETRATING INJURY PROCESS

To harm a patient, a projectile must exchange its energy with the human tissue it contacts. To better understand the process of this exchange, and the resultant bodily injury, we investigate the principles of kinetic energy and aspects of projectile travel that effect the rate of energy exchange. This energy exchange results in injury and depends on both the nature of the projectile and the tissue it strikes. By examining projectile kinetic energy, the physical characteristics of energy exchange, the damage pathway, and the relative devastation projectile passage has on various body tissues and structures, we can better appreciate and care for projectile wounds.

The Bullet's Travel

When the firing pin of a gun strikes the primer of a shell casing, the resulting flash ignites the powder charge. The explosion pressurizes the space behind the bullet and pushes it forward. The gun barrel, which is slightly smaller than the bullet, resists its movement while the explosive pressure behind it grows. As the bullet travels down the barrel, its speed rapidly increases. The bullet also turns, following the small grooves, called rifling, in the gun's barrel. As it leaves the end of the gun barrel, it is spinning rapidly and is pushed by the barrel exhaust, often resulting in a slight wobble. For the first several inches, the bullet is followed by the very hot exhaust gasses, which drove the bullet down the gun barrel, and spent explosive charge residue (Figure 2-1).

While the bullet moves down the gun barrel, the rifle is propelled in the opposite direction. The energy of motion, called kinetic energy, is equal between the two objects; however, the bullet, being of much less weight, travels at a much, much

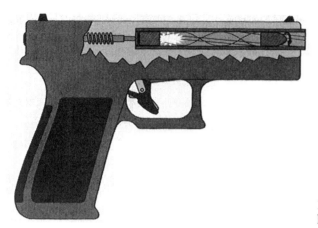

*higher speed. The force of the gun moving away from the target is called recoil and is
absorbed by the shooter.*

*The bullet spin, induced by the rifling, causes it to track very straight and generally
prevents serious wobble (called yaw) during flight. The bullet's speed slows gradually as
it meets resistance from the air it must push out of its way. It also is accelerated toward
earth by gravity, dropping faster and faster with time. This effect gives a bullet's travel
(called trajectory) a curved shape. The **trajectory** of a very fast bullet is much less
curved or flatter than that of a slower projectile.*

*As the bullet impacts its target, it exchanges its energy of motion by deforming the
target and creating a shock wave within it. This transfer of kinetic energy causes the
damage associated with projectile injury.*

PROJECTILE KINETIC ENERGY

When a projectile strikes a target, it exchanges its energy of motion, **kinetic energy**,
with the object struck. This kinetic energy is the energy any object has when it is moving. It is related to two aspects of the object: its mass and its velocity. An object's **mass**
(weight is the object's mass as pulled by gravity) has a direct, and linear, relationship to
its kinetic energy; the greater the mass, the greater the energy. If you double the mass of
a bullet, it has twice the kinetic energy if the speed remains the same (Figure 2-2). The
speed (or velocity) of a projectile demonstrates a squared relationship to its energy. As
the speed doubles, the energy increases by fourfold. As the speed triples, the energy
increases by ninefold (Figure 2-3), and so on. The formula that describes this relationship is as follows:

$$\text{Kinetic Energy} = \frac{\text{Mass} \times \text{Velocity}^2}{2}$$

Kinetic Energy

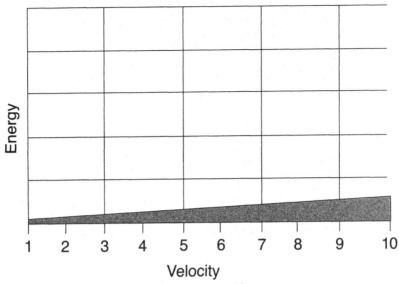

Figure 2-2 Linear relationship between mass and kinetic energy.

Kinetic Energy

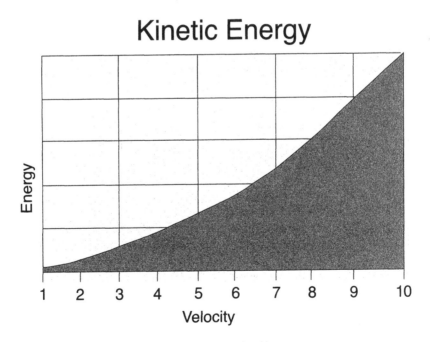

Figure 2-3 Squared relationship between speed and kinetic energy.

This relationship between mass and velocity explains why a very small and relatively light bullet, traveling very fast, has the potential to do great damage. It also identifies that faster, and to a lesser degree, heavier bullets have the ability to do greater damage. The handgun bullet is generally smaller and much slower (250 to 400 meters per second) than the rife bullet. The rifle, on the other hand, expels a slightly heavier bullet at speeds of 600 to 1000 meters per second. Hence, the kinetic energy of the rifle bullet is three to nine times greater and can be expected to do significantly more damage. Experience in Northern Ireland suggests that *rifle bullets are between two and four times more lethal than handgun bullets*.

ENERGY EXCHANGE

Objects traveling relatively slowly, and without much kinetic energy, will affect only the tissue they contact. High-velocity projectiles, however, set a portion of the semifluid body tissue in motion, creating a shockwave and a temporary cavity. This dynamic change in the destruction process depends on how fast the bullet is traveling and how quickly it gives up its energy. The rate of bullet energy release is determined by the size of the contacting surface, called bullet profile, and its shape.

Profile

Profile is the portion of the bullet you see if you look at it as it travels toward you. The larger this surface, the greater the energy exchange rate, the more quickly the bullet slows, and the more extensive the damage to surrounding tissue. For the bullet that remains stable in its travel and does not deform, the profile is the diameter (or **caliber**) of the bullet. To increase the rate of energy exchange, bullets are designed to become unstable as they pass from one medium to another, or to deform, through expansion or fragmentation (Figure 2-4).

Stability

The location of a bullet's center of mass affects its stability during flight and when it impacts a solid or semisolid object. The longer the bullet, the further the center of mass is from the leading edge. If the bullet is deflected from straight flight, such as by the barrel exhaust or a gust of wind, the lift created by the projectile tip passing through air at an angle will cause it to tumble. Once tumbling, it will continue to do so, slowing the bullet and reducing its accuracy. To prevent tumbling, the bullet is sent spinning through the air by the rifling of the gun barrel. This rotation gives the bullet gyroscopic stability like a spinning top. If the bullet is slightly deflected, it will wobble, called **yaw**, then slowly return to a straight orientation. When the bullet impacts a substance denser than air, several things happen. If there is already a yaw, it is greatly increased as the bullet strikes the denser medium. This occurs because the mass of the bullet tries to overrun the leading edge. Second, the gyroscopic spin designed for air becomes insufficient. *A bullet would need to spin at a rate 30 times greater in body tissue than air to maintain the same stability.* The result may be tumbling and a great increase in the bullet's present-

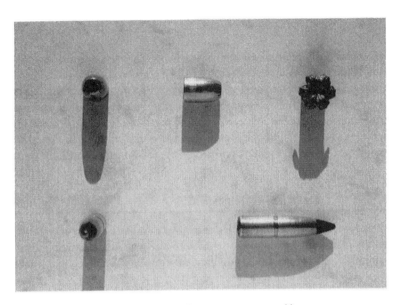

Figure 2-4 Different views of a bullet showing presenting profiles.

ing profile . Since rifle bullets are generally longer with their center of mass farther back from the leading edge, they are more prone to tumble once they hit body tissue. Tumbling greatly increases the bullet's presenting profile, its kinetic energy exchange rate, and its damage potential. Generally, in human tissue, a rifle bullet will rotate 180 degrees and then continue its travel, base first.

Expansion and Fragmentation

Projectiles also increase their profile and energy exchange rate by deforming when they strike a medium denser than air. As the bullet nose contacts the target, it is compressed by the weight of the following portion of the bullet. It mushrooms outward as the rear of the bullet pushes into it, increasing the projectile diameter. In some cases the forces of initial impact are so great that the bullet separates into several pieces or fragments. This fragmentation increases the rate of impact energy exchange because the fragment surface area is much greater than the original bullet profile. Although handgun bullets are made of relatively soft lead, their velocity, and hence kinetic energy, is generally not sufficient to cause significant deformity. Rifle bullets have much greater velocities and much more kinetic energy. They are more prone to deform when contacting human tissue, especially bullets used for large game hunting. Most military ammunition is fully jacketed with impact-resistant metal and seldom deforms solely with soft tissue collision.

Secondary Impacts

The energy exchange between a projectile and body tissue can also be affected by objects it strikes earlier in its travel. Branches, window glass, or articles of clothing may deflect the bullet and induce yaw and tumble. They may also cause bullet deformity, and thereby increase the energy exchange rate once the bullet impacts the victim.

Shape

Bullet shape affects its rate of energy exchange and the damage it will likely do. Handgun ammunition is rather blunt and releases kinetic energy more quickly as it moves through human tissue. Rifle bullets have more of a point and cut through the tissue more efficiently. However, since the rifle bullet velocity is high, the wound will be as or more severe, and penetration will be deeper than the slower, blunt, pistol bullet. The shape of shrapnel, bullet fragments, and explosive debris is frequently irregular, allowing the projectile to give up its energy rapidly through a more unpredictable pathway than either style of bullet.

SPECIFIC WEAPON CHARACTERISTICS

Each type of weapon encountered on the streets and associated with military deployment results in specific types of injuries. These weapons include the handgun, domestic rifle, assault rifle, shotgun, machine gun, artillery and cannon, small antipersonnel explosives, and knives and bayonets (Figure 2-5).

Handgun

The handgun is often a small caliber, medium velocity, weapon with limited accuracy. It is effective only for close range and does not produce the high-velocity, high-energy projectile of the rifle. Hence, its damage potential is limited. The blunter bullet shape and, in rare cases, the softer composition and associated mushrooming and fragmentation may expend the bullet's energy more rapidly. The damage is still, however, much less than the higher-energy rifle bullet. Serious injury usually depends on the organs damaged as a direct result of the bullet's passage.

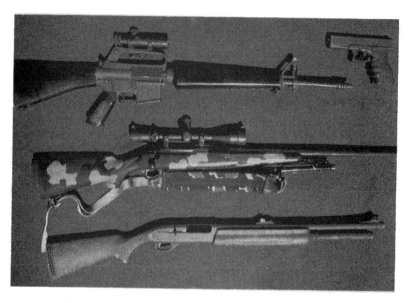

Figure 2-5 Photo of various guns (handgun, assault rifle, rifle, shotgun).

Some handguns fire automatically (machine pistol). That is, they continue to discharge bullets until the trigger is released or the magazine empties. Although the projectile energy remains the same, multiple impacts or multiple victims increase the seriousness associated with automatic weapon discharge.

Rifle

The domestic hunting rifle fires a heavier projectile than the handgun and with much greater muzzle velocity. It is a manually loaded, single-shot weapon with some loading action to advance the next shell, or semiautomatic, where the next shell is fed into the chamber by recoil or exhaust gases. However, no more than one bullet is expelled per squeeze of the trigger. Its high-energy missile travels much farther, more accurately, and retains much more of its kinetic energy than does the handgun projectile. Owing to the high speed and high energy of the projectile, great damaging power is expended in the target. This results in extensive wounds with injury far beyond just the missile track. Domestic hunting ammunition is especially lethal. It is often designed to expand on impact, greatly increasing the rate of energy exchange and expanding the temporary cavity size and the injury pathway.

Assault Rifle

The assault rifle differs from the domestic hunting rifle in that it has a larger magazine capacity and will fire in both the semiautomatic and automatic mode. The resulting injuries are similar to domestic rifle injury though multiple wounds and casualties are expected. The ammunition is not designed for expansion, and though still very deadly, the energy delivery is not as severe as with hunting ammunition.

Shotgun

The shotgun may expel a single projectile (a slug) or numerous spheres. The shell is loaded with a particular size of lead shot, varying from 00 (about 1/3 inch in diameter) to #9 shot (about the size of a pinhead). The projectile compartment is relatively the same between various loads, so the larger the shot, the smaller the number of projectiles. Each projectile shares a portion of the total energy and adds to the resistance as it moves through air. The shotgun is limited as to its range and accuracy; however, the injuries sustained at close range can be very severe or lethal.

Machine Gun

The machine gun is a heavy gun that sends large, very high energy projectiles at the enemy. They fire a great number of rounds per minute and are boat, ship, vehicle, or plane mounted or carried in pieces by several personnel, and then assembled to fire on a tripod. Small machine guns may be used against personnel, whereas larger weapons are effective against equipment. The larger weapon caliber, weight of projectile, and projectile velocity give the bullet very high energy. Fifty-caliber machine gun bullets can penetrate several inches of aluminum armor or 1" to 2" of steel plate. The energy exchange of these large-caliber, high-velocity projectiles in human tissue will be devastating.

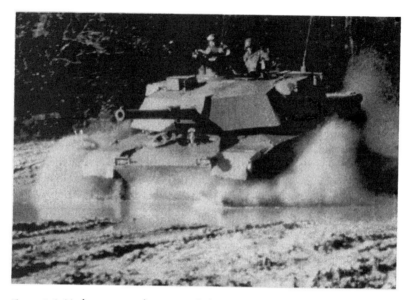

Figure 2-6 Tanks carry great firepower with their main gun.

Artillery and Cannon

Artillery is an even larger projectile gun or may be a self- propelled projectile (rocket) launcher. The shell is usually explosive and designed to compromise armored vehicles or distribute shrapnel among personnel. It can be fired line of sight to its target or carry a high trajectory to permit its firing over obstacles such as a hill or mountain. Artillery can also be fired from great distances (Figure 2-6).

Antipersonnel rounds are generally designed to explode a few meters above the ground, spraying shrapnel horizontally away from the detonation point. This maximizes the rounds' ability to produce injury. Injuries may occur over the entire body and especially to the head, upper extremities, and upper torso. Lying down reduces the troops' profile to the blast and the incidence of injury. Overhead, or horizontal, cover such as lying in a shallow ditch reduces shrapnel injury but does not protect the casualty against blast pressure-wave injury.

Antiarmor rounds are of two types: high-energy antitank (HEAT) rounds and armor-piercing rounds. HEAT rounds use shaped charges to direct and focus the explosive energy as a superheated jet of gas. This melts and penetrates the armor, sending a blast of molten metal and very hot gasses into the armored bunker, vehicle, or ship. Personnel within may suffer serious airway burns and extensive exterior burns as well as pressure injury. They may also suffer injury from projectiles released from the interior as the shell impacts the exterior of the bunker, vehicle, or ship (spalling).

Armor-piercing rounds use high-impact energies from heavy shells fired at great velocities from large cannons aboard ships, planes, or tanks. The kinetic energy of each shell may exceed that of a railroad locomotive, traveling at 50 miles per hour.

The penetrator, a small metal rod, directs the energy of the shell against the armor and creates a small hole. This induces a metal fragment shower from the interior of the armor. This **spalling** causes serious, high-velocity, penetrating injury from close range shrapnel.

Small Antipersonnel Explosives

Land mines, hand grenades, and terrorist bombs all have the potential to do great harm to the human body. To do damage, they must detonate in proximity to personnel and cause injury via projectile wounds, blast pressure injuries, or personnel displacement. Because of the small amount of explosive charge, the most frequent and severe injuries result from projectiles. The projectile injury is usually related to shrapnel, damaging tissue directly as the projectile penetrates the human body.

Knives and Bayonets

In contrast to other mechanisms of injury mentioned in this chapter, bayonet and knife wounds are low-velocity and low-energy wounds. Damage is limited to physical injury caused by direct contact between the blade and tissue. However, the wound is difficult to assess because the depth and angle of insertion are unknown. Additionally, the penetrating object may be moved about inside the casualty, then left in place or withdrawn. The penetration can result in serious internal hemorrhage or injury to individual or multiple body organs.

The Projectile Injury Process

The spinning bullet smashes into a semisolid target (such as human tissue) with great speed. The bullet front impacts tissue, pushing it forward and to the side along the pathway of its travel. This tissue collides with adjacent tissue, ultimately creating a shockwave of pressure moving forward and lateral to the projectile. This shock wave continues perpendicular from the bullet's path as it passes. The rapid compression of tissue laterally and the stretching of it as it moves outward from the bullet path tears and crushes its structure. The motion creates a pocket, or cavity with a reduced pressure, or suction within. This suction draws air and debris into the cavity from the entrance and, if present, the exit wound. The elastic nature of body tissue then draws the cavity back inward causing the entrance wound, exit wound, and wound pathway to close completely or remain only partially open.

DAMAGE PATHWAY

The damage pathway inflicted by a high-speed projectile results from a phenomenon called **cavitation** and its three specific processes: direct injury, pressure shockwave, and temporary cavity. The events of the projectile passage create a permanent cavity and a zone of injury (Figure 2-7).

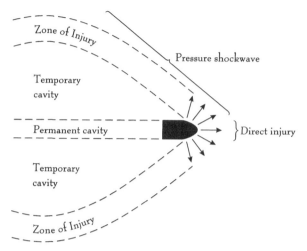

Figure 2-7 Illustration of the bullet injury process.

Direct Injury

Direct injury is the damage done as the projectile strikes tissue, contuses and tears it, and pushes it out of its way. The direct injury pathway is limited to the bullet profile as it moves through the body or the profiles of resulting fragments as the bullet breaks apart. Except for magnum rounds (generating particularly high velocities), handgun bullet damage is usually limited to direct injury (Figure 2-8).

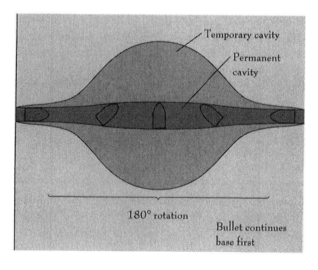

Figure 2-8 Illustration of the cavitation wave caused by a bullet travelling through soft tissue.

Pressure Shockwave

When high-speed and high-energy projectiles strike human flesh, they create a shock-wave of pressure. Since most human tissue is semifluid and elastic, impact transmits energy outward very quickly. The cells in front of the bullet are pushed forward and to the side at great speed. They, in turn, push adjacent cells forward and outward, creating a wave of pressure and moving tissue. The faster the bullet, the greater the effect. With high-speed rifle bullets, the pressures are extreme, approaching 100 times normal atmospheric pressure. The pressure wave travels very well through fluid, such as blood, and may injure blood vessels distant from the wound pathway. Air-filled cavities, such as the small air sacs (alveoli) of the lung, compress very easily and absorb the pressure wave, limiting the shock wave pressure magnitude and the resulting temporary cavity.

Temporary Cavity

The temporary cavity is a space created behind the high-energy bullet as tissue moves rapidly away from the bullet's path. The cavity size depends on the amount of energy transferred during the bullet's passage. With rifle bullets, the temporary cavity may be as large as 30 times the profile of the projectile. After the bullet's passage, tissue elasticity causes the cavity to close.

The process creating the cavity also results in a subatmospheric pressure as the cavity expands. Air is drawn into this cavity from the entrance wound, and the exit wound if it exists. Debris and contamination may enter the cavity with the inflowing air, adding to the risk of infection.

Permanent Cavity

The tissue movement creating the temporary cavity crushes, stretches, and tears the affected tissues. This seriously damages the area most adjacent to the bullet path and may also damage the tissue's elastic recoil. The tissue may not return to its normal orientation, resulting in a permanent cavity that is in some cases larger than the bullet's diameter. This cavity is not a void but is filled with disrupted tissues, some air, fluid, and debris.

Zone of Injury

Associated with most projectile wounds is a zone of injury extending beyond the permanent cavity. This zone contains contused tissue that will not function normally and may be slow to heal because of cell and tissue damage, disrupted blood flow, and infection.

TISSUE/ORGAN SPECIFIC INJURY

The extent of damage caused by a passing projectile depends primarily on the particular tissue it encounters. The density of an organ affects how efficiently the energy of projectile passage is transmitted to surrounding tissues. The connective strength and elasticity, called **resiliency**, also determine how much tissue damage occurs with the transfer of kinetic energy. Air is compressible and will absorb the pressure wave energy, whereas fluids, which are not compressible, will transmit energy efficiently away from the point of impact. Structures and tissues within the body that behave differently during projectile passage include connective tissue, solid organs, hollow organs, lungs, and bone.

Connective Tissue

Muscle, the skin, and other connective tissues are dense, elastic, and held together very well. When exposed to the pressure and stretching of the cavitational wave, these tissue characteristics absorb energy while limiting tissue damage. The wound track closes because of tissue resiliency, and frequently, injury is limited to the direct bullet pathway.

Solid Organs

Solid organs such as the liver, spleen, kidneys, and pancreas have the density but not the resiliency of muscle and other connective tissues. When subjected to bullet impact forces, the tissue compresses and stretches, resulting in greater damage, more closely associated with the size of the temporary cavity. The tissue returns to its original location, not due to its elasticity but to that of surrounding tissues or the organ capsule. Hemorrhage associated with solid organ damage can be severe.

Hollow Organs

Hollow organs such as the bowel, stomach, urinary bladder, and heart are muscular containers holding fluid. The fluid within is noncompressible and will rapidly transmit the energy of impact outward. If the container is filled and distended with fluid at the time of impact, the energy released can tear the organ apart explosively. Large blood vessels respond to projectile passage much like hollow, fluid-filled, organs. If the container is not distended, it is more tolerant of cavitational forces. If a hollow organ, such as the bowel or stomach, holds air, the air compresses with the pressure wave passage and somewhat limits the extent of injury.

Lungs

The lungs consist of millions of small, elastic air-filled sacs. As the bullet and its associated pressure wave passes, the air is compressed, thereby slowing and limiting the transmission of the cavitational wave. *Injury to lung tissue is generally less extensive than expected with any other body tissue.* The bullet may open the chest wall or disrupt larger airways permitting air to escape into the thorax (pneumothorax), or the injury may form a valvelike opening, accumulating pressure within the chest (tension pneumothorax).

Bone

In contrast to lung tissue, bone is the densest, most rigid, and least elastic body tissue of all. When impacted by a projectile or its associated pressure wave, bone resists displacement until it fractures, often into numerous pieces. These bone fragments then may absorb the energy of impact and become projectiles themselves, extending the area of tissue damage.

The particular organ involved in a penetrating injury also has profound effects on the casualty's potential for survival. Some organs, like the heart, are immediately necessary, and serious injury may not be survivable. When large blood vessels are involved, the hemorrhage can be rapid and severe. Penetrating injury of the urinary bladder, on the other hand, may allow survival for many hours without surgical intervention. When evaluating the seriousness of a wound, anticipate the organs injured and their impact on the casualty's condition and survivability.

GENERAL BODY REGIONS

Several body regions are of importance regarding projectile wounds. They include the extremities, abdomen, thorax, and head. Projectile passage also has a special effect on the initial and last tissue it contacts, the entrance and exit wound.

Extremities

The extremity consists of skin, covering muscle, surrounding a large long bone. Its injury may be debilitating but does not immediately threaten life unless there is associated severe hemorrhage. The injury is confined by the resiliency of the skin and muscle, though if the bone is involved, it may extend the degree of soft tissue damage. Extremity injuries account for between 60% and 80% of battlefield injuries yet result in less than 10% of the fatalities. The remaining 20% to 40% of penetrating injuries are divided among the abdomen, thorax, and head, and account for more than 90% of mortality.

Abdomen

The abdomen (including the pelvic cavity) is a major body cavity containing most human organs and is not well protected by skeletal structure. Bullet passage, especially that of a rifle bullet, induces a pressure wave throughout the cavity. Organs especially susceptible to injury include the liver, spleen, pancreas, and urinary bladder. The missile may perforate the small and large bowel in several locations, causing them to spill their contents into the abdominal cavity. If larger blood vessels are affected by the pressure wave, injury may extend along their path and result in rapid and severe blood loss. The release of bowel or bladder contents or free blood into the abdominal cavity can contribute to the injury process. Blood, urine, or bowel contents irritate the delicate abdominal lining and result in serious inflammation or infection.

Thorax

The chest is a cavity contained by the ribs, spine, sternum, clavicles, and the strong muscle of the diaphragm. It houses the lungs, heart, and major blood vessels as well as the esophagus and part of the trachea. Bullet impact with the ribs may induce an explosive energy exchange, injuring the surrounding tissue with numerous boney projectiles. The lung tissue absorbs much of the cavitational energy while sustaining limited injury itself. The heart and great vessels, as fluid-filled containers, may suffer greatly from the energy of bullet passage. Because of the dynamics of chest movement and respiration, any large chest wound may compromise breathing. Air may pass through a wound instead of the normal airway or may build, under pressure, within the chest wall.

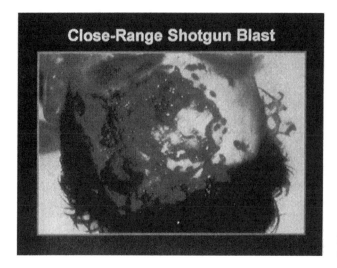

Close-Range Shotgun Blast

Figure 2-9 Projectile wound to the head.

Head

The skull is a hollow, strong, and rigid container, filled with the delicate, semifluid tissue of the brain. It is highly susceptible to projectile injury. If a bullet penetrates the skull, its cavitational energy is trapped within the cavity and subjects the brain to extreme pressures. If the released kinetic energy is great enough, the skull may explode outward. The destructive forces of projectiles may also disrupt the airway or the casualty's ability to control his or her own airway. *Bullet wounds to the head, particularly those penetrating the skull, are especially lethal* (Figure 2-9).

When evaluating the gunshot wound victim, try to determine the bullet pathway and the organs involved in the wounding process. Anticipate the impact their injury will have on the casualty, and use this information to determine the casualty's priority for care and rapid transport and to direct your care. Remember, however, that the bullet may not travel in a direct and straight line between the entrance and exit wound. And a very small shift in pathway may mean the difference between tearing open a large blood vessel or missing critical organs completely.

Entrance Wound

Entrance wounds are usually the size of the bullet or shrapnel profile. The energy of the cavitational wave has not yet had time to develop and contribute to the wounding process. The exception to this is with missiles that have deformed or are tumbling during flight. Here the impact can be especially violent with a much larger and more disrupted wound. If a bullet wound is sustained at close range, a few feet or less, the wound may be marked by elements of the barrel exhaust. Tattooing from the propellant residue may form a circle or oval around the wound entrance and contaminate the wound itself (Figure 2-10).

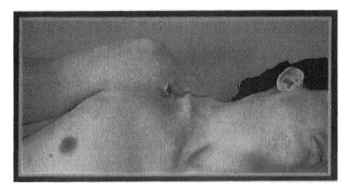

Figure 2-10 Close range entrance wound with residue.

Exit Wound

The exit wound is caused by the physical damage of the bullet's passage and the cavitational wave. Since the wave of pressure is moving forward and outward, the wound may have the appearance of being "blown outward." Because the cavitational wave has had time to develop, *the exit wound may more accurately demonstrate the wounding potential of bullet passage* than the entrance wound. If the projectile expends all its kinetic energy before it can exit the body, there is no exit wound. If it does exit, the kinetic energy expended within the body is equal to the kinetic energy before impact less that which it has after leaving the body (Figure 2-11).

It is often hard to anticipate the seriousness of a projectile wound. The exact wound pathway and precise organs involved may be difficult to determine. Further, injury to the large blood vessels, heart, and brain may be immediately or rapidly fatal, whereas injury to the solid organs (liver, pancreas, kidneys, or spleen) may have the same result though the process may take more time. On the other hand, bullet wounds that appear to impact vital areas may miss the critical organs. In bullet wounds that involve the head, chest, or abdomen, suspect the worst, provide rapid transport when possible, and treat aggressively.

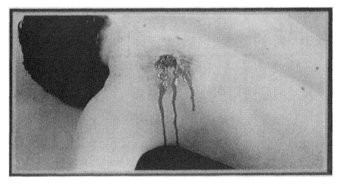

Figure 2-11 High-powered rifle exit wound.

SUMMARY

In the tactical engagement, the patient is a casualty with a greater incidence of penetrating trauma caused by the high-speed bullet or from the results of an explosive detonation. Here the principles of physics, specifically ballistics, apply. The projectile's kinetic energy determines the potential for injury, whereas the profile, stability, and projectile shape determine how quickly that energy is delivered to the human tissue. The various tissues and body organs react differently to the energy exchange (direct injury, cavitational wave, formation of a temporary cavity, permanent cavity, and zone of injury), and vary with regard to their degree of damage. These principles, when applied to the battlefield or tactical casualty, determine the seriousness of the penetrating injury and the care it requires.

FOR FURTHER READING

Textbook of Military Medicine (Part 1, Volume 5) Conventional Warfare; Ballistic, Blast and Burn Injuries. Office of the Surgeon General, Washington, DC, 1990.

GROSS GM, Leeming DW, Farrar CL: Military Ballistics, A Basic Manual. Royal Military College of Science, Brassey's Limited, London, UK, 1995.

WILBER, CHARLES G, PhD: Ballistics for the Law Enforcement Officer. Charles C. Thomas, Springfield IL, 1977.

3

CARE OF BALLISTIC AND MISSILE CASUALTIES

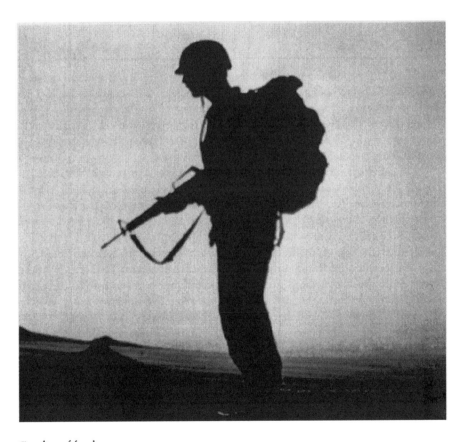

Guardian of freedom

OBJECTIVES

After reading this chapter, you will be able to:
1. Identify important elements of the scene size-up associated with the tactical engagement.
2. Explain conventional casualty assessment, including your responsibilities during the initial, focused, detailed, and ongoing assessments.
3. Identify the wounds most frequently experienced during the battlefield or tactical deployment.
4. Define the care associated with conventional casualties, including general trauma care, projectile injury care, fluid resuscitation, pleural decompression, blast injury care, pain medication, and antibiotic therapy.
5. Given several preprogrammed and simulated conventional casualties with projectile and other penetrating wounds, provide the appropriate scene size-up, initial assessment, focused assessment, detailed assessment, and patient care.

CASE

Your unit is assigned to patrol for insurgent activity along a disputed border. A single rifle report is heard, and word comes back to you that the scout was hit by enemy fire. You move forward to the lieutenant, where several soldiers are working the area to locate the sniper. Two soldiers emerge from the brush with the casualty and set him down before you. Though conscious and alert, he is having trouble speaking and has a small bleeding wound of the right upper anterior chest.

You find the patient conscious and able to speak in broken but intelligible sentences. His airway is clear, but he is breathing with great effort, and his dyspnea is getting much worse. You quickly auscultate breath sounds and find that they are absent on the right. Exposing the chest, you notice a small wound with limited hemorrhage in front, and a much larger wound, with air bubbling through the blood in back. You also notice the right side of his chest is not moving as much as the left, and your palpation of the area reveals a crackling sensation just beneath the skin. You quickly insert a large bore needle just above the third rib and directly below the center of the clavicle. Air escapes through the needle, and the patient's respirations improve some. You withdraw the needle, leaving the catheter in place and continue your assessment.

There are no other apparent wounds or signs of injury though the casualty appears anxious, and his level of consciousness is diminishing. You initiate an IV with a saline lock and immediately infuse 1000 ml of normal saline. You call for a medical evacuation by helicopter and continue to monitor your patient. Ten minutes later, you notice your patient's respirations are again deteriorating. Auscultation of the chest reveals diminished breath sounds on the right. You insert a second needle, hear an escape of air, and notice your patient's breathing again improves. Finally, the helicopter arrives, and you, with great relief, transfer your patient responsibilities to the helicopter medic.

INTRODUCTION

Both the military engagement and the civilian tactical situation change the rules by which you provide emergency medical care. In combat, the mission is the first priority followed by personal safety and defense. The tactical police action maintains the same priorities as normal civilian care, but both may place the medic in a real-time and ongoing casualty-generating situation. That situation has concurrent life-threatening dangers that are not under the control of either the medical contingent or the engagement command authority. Hence, when casualties occur, care is withheld until hostile fire can be eliminated, the casualty can be safely evacuated to cover or concealment, or if the mission demands, limited stabilization is provided while under fire. Once the patient is remote from danger, field care, resembling normal prehospital care, can be instigated. Here, however, limited resources and prolonged evacuation times to the next echelon of care may also change the way out-of-hospital care is administered.

CONVENTIONAL CASUALTY ASSESSMENT

Conventional casualty assessment, and the care to follow, are applied under very different circumstances than prehospital care in the civilian setting. However, the format for offering that assessment and care is the same. The assessment begins with a scene size-up to determine the mechanism of injury and assure the scene is safe. It follows with the initial assessment and the employment of immediately life-saving care. After the initial assessment, a focused assessment and, if conditions merit, a detailed assessment are provided; finally, periodic ongoing assessments are provided.

SCENE SIZE-UP

The military or tactical scene size-up differs greatly from its civilian counterpart. Civilian scene size-up is directed at one incident that has already happened and usually involves but one patient. Further, civilian care does not occur until the scene is completely secure. Your size-up, as a medic, examines the battlefield or fire zone before and while the engagement continues. Casualties occur over time, changing the demands on your services and resources. These differences make the scene size-up a critical element of any deployment (Figure 3-1).

As you enter a fire zone, seek safe cover, or at least concealment, and carefully view the area. Examine factors that will affect your actions, including the terrain; nature of the hostile fire; cover and concealment available; the relative danger associated with care under fire and evacuation; any special considerations such as light or NBC discipline; the number of casualties and the nature of their expected wounds; the equipment, supplies, and personnel resources available for evacuation and care; and the time between the casualty-generating injury, your arrival at the casualty's side, and his or her arrival at the next echelon of care.

Analyze the information you gather on terrain, cover, and concealment to identify the safest and quickest egress to any current or future casualties. Plan to move any

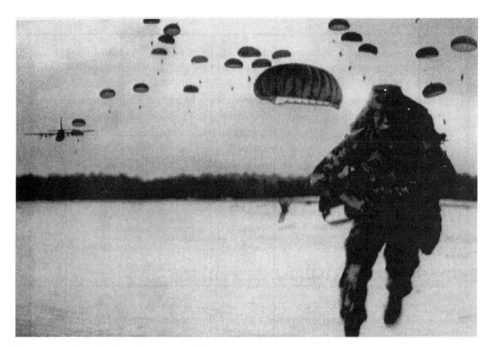

Figure 3-1 The battlefield offers unique challenges to sizing up the scene.

casualties using whatever cover is available, and note the locations from which enemy fire originates. Consider requesting covering fire to reduce the risk to you and your patient during travel to and from his or her location. Be sure that the location to which you will transport a casualty provides optimum cover, or at least concealment, allowing you to render safe assessment and care.

Anticipate the care you will offer at the casualty's side in the context of the relative danger and what effect that care will have on drawing fire (movement, noise, or light). Determine what care, if any, is best offered at the casualty's side and what is best given after evacuation to safe cover. Anticipate the care steps you will employ, and leave nonessential equipment where you will care for the patient after evacuating him or her from fire.

Carefully plan your extraction to safe cover, including the route, movement technique, equipment, and personnel needed. Determine what movement technique the terrain, hostile fire, and resources at hand allows, while exposing you and other rescuers to the least amount of danger. Brief fellow rescuers about what you intend to do and what is expected of them (see chapter 8, Tactical Evacuation).

You may also begin planning for care of the total complement of casualties during the scene size-up. Anticipate the nature, severity, and number of casualties, and match them against the care resources you have at hand. Determine how best to use the resources available to you, and request support and supplies as necessary. Communicate your assessment and evaluation to the next echelon of care so that they can prepare and allocate resources appropriately. This information may begin to define the nature of triage necessary for the action. Will resources have to be rationed? Will more serious casualties be tagged expectant because medical supplies and personnel are limited? How can your time best serve the most casualties?

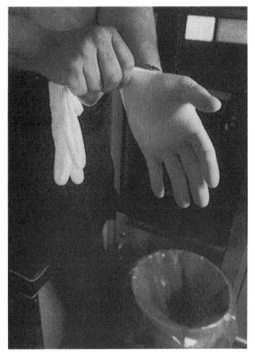

Figure 3-2 Donning of sterile gloves.

As you prepare for assessment and care, don protective gloves and be ready to employ body-substance isolation procedures. The deployment area is anything but sterile, and you may be in contact with several patients and their blood and other body fluids. It is important to protect a patient from cross contamination with blood and body-fluid-borne pathogens acquired by caring for other patients. Change gloves when they become soiled or contaminated, especially as you move from one patient to another. You may consider wearing multiple gloves and peeling one pair after another as you care for each patient. Be sure glove disposal is safe and does not give the enemy potential intelligence clues. In dire and austere circumstances, gloves and sterile dressings may be in short supply. Use whatever materials are available, and maintain as clean an environment as is possible. Remember, *infection is a lethal potential with any serious wound* (Figure 3-2).

The short time you use to plan your actions during the scene size-up assures efficient and expeditious casualty evacuation, assessment, and care. It may better assure your safety, the safety of your patient, and your ability to provide optimum care under less than ideal conditions.

ASSESSMENT UNDER FIRE

Unless it is mission essential, *do not offer extensive assessment and care until you can move the casualty to cover or at least concealment.* Such activity exposes both the casualty and you to hostile fire. If immediate movement is necessary, select a rapid movement technique based on the terrain and the equipment and manpower available, as described in chapter 8. When possible, move the casualty along the long axis of his or her body, head first, to limit any aggravation of initial injuries. Direct assessment and any care you offer under fire at manually maintaining the airway and locating and stopping any serious hemorrhage. Proper head positioning and direct pressure or tourniquet application may be necessary. Once the patient is moved to cover or the hostile fire has been neutralized, begin tactical field assessment and care.

TACTICAL FIELD ASSESSMENT

Assessment consists of the same initial assessment steps employed in the civilian theater, including the level-of-consciousness evaluation, the ABCs, and a quick exam for serious hemorrhage or injury to the head or trunk. Follow the initial assessment with the focused physical assessment, examining areas where injury is expected from information you gather during the scene size-up or initial assessment. Only if time permits do you provide a detailed assessment (a complete head-to-toe exam), and then only after you address any life-threatening injuries and provide the initial and focused assessment for other casualties. Follow your assessment with a regular ongoing assessment, reexamining the vital signs and any serious injuries frequently while the casualty remains in your care.

Initial Assessment

The initial assessment evaluates critical signs and symptoms that identify life-threatening injuries and problems. The major elements of this assessment evaluate the casualty's level of consciousness, airway, breathing, and circulation, as well as any other severe hemorrhage and major injury sites on the head and torso. During the initial assessment, treat only life-threatening problems that you can quickly correct.

Level of Consciousness

The casualty's level of consciousness is a quick and accurate indicator of his or her respiratory and cardiovascular systems' status. Without good respiration, heart action, adequate vascular tone, and blood volume, the casualty does not maintain consciousness. Quickly determine if the casualty can answer simple questions in complete, coherent, and appropriate sentences. If not, establish whether the problem is due to an airway, respiratory, cardiac, or vascular problem, and be ready to intervene. Note how well the casualty responds to questioning to determine, later in care, if his or her level of consciousness is improving or deteriorating.

Airway

Assure that the airway is open and unobstructed, and that the casualty is moving air through it. If any problem is noted, protect the airway with head and neck positioning, using the chin lift-head tilt. Neck injury, involving the spine, is usually associated with blunt trauma and rarely with projectile wounds. If there is a possibility of neck injury, use the chin lift without head tilt or the jaw thrust. Employ spinal precautions if indicated and continue them throughout the casualty's care.

Determine if the patient is conscious and is otherwise able to control his or her airway. The oral airway is indicated in the completely unresponsive patient, whereas the nasal airway is helpful in the patient with potential airway problems who has some gag reflex. If oral fluids or blood endanger the airway, place the patient on his or her side, in the recovery position, and suction as necessary (Figure 3-3). If simple airway procedures do not provide a secure airway, consider intubation.

Endotracheal intubation is the only definitive way to keep the airway open and protect the lungs from fluid aspiration. It also increases the efficiency and effectiveness of artificial respiration. The procedure uses a lighted tongue blade, called a **laryngoscope**, to open the mouth and visualize the opening of the trachea. Then an **endotracheal tube** is inserted into the opening. The space between the inside of the trachea and outside of the endotracheal tube is sealed with an inflatable cuff. Once sealed, the tube provides a secure airway from the trachea outward (see Appendix D, Advanced Airway Procedures).

In the nighttime tactical operation, where light discipline must be observed, consider an alternative procedure called digital intubation. This procedure introduces the endotracheal tube blindly and without the laryngoscope. During intubation, you hold the oral cavity open with a bite block or oral airway while your fingers walk down the tongue until you feel the tip of the epiglottis. Stiffen the endotracheal tube with a stylet and prebend into a J shape. Then guide it along the tongue, then the epiglottis, until it enters the trachea (see Appendix D, Advanced Airway Procedures).

Once the endotracheal tube is placed, assure its correct location. Carefully listen to both sides of the chest and assure adequate, clear, and equal sounds are heard with each ventilation. If breath sounds are stronger on the right side, suspect the tube has been introduced too far into the trachea and has lodged in the right mainstem bronchus. Withdraw the endotracheal tube slightly, and check the sounds again. Also listen for sound at the epigastric region of the abdomen (just below the sternum). If you hear a gurgling sound with each breath, the endotracheal tube has been placed in the esophagus. Withdraw it and reattempt placement.

In the tactical environment, the noise level may be such that auditory confirmation of endotracheal placement is unreliable. Then carefully assess chest rise and assure it is bilaterally equal. Watch for condensation on the inner surface of the tube, increasing and decreasing, synchronized with each inspiration and expiration. Patient skin

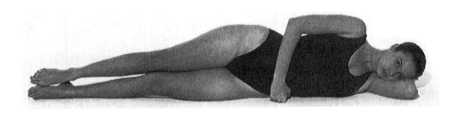

Figure 3-3 Recovery position.

color and level of consciousness may also help in assessing in the effectiveness of artificial respiration and proper endotracheal tube placement. Consider using an **end-expiratory CO_2 detector** (electronic devices register the CO_2 level of expired air while colormetric devices change color in the presence of CO_2).

It is essential that you carefully confirm the placement of the endotracheal tube. If it is lodged in the esophagus, the casualty will not be ventilated by your bag-valve-masking attempts. The absence of respiration for just a few minutes results in death. If in doubt, revisualize its entry into the trachea using the laryngoscope. *If you are not absolutely sure the endotracheal tube is properly placed, remove it, hyperventilate the casualty, and reattempt its placement.* Remember, each time you move the patient, you may dislodge the endotracheal tube from the trachea, so it is essential that you reassess tube placement after every patient move.

Once you are certain the endotracheal tube is placed properly in the trachea, note the depth of insertion (denote the centimeter markings on the side of the tube) and secure it firmly in place. Do so by wrapping the tube with tape, which is then secured to the chin or upper lip and around the neck. Frequently monitor the depth and other signs of correct endotracheal tube placement.

Past experiences with modern warfare denote a relatively high incidence of trauma-induced airway obstructions. These injuries, usually related to severe facial trauma, may be impossible to relieve with airway positioning and attempts at endotracheal intubation. Two related techniques that can restore the airway, at least long enough to obtain more definitive care, are the **cricothyrotomy** and **cricothyrostomy**. These emergency (and surgical or needle) airway procedures perforate the membrane between the thyroid and cricoid cartilages, providing a route for ventilation directly into the lower airway (see Appendix D, Advanced Airway Procedures).

Breathing

Make sure the casualty is moving an adequate volume of air with each breath and the respiratory rate is between 12 and 28 times per minute. Respiration outside this range suggests serious respiratory problems. Quickly expose the chest and examine its movement associated with breathing. Look for equal motion on both sides and determine if excursion is minimal, normal, or exaggerated. Then look for entrance and exit wounds and other signs of trauma. Anticipate projectile travel through the body and the structures and organs it may have injured. If the casualty is experiencing dyspnea, auscultate the lungs and assure breath sounds are equal throughout the chest. Carefully record your findings so that you or others can determine if the casualty's condition is changing with time.

If the casualty has received anything but minor injuries, administer supplemental oxygen at 15 liters per minute (LPM) via the nonrebreather mask. However, if oxygen is in short supply and time until evacuation may be prolonged, conserve oxygen for administration to casualties exhibiting signs of serious respiratory problems. One method to conserve oxygen is to use the nasal cannula. It will enhance the oxygen content of air by about 4% for every liter of flow up to 6 liters per minute (1 LPM = 24%, 2 LPM = 28%, 3 LPM = 32%, ... 6 LPM = 44%). *If pulse oximetry (a device that measures oxygen delivery to distal tissues) is available, adjust the oxygen flow to maintain an oxygen saturation of at least 95%.*

If the casualty is not moving an adequate volume of air or the respiratory rate is overly slow, consider overdrive ventilation. (Rapid, shallow respirations may also deliver inadequate respiratory volumes and may require overdrive ventilation.) Overdrive ventilation requires bag-valve-masking the patient at between 20 and 24 full breaths per minute. Remember, this task takes at least one trained person, providing constant care, until the casualty arrives at the next echelon of care. If resources are austere, place a battlefield casualty needing artificial ventilation in the expectant triage category.

If the casualty is experiencing any serious dyspnea, search out a cause. Look for entrance and exit wounds or signs of blunt chest trauma. Examine all open wounds for any evidence of air flowing in or out, and cover them with dressings. If any bubbling or frothy blood is associated with the wound, consider the patient to have a pneumothorax and carefully monitor him or her for tension pneumothorax. The frothing blood suggests the blood is being pushed out of the wound. Completely sealing it may permit pressure to build within, creating a tension pneumothorax.

The chest wall is rather thick and resilient. It takes large wounds to open a track to permit air to move freely through the chest wall. Small caliber handguns usually result in no air movement, whereas shotgun and high-velocity exit wounds are more commonly associated with such injury. When tension pneumothorax develops from an internal defect, the pressure may move air outward, creating a bubbling or frothy wound.

Blunt wounds can suggest internal bleeding and, if extensive, may disrupt chest integrity. If a chest segment is free to move on its own, it moves opposite of the rest of the chest wall (paradoxical respiration). This motion compromises the casualty's breathing effort and is called flail chest. If you observe paradoxical respiration, stop the segment's motion with gentle hand pressure and assume that gentle pressure with bulky dressings and bandage materials. Do not restrict chest excursion with your bandage application.

Consider the possibility of heart and great-vessel injury. These injuries may lead rapidly to severe internal hemorrhage and death. Pericardial tamponade occurs when an object or projectile perforates the heart and permits blood to leak into the pericardial sac. As blood accumulates in the sac, the heart can no longer fill with blood, and circulation slows. This condition, if uncorrected, carries a very poor expected outcome (**prognosis**). However, rapid care, usually available at the military aid station or civilian hospital, can quickly alleviate the life threat. Therefore, if you suspect this condition, arrange for rapid evacuation if possible.

Circulation/Hemorrhage Control

Check the casualty's pulse, feel for skin temperature, examine for capillary refill, and look at the casualty's general appearance. A rapid strong pulse may suggest only excitement or exertion, whereas a rapid weak pulse may suggest impending shock. A slow bounding pulse in an unconscious casualty may suggest head injury. Cool skin temperature may be an early sign of shock. Capillary refill returns in under 3 seconds after you release blanching pressure. If it does not, suspect circulatory compromise and shock, exposure to a cold environment, or possibly a preexisting condition. Look carefully at the casualty's general appearance. If he or she is pale, ashen (gray), or cyanotic (bluish) and appears anxious, frightened, or restless, suspect shock. If the signs and symptoms of circulatory compromise and shock are present, you may wish to initiate an IV and infuse fluids at the conclusion of the initial assessment.

Quickly survey the body for any signs of serious hemorrhage. Sweep the hidden body regions, under the head, neck, back, buttocks, and legs. Immediately stop any serious and continuing hemorrhage by quickly applying a pressure dressing or, in dire circumstances, a tourniquet.

The initial assessment ends with a quick examination of the areas not already surveyed and most likely to induce life-threatening injury. In conventional casualties, these areas are the head and abdomen. (You have already extensively assessed the thorax during earlier steps of the initial assessment.)

Head

Projectile wounds penetrating the skull are often immediately fatal. Other wounds may damage the facial structure and endanger the airway. *Focus your care for head injuries on assuring a patent airway, adequate respiration, and hemorrhage control.* Consider supplemental oxygen, and bag-valve-mask the patient if needed to assure good ventilation. Endotracheal intubation may be necessary if the airway is difficult to control.

The head is highly vascular, and wounding often causes serious bleeding. Although head wounds alone infrequently account for shock (except in pediatric patients), the blood loss can significantly contribute to it. Use care in applying direct pressure since the wound may damage the stability of the skull, and fracture site pressure may produce physical brain injury.

Abdomen

The major immediate life-threat from abdominal wounds is internal hemorrhage. Examine for signs of blunt or penetrating injury, and carefully monitor for the signs and symptoms of shock. Again, anticipate the organs affected by injury, and consider fluid resuscitation.

Results of the Initial Assessment

With the conclusion of the initial assessment, you have quickly corrected all easily reversed life-threatening problems. You also know enough about your patient's wounds to identify what care steps and continuing treatment are necessary for his or her survival. Use this information to plan care and to determine the patient's triage status. Integrate the nature and seriousness of your casualty's injuries with the nature and scope of the engagement as determined from your scene size-up. The result is a triage format to assure the placement of salvageable casualties in an appropriate (immediate, delayed, minimal, or expectant) category so that they receive the needed care. If practical, make patients who are determined as expectant comfortable during your time at their side.

In the prolonged and extensive tactical engagement, you may care for the walking wounded first to return them to duty quickly so as to accomplish the mission. This recognizes that many seriously injured casualties cannot be salvaged because of austere resources and lengthy time to definitive care. In other circumstances, and in the civilian theater, you care for those who, with more intense care, will survive otherwise mortal wounds first. Where the number of casualties is well matched to the resources, you may care for the most serious patients first, excepting those with mortal wounds not affected by the degree of care (see chapter 10, Tactical Triage).

Establish the appropriate triage for casualties under your care, and then begin care for the immediate category patients first, then the delayed category patients. In multi- or mass-casualty situations, spend only a few moments with each patient when deciding a triage category.

Focused Physical Assessment

Once you initially assess the casualty, and life-threatening problems have been corrected, employ the focused assessment. This assessment step more carefully examines specific body areas for further, though less life-threatening, injuries.

Examine any wounds to the head, chest, and abdomen located during your initial assessment. Identify entrance wounds, and search for any associated exit wounds. Quickly examine the wound nature to determine the impact energy associated with the exit wound (which will be generally more extensive and "blown out" in appearance), if one exists. This probably represents the wound's damage potential once it began to generate the cavitational wave. Visualize the missile's travel through the body, and anticipate the structures and organs it affects. Suspect the bearing the injury may have on the patient's overall condition (Figure 3-4).

Question the casualty on any signs or symptoms associated with the wound. Ask specifically about breathing difficulty, and question about the symptoms of developing shock: thirst, anxiety, weakness, dyspnea, coldness, and so on. Also ask about any limits to mobility or pain on motion. Although you may anticipate many casualty complaints, your questioning may reveal otherwise hidden or unexpected injuries.

Quickly scan all four extremities for injury. Extremity wounds do not frequently result in casualty death, but they are often severe and lead to disability. Assure they are not associated with severe hemorrhage, and control any moderate or serious blood loss with direct pressure, elevation, pressure points, or if necessary, a tourniquet. Often severe amputations associated with land mines and other explosive detonation result in mangled wounds with blood loss from nonspecific locations. Here the tourniquet may be your only choice for adequate hemorrhage control.

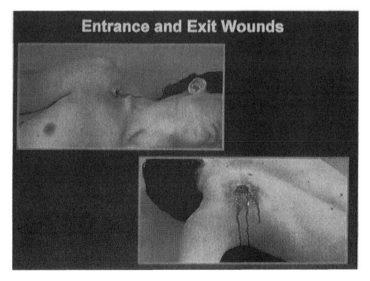

Figure 3-4 Entrance-exit wound.

Detailed Assessment

The detailed physical assessment is not indicated while under fire or while providing field care unless all patients are stable and time permits. Then conduct a complete head-to-toe assessment, and question the patient about all signs and symptoms as well as his or her medical history. Be certain to inquire about allergies to the drugs associated with emergency trauma care-antibiotics, narcotics, anesthetics, and the like. Look for additional penetrating and blunt injuries and any associated trauma.

Ongoing Assessment

The ongoing assessment periodically evaluates the patient's vital signs, level of consciousness, and signs of injury to determine whether the patient's condition improves, deteriorates, or remains the same. Watch the casualty for increasing pulse rate, deteriorating level of consciousness, increasing capillary refill time, or respirations moving outside the 12- to 28-breath-per-minute range. Also examine any previously noted serious injuries for continued hemorrhage or other indications of problems associated with the wounds (see chapter 9, Evacuation Care).

Ask about symptoms, and compare the casualty's answers to previous descriptions of his or her condition. The body's response to trauma often masks serious injury symptoms. With time, the signs and symptoms of injury may become more apparent. Consequently, further symptom questioning may reveal patient complaints not reported earlier. Investigate any changing casualty complaints.

In a critical patient, the ongoing assessment occurs about every 5 minutes or shortly after any significant intervention. In stable patients, this occurs every 15 minutes or so. However, during an engagement, your attention may be rationed between several casualties, limiting your ability to provide timely ongoing assessments.

CONVENTIONAL CASUALTY CARE

Conventional casualty care employs the same skills as civilian care though you offer them under much more severe and constraining conditions. The care is also directed more frequently toward penetrating, high-energy trauma caused by assault rifles and exploding ordinance. Conventional casualty care procedures, in addition to those provided during the initial assessment, include general trauma care, projectile wound care, fluid resuscitation, pleural decompression, blast injury care, pain medication, and antibiotic therapy. Burn therapy is frequently a required part of battlefield injury care but will be addressed in chapter 4, Care of Blast and Burn Casualties.

GENERAL TRAUMA CARE

Trauma care for the casualty of an engagement resembles standard prehospital care (Figure 3-5). You bandage wounds and splint limbs with suspected fractures using the techniques associated with the basic EMT. Package the patient for transport by securing the head, trunk, and legs to a spine board or stretcher and by tying the hands together. If

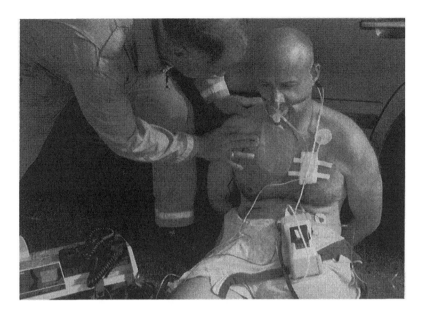

Figure 3-5 General penetrating trauma care.

you suspect spinal injury, employ the cervical collar and other spinal precautions from the moment you recognize the injury until the casualty arrives at the next echelon of care. Monitor the patient for signs of shock, including rising pulse rate, increasing capillary refill time, cool and clammy skin, anxiety and restlessness, and dropping blood pressure. Investigate any reasons for a patient's changing signs and symptoms as soon as you note the change.

PROJECTILE WOUND CARE

You located and arrested all serious hemorrhage and hidden bleeding during the initial assessment. Now care for all remaining moderate and minor hemorrhage with the quick application of direct pressure and bandages. Though civilian care limits the amount of wound cleansing, your circumstance may require some decontamination. Battlefield contamination accounts for serious infection risk and, ultimately, some mortality. This is of special concern if the patient will not arrive at the next echelon of care for more than an hour or so.

When time permits and when serious bleeding is not a problem, remove the wound dressing and examine for large contaminants such as grass, soil, glass, and other debris. Physically remove any large pieces from the wound if you can do so without further patient injury. Follow gross contaminant removal with **irrigation** to "wash" smaller contaminants, debris, and potentially infectious material from the wound. Flush from the center of the wound outward using a bulb or ordinary syringe filled with sterile normal saline solution. Then, starting from the wound center, pat the area dry with sterile gauze pads. Replace the dressings with new sterile gauze or other dressing, and bandage the wound.

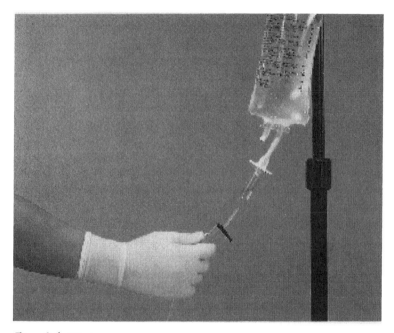

Figure 3-6 IV setup

FLUID RESUSCITATION

Provide an intravenous (IV) line for any casualty with serious penetrating trauma, and if any signs of shock develop, administer an initial bolus of 1000 ml of normal saline (20 ml/kg in the pediatric patient). Start an IV line with a large **catheter** (14 or 16 gauge), and maintain the administration site with a nonrestrictive **saline lock**. When attempting an IV site under light discipline, locate a vein by feel and watch for fluid flashback and flow by very subdued red or blue light (Figure 3-6).

Be judicious in the administration of fluids in battlefield conditions. Resources may be limited, and research has shown that large volume infusions in uncontrolled hemorrhage (such as penetrating chest and abdominal wounds) may actually increase the internal fluid loss and reduce patient survival. The objective of fluid resuscitation in the field is not the return to a preshock blood pressure but a stabilization or slight improvement in vital signs-heart rate, blood pressure, or level of consciousness.

After the initial bolus of IV fluid, disconnect the administration set and depleted fluid bag and seal the saline lock. If the casualty will not arrive at the next echelon of care for some time, provide him or her with fluid boluses of 1000 ml. Rebolus the patient if and when the vital signs suggest the patient's condition is deteriorating, or as directed by your medical control authority. In the tactical setting, avoid maintenance infusion of fluids because it requires constant attention, the administration set is cumbersome, and it requires either elevation or a pressure infuser. Remember, *the object of fluid administration is to maintain the casualty's blood pressure and other signs, not to return him or her to preshock levels.*

PLEURAL DECOMPRESSION

In the presence of severe dyspnea, suspect tension pneumothorax and consider pleural decompression (Table 3-1). Auscultate both lung fields and evaluate jugular vein distension. If breath sounds are greatly diminished on the injured side and the jugular veins (veins on both the sides of the neck) are noticeably distended, suspect tension pneumothorax. (Jugular vein distention is a late sign and may not appear in the hypotensive patient.) In a noisy environment, carefully examine the chest for excursion. In tension pneumothorax, chest rise and abdominal motion are minimal; the patient displays limited air movement and is very short of breath. You may also notice tracheal deviation, the trachea displaced away from the injured side, though this is a very late sign. If you have covered an open chest wound, uncover it. If the patient's dyspnea improves, you have corrected a tension pneumothorax. If the dyspnea does not improve or there is no open wound, employ pleural decompression (Figure 3-7).

When attempting pleural decompression, place the casualty in a semiseated position, if possible. Then locate the second or third intercostal space on the affected side by counting down two or three intercostal spaces from the top of the rib cage. You may also locate the proper position by palpating the small bump about 1" from the top of the sternum (called the **Angle of Louis**) and selecting the intercostal space above (2nd intercostal space) or below (3rd intercostal space) this bump. Then, at a location down from the middle of the clavicle, insert a long (2 1/2" to 3 1/2") large bore (14 gauge or larger) catheter. Insert the needle just over the rib to avert injuring the blood vessels and nerves that travel below each rib. Advance the needle until you feel it "pop" through the rib cage. You may hear air rush out of the catheter if the needle is releasing the pressure.

TABLE 3-1 SIGNS AND SYMPTOMS OF TENSION PNEUMOTHORAX

Respiratory	Increasing dyspnea
	Decreasing tidal volume
	Increasing respiratory rate
	Reduced chest excursion
Vascular	Jugular vein distension
	Pulsus Paradoxus
	S&S of Shock
Assessment	Diminished breath sounds, affected side
	Hyper-resonant chest, affected side
	Tracheal deviation (late)
	(away from affected side)
	Subcutaneous emphysema
	Increasing anxiety & restlessness
	Decreasing level of consciousness
	Ashen or cyanotic skin color

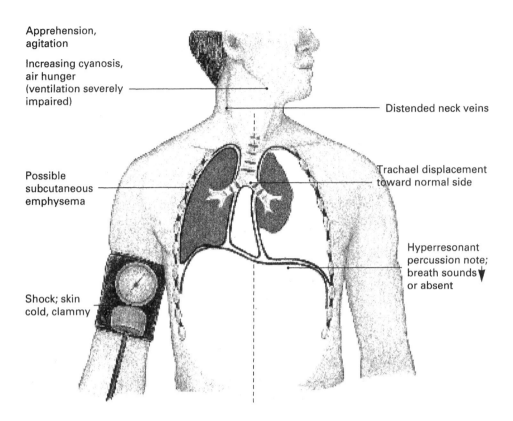

Apprehension, agitation

Increasing cyanosis, air hunger (ventilation severely impaired)

Possible subcutaneous emphysema

Shock; skin cold, clammy

Distended neck veins

Trachael displacement toward normal side

Hyperresonant percussion note; breath sounds ▼ or absent

Figure 3-7 Pleural decompression.

Remove the needle, leaving the catheter in place, and continue to monitor the patient for further signs of increasing respiratory difficulty. If the dyspnea increases, or breath sounds again diminish on the injured side, you may need to insert a second or third catheter (near the first). Over time, catheters may clog with clotting blood or bend inside the chest wall, necessitating another decompression.

Some systems employ the use of a flutter valve, either commercially available or cut from the finger of a sterile glove, to attach to the inserted needle. There is some concern that the needle may contribute to any existing pneumothorax, and the valve may prevent this. However, in the tactical setting, this danger must be weighed against the time to affix the valve and the relative risk of a simple pneumothorax.

PAIN MEDICATION

Morphine sulfate is a potent narcotic that depresses the central nervous system (a sedative) and reduces pain (an analgesic). It is used primarily to reduce or alleviate the pain associated with serious traumatic extremity wounds and severe pain affecting the expectant triage category patient. It acts on pain receptors in the brain providing both pain relief and sedation. It also relaxes peripheral venous tone, reducing blood return to the heart and blood pressure. Administer morphine with great care, to patients with head or abdominal trauma. It reduces the level of consciousness and may mask the signs if internal injury. Because of its effects on blood pressure, morphine also is given with great care, or not at all, in patients with serious hemorrhage, the signs of shock, or low blood pressure.

Be careful in the administration of *morphine sulfate* because it *may cause respiratory depression and hypotension*. Administer it in 2-mg IV increments every few minutes up to 10 mg until the patient experiences pain relief or the signs of respiratory depression or hypotension develop. If an IV route is unavailable, administer 2 mg IM. Repeat the dosing every 4 hours, as needed. Be cautious of nausea and vomiting. These side effects are common and may endanger the patient's airway, especially with the sedating effects of morphine. For this reason, it is good to place the casualty in the recovery position, if possible, when administering morphine and have suction ready in case vomiting occurs.

ANTIBIOTIC THERAPY

Infection has long been a serious life threat associated with combat. Only since the advent of antibiotic therapy has this hazard been effectively controlled. Today, antibiotic therapy is used aggressively in serious penetrating wounds such as those caused on the battlefield. High-velocity wounds and those caused by shrapnel are likely to introduce infectious agents into the wound. The wound itself consists of damaged tissue and compromised circulation. This provides an excellent growth medium for infection. Only with the assistance of potent antibiotics can this life threat be reduced. However, it is essential that antibiotic therapy be initiated within the first few hours after the introduction of the agent. This time constraint can usually be met in the police tactical operation by the patient's hospital arrival. However, in the military engagement, it may be many hours before the casualty is treated at the next echelon of care. Here the use of antibiotics becomes very important.

The chief antibiotic agents used in the military deployment are Cefazolin (Ancef) and Cefoxitin (Mefoxin). Both are potent antibiotics that fight bacterial infections. They both are administered in a single dose of 2 gm IV or IM (50 mg/kg for the pediatric patient). Contraindications include known allergy to penicillin or cephalosporin-type antibiotics. Administer Cefazolin or Cefoxitin after you offer the patient all emergent care and stabilize other serious casualties.

Closely coordinate the administration of antibiotics, analgesics, and other drugs with the next echelon of care. The supervising physician (for example, flight surgeon or battalion surgeon) must authorize and supervise all aspects of medication administration. This is usually done through protocols or unit standard operating procedures.

SUMMARY

In responding to the engagement, you are faced with different hazards than your civilian counterpart. You must protect yourself and your patients from fire by the use of cover or concealment, wait until hostile fire is neutralized, or move the casualty quickly to safety.

Once risk is removed, your treatment resembles normal prehospital care. Care centers on the scene size-up; initial, focused, and ongoing assessments; and general trauma care with a focus on hemorrhage control, respiratory stabilization, and fluid resuscitation. Endotracheal intubation secures the airway in patients with airway problems, and possible tension pneumothorax, if found, is relieved by pleural decompression. You will employ pain medication and antibiotic therapy to help comfort the patient and to combat infection, respectively, in the seriously wounded casualty. The application of these assessment and care steps assures optimum field treatment of the battlefield or tactical engagement casualty.

FOR FURTHER READING

Textbook of Military Medicine (Part 1, Volume 5) Conventional Warfare: Ballistic, Blast and Burn Injuries. Office of the Surgeon General, Washington, DC, 1990.

DI MAIO, VINCENT J.M., Gunshot Wounds: Practical Aspects of Firearms, Ballistics, and Forensic Techniques. CRC Press, New York, NY, 1993.

BLEDSOE B, Shade B, Porter R: Paramedic Emergency Care, 3rd ed. Brady, Upper Saddle River, NJ, 1996.

BUTMAN A, Martin S, Vomacka R, McSwain N: Comprehensive Guide to Pre-Hospital Skills: A Skills Manual for EMT-Basic, EMT-Intermediate, and EMT-Paramedic. Mosby-Yearbook, Inc. St. Louis, MO, 1996.

Prehospital Trauma Life Support, 3rd ed.: National Association of EMTs & American College of Surgeons—Committee on Trauma: C. V. Mosby, St. Louis, MO, 1994.

CAMBELL J : Basic Trauma Life Support: for Paramedics and Advanced EMS Providers, 3rd ed. Brady, Englewood Cliffs, NJ, 1995.

4

CARE OF BLAST AND BURN CASUALTIES

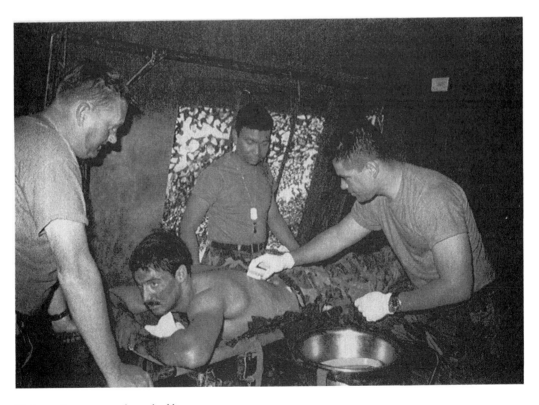

Medics perform care to a burned soldier.

OBJECTIVES

After reading this chapter, you will be able to:

1. Describe the basic mechanisms of blast injury and outline the medical effects.
2. List the signs and symptoms of blast injury, and describe the tactical management of these casualties.
3. Describe the effects of blast effect munitions and how they differ from traditional explosives.
4. Describe the basic mechanisms of burn injury and outline the medical effects.
5. List the signs and symptoms of burn injury, and describe the tactical management of these casualties.
6. Describe the effects of flame and incendiary weapons, and how casualties are managed.
7. Describe the basic mechanisms of lasers, masers, and other directed energy weapons, and outline their medical effects.
8. List the signs and symptoms of the different types of directed energy weapons, and describe the tactical management of these casualties.

CASE

You are a naval corpsman supporting a marine expeditionary force conducting an amphibious assault. Your unit's mission is target acquisition and range finding. To perform the mission, marines use several low- and medium-powered laser range finders. While working with the laser equipment, a marine notices blurred vision. Fearing an accidental laser exposure to the eye, she reports to you, the corpsman. Her complaint is severe blurring of vision in the right eye only. She denies pain or discomfort. Other symptoms are absent. She does not wear spectacles and was not wearing laser safety eye wear at the time of symptom onset. Examination of the external eye reveals no obvious injury. However, the marine has great difficulty reading even large printed letters held only a few feet away. The remainder of the focused and detailed assessment reveals no new information.

You immediately recognize possible laser burns to the right eye. You patch the affected eye with gauze and tape, taking care to leave the unaffected eye uncovered. The casualty will need to see to find her way back to the rear for definitive treatment. You document your findings appropriately, and then arrange for evacuation, which in this case is conveniently performed by empty supply trucks heading back to the beachhead.

In the rear, the casualty will be evaluated first by a generalist physician, who will confirm the diagnosis of retinal burns by ophthalmoscopy. Later, an ophthalmologist on board a hospital ship will perform a more extensive evaluation. Unfortunately, burns of the retina heal poorly or not at all, and the casualty will likely suffer vision deficits in the affected eye. The competent and compassionate care rendered in the field, however, will go a long way toward restoring the marine's confidence and speeding rehabilitation.

INTRODUCTION

This chapter introduces the care of casualties caused by blast and burn. Many traditional weapons and threats use explosives and fire to inflict injury. All tactical medics need to be familiar with the effects of these common threats. Newer weapon systems that enhance **blast** or harness the power of lasers and similar energy beams are fast emerging as additional threats. Knowledge of the care of casualties produced from these weapons and devices is increasingly important.

BLAST INJURIES

Blast injuries are generally caused by explosive-containing devices such as bombs, shells, mines, or missiles. Explosives function by the extremely rapid (explosive) burning of special fuels. The burning or combustion process occurs so rapidly that the hot gases produced are pushed outward in a violent fashion. This compresses the air surrounding the explosion and forms a shock wave. This shock wave propagates or moves outward at the speed of sound in all directions. This shock wave or blast effect is what causes blast injury (Figure 4-1).

Blast Characteristics

Near the site of the explosion, the shock wave can be very powerful. Blast overpressure is a term used to describe how powerful the shock wave is. Conventional explosives such as trinitrotoluene (TNT) can produce enormous peak overpressures measuring thousands of pounds per square inch near the point of detonation. Fortunately, this peak overpressure lasts only a few milliseconds and dissipates rapidly with distance. However, even 2 ounces of TNT can be lethal up to 1 meter (yard) away. Table 4-1 lists several types of explosives and their power as compared to TNT.

Underwater Blast

Underwater blasts differ from air blasts in the speed, pressure, and duration of the explosive impulse. The higher density of water extends the lethal range of underwater charges threefold as compared to air detonations. Two ounces of TNT detonated underwater can be lethal at over 2 meters (yards).

Modifying Factors

A number of factors can modify the effects of explosive blasts. Obviously, distance is the most important factor. *The greater the distance from the detonation, the lower the peak overpressure, and thus the effects.* Sturdy barriers between the detonation and the target will afford some protection. Conversely, a detonation in a closed room or space will greatly amplify the effects of the blast. This has practical implications for the tactical medic: seeking shelter in a bunker, foxhole, ship's compartment, or armored vehicle provides excellent protection against external blasts, but can become perilous in an internal explosion (for example, grenade tossed into a bunker or magazine explosion aboard ship).

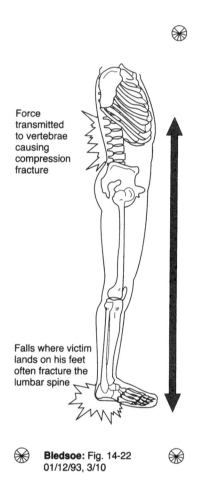

Force
transmitted
to vertebrae
causing
compression
fracture

Falls where victim
lands on his feet
often fracture the
lumbar spine

Bledsoe: Fig. 14-22
01/12/93, 3/10

Figure 4-1 Blast can cause injury from a variety of factors.

TABLE 4-1

RELATIVE EXPLOSIVE POWER OF COMMONLY USED EXPLOSIVES

EXPLOSIVE	RELATIVE POWER
TNT	1
Dynamite	0.9
C4	1.4
Ammonium nitrate/fuel oil	0.8
Sheet explosive	1.3

Body Position

Body position plays an important role in determining the extent of blast injury. Victims who are standing up or lying perpendicular to the blast will suffer the greatest injury, whereas victims facing directly toward or away from the blast suffer the least. Thus, if threatened by an imminent blast, immediately drop prone (on your stomach, face down) and face away from the expected detonation. This position minimizes blast effect and also creates a small cross-sectional profile, reducing associated **shrapnel** injury. For underwater blasts, floating on the surface is preferable to treading water because body parts deeply immersed suffer the greatest effects.

Medical Effects

The effects of a serious blast can induce injury to the lungs, abdomen, and ears (Figure 4-1). These injuries require special considerations regarding tactical care.

Lungs

The history of exposure to the effects of a detonation should leave you suspicious of lung injury. Since it occurs more frequently and is more serious than abdominal and ear injury, any time you note such in a patient, suspect and rule out any lung involvement. The patient will frequently experience disturbances in the level of consciousness or small strokelike symptoms. The patient may have dyspnea and, in extreme cases, may display blood-tinged sputum or cough up frank blood (hemoptysis).

If it becomes necessary to ventilate the blast injury casualty, do so with caution. The mechanism of injury may damage the alveolar-capillary wall and open small blood vessels to the alveolar space. Positive pressure ventilation may push small air bubbles into the vascular system creating emboli. These emboli may quickly travel to the heart and brain, where they can cause further injury or death. The pressure of ventilation may also induce pneumothorax by pushing air past blast-induced defects in the lungs and into the pleural space.

Despite the potential risks of causing air emboli or pneumothorax, you should always provide artificial ventilation to blast injury casualties with serious dyspnea. Use only the pressure needed to obtain moderate chest rise and respiratory volumes. High-flow oxygen, as supplied with a reservoir, is also helpful because bubbles of oxygen in the bloodstream are absorbed by the blood and less likely to cause injury than is the nitrogen of room air.

Abdomen

Blast injury to the abdomen calls for no special attention in the early stages of care. The associated injuries, the bowel hemorrhage and spillage of bowel contents, will take some time before their impact is felt on the patient's overall condition. The only exception to this is when the blast is extremely powerful or the casualty was very close to the detonation. In this case, look for evisceration of abdominal contents, and provide rapid evacuation and fluid resuscitation as needed.

Ears

The ears suffer greatly from the blast-wave forces associated with ordinance explosion, artillery fire, and even repeated small arms fire at close range. The outer ear focuses the blast impact on the ear drum casing irritation or rupture. If the blast is forceful, the delicate bones that transmit sound may fracture or dislocate. The casualty may experience hearing loss on either a temporary or permanent basis. Provide psychological support and reassurance. Place a loose dressing over the ear to assure the ear canal remains uncontaminated. Often these injuries, even with as much as 1/3 the ear drum torn, will improve over time without much attention. The loss of hearing, however, may reduce the casualty's ability to rejoin the team because of his or her inability to understand commands and recognize danger.

Blast injury can also result in extensive burn injury due to either the explosive charge ignition or ignition of fuels, clothing, or other munitions. Care of serious burn injury is discussed later in this chapter. Blast injury is frequently associated with shrapnel and missile injury. Care of these wounds is discussed in the chapter 3, Care of Ballistic and Missile Casualties.

Approach

Pressure injuries needing your greatest concern and care are those affecting the lungs. The damage and tearing of the alveoli causes swelling, fluid accumulation, and possibly pulmonary emboli. Progressive swelling and fluid accumulation makes breathing more and more difficult and less efficient with time. Oxygen has a more difficult time getting into the bloodstream, and the patient becomes hypoxic. If any lung pressure injury signs are present, administer 100% oxygen. Use positive pressure ventilation only when necessary and then only to obtain moderate chest rise and air movement. Lung tissue damage may allow air to enter the bloodstream directly and seriously threaten life. *If pulmonary emboli are suspected, place the patient in a head-down position on his or her left side (Figure 4-2). This will slow the movement of air bubbles into the systemic circulation.* Also monitor respirations and watch for developing dyspnea and possible tension pneumothorax. If it appears, consider pleural decompression.

Ear and bowel injury caused by the blast pressure wave require only supportive care. Bowel injury presents with abdominal pain and needs no immediate field treatment other

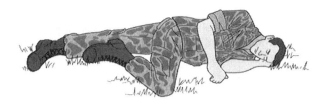

Figure 4-2 If pulmonary air embolus from blast injury is suspected, place the casualty on the left side with the head down.

than making the casualty as comfortable as possible. If there is ear pain and/or hearing loss, keep the ear (auditory) canal clean, make the patient as comfortable as is possible, and suspect possible lung damage. Remember that casualties with diminished hearing cannot recognize danger. Their duty should be limited accordingly.

Assessment

The most immediately life-threatening result of blast injury is respiratory failure from lung injury. Lung tissue injury may result in bleeding, pulmonary edema, or pneumothorax. Signs and symptoms include pain on respiration, dyspnea, hemoptysis, and ultimately, respiratory failure. Auscultation may reveal crackles, diffusely decreased breath sounds and if pneumothorax is present, decreased breath sounds over the affected lung.

Hollow organ (stomach, intestines, bladder) injury presents with abdominal pain, nausea, vomiting, hematemesis (bloody emesis), and ultimately, shock. Tympanic membrane (ear drum) damage presents with ear pain, loss of hearing, tinnitus (ringing in the ears), and perhaps a trickle of blood in the external ear canal. Rarely, loss of balance or ataxia will occur.

Blast injury is rarely found in isolation. Instead, most casualties will have associated injuries from falls, shrapnel, burns, and being struck by flying debris. Each of these possibilities must be considered and sought during the focused and detailed assessment. The signs and symptoms of these associated injuries are discussed later in this chapter and in other chapters of this text.

Management

Treatment of primary blast injury is directed first at correcting imminent respiratory failure. Clear the airway with manual maneuvers, taking care to maintain cervical immobilization. Depending on the degree of airway compromise present, oral or nasopharyngeal airways, suction, or orotracheal intubation may be indicated. If available apply high-flow oxygen by nonrebreather mask to all casualties with dyspnea. Casualties with severe respiratory distress or significant hypoxia require assisted ventilation with a bag-valve-mask. Unfortunately, such blast-injury casualties have a poor survival rate even with aggressive tactical care.

Simple pneumothorax is a significant risk of primary blast injury. However, tension pneumothorax is uncommon in this setting. Nonetheless, the signs of tension pneumothorax (including severe respiratory distress, hyperresonance to percussion and absent breath sounds on the affected side, tracheal deviation, distended neck veins, and hypotension) must be sought. If present, tension pneumothorax is immediately treated with needle decompression (see chapter 3, Care of Ballistic and Missile Casualties). Simple pneumothorax (absent or decreased breath sounds on the affected side without other serious signs) is treated with oxygen, nonocclusive dressings, reassurance, and close monitoring for any changes.

Hollow organ injury requires no specific treatment beyond good supportive care and rapid evacuation to definitive care. Administer high-flow oxygen, initiate a large-bore saline lock, and keep the casualty warm. If signs of uncompensated shock are present, administer 1000 ml normal saline bolus (20 ml/kg for children). Antibiotics and narcotic analgesics are withheld until directed by a physician. Do not give anything by mouth (npo) since the casualty may require anesthesia and surgery for definitive management.

Tympanic-membrane injury requires no specific therapy in the tactical environment. The casualty will require reassurance, however, because sudden hearing loss can create a sense of isolation and fright.

Triage

Triage of primary blast injury depends on the severity of injury and presenting problem. Casualties with airway obstruction, respiratory distress, and signs of uncompensated shock should be categorized as immediate. Hollow organ injury, with or without compensated shock are considered delayed. Most ambulatory casualties, including those with tympanic-membrane damage and hearing loss, will be categorized as minimal. Respiratory failure, apnea, and pulselessness are indications of poor survival in the face of primary blast injury and are therefore categorized as expectant.

BLAST EFFECT MUNITIONS

Blast effect munitions (BEM) are a relatively new form of weapon. They use traditional materials (such as flammable liquids) to multiply or enhance the explosive power of the device. The prototypical BEM is the fuel-air mixture bomb. In this device, a fuel such as propane or ethylene oxide is dispersed over the target by an aircraft, missile, or artillery shell. The dispersal and cloud size of the fuel is carefully controlled so that the fuel becomes explosive in the air (atmosphere). This cloud of fuel and air is then detonated, resulting in an enormous explosion.

BEMs differ somewhat from conventional bombs and explosives. First is the enormous power potential of a BEM. The bomb "size" is not limited to its casing but rather can be many dozens of meters in diameter (the size of the fuel-air cloud is limited only by the amount of fuel and the dispersal means). This allows for an enormous release of explosive energy and accounts for the large blast overpressure produced by these weapons. The second important difference between BEMs and conventional explosives is that a BEM explosion emanates not from a single point, but from a large volume (the cloud diameter). This, too, enhances the blast overpressure produced by the weapon. Last, BEMs produce little shrapnel because there is no bomb casing. BEMs can, however, hurl dust, dirt, and other objects on the ground at great speeds and cause damage in this manner.

Medical Effects

The primary effect of a BEM is to produce strong blast overpressure. This blast overpressure is no different from that produced by conventional munitions; it is only stronger. In fact, over shorter ranges, a BEM may rival a small nuclear weapon in the blast effects it produces. Thus the medical effects of a BEM are the same as those produced by the blast of a nuclear weapon (see Chapter 7, Care of Nuclear Casualties).

The body systems most susceptible to BEMs are the hollow and air-filled organs. The lungs, digestive tract, and middle ear are most commonly affected. Immediate life threats include tension pneumothorax and respiratory failure from widespread lung damage. Delayed life threats from ruptured viscous (for example, small or large intestine) are also possible. Eardrum rupture is likely, and the casualty may experience acute hearing loss and ear pain.

Thermal burns and missile wounds are also possible from BEMs. However, casualties close enough to the detonation to experience these effects will likely suffer lethal blast overpressure. Nonetheless, burns and shrapnel wounds should be sought in any casualty of a BEM explosion.

Assessment

Tactical management of BEM casualties is straightforward. *The focus of the initial assessment falls on airway and breathing function. In the focused assessment, seek evidence of pneumothorax and respiratory failure.* Abdominal tenderness may reflect hollow viscous injury. In the detailed assessment, seek evidence of skin burns and missile wounds.

Treatment

Casualties exhibiting dyspnea require high-flow oxygen and, possibly, assisted (over-drive) ventilations. A large-bore saline lock should be initiated. Fluid resuscitation should be administered only if signs of shock are present (see chapter 1, Tactical Environment of Care). Perforated viscous is difficult to assess in the field, and therefore prophylactic antibiotics should be withheld unless ordered by the physician. Most BEM casualties will suffer hearing loss, so reassurance is particularly important.

Triage

Triage of BEM casualties depends on the presenting signs and symptoms. Serious, unrelieved airway obstruction and dyspnea should be categorized as immediate. Most other seriously injured casualties will be delayed. Apneic and pulseless casualties are considered expectant. Virtually all ambulatory casualties will fall into the minimal category.

BURN INJURIES

Many weapons and munitions cause burn injury. Some, such as incendiary and flame munitions, are designed to cause high heat and burning (see discussion of these weapons later in this chapter). Others, such as high explosives, bombs, and mines cause burns incidental to their primary effects. In either case, the tactical medic must be familiar with the mechanism of burns and the tactical management of burn injuries.

Mechanism of Burns

Thermal burns are caused by contact with material sufficiently hot to cause damage. It can also be caused by exposure to energy of sufficient strength. (Burns are also caused by contact with chemicals, which is discussed in chapter 5, Care of Chemical Casualties.) Hot gases, including steam, flames, electricity, laser beams, and microwave energy are examples of burn-causing agents. The common result of these agents is damage and destruction of the skin and other bodily structures.

Medical Effects

The medical effects of burn-causing agents in the tactical environment are no different from those found in traditional prehospital care. The primary organ system affected by burns is the skin (Figure 4-3). Initially, the skin reddens (erythema) and becomes painful

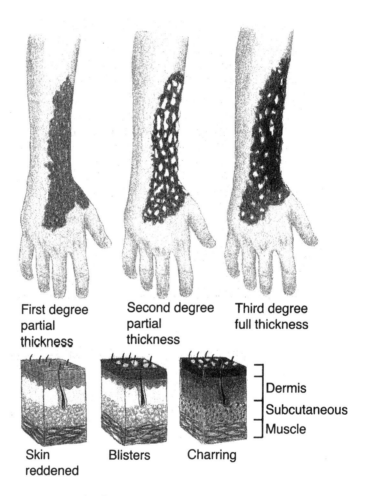

Figure 4-3 Burn classification system.

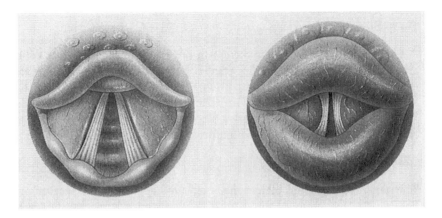

Figure 4-4 Laryngeal edema from airway burns can be immediately life-threatening.

(first-degree burn). As damage progresses, the skin blisters and swells (second-degree burn). Because only the outer layers of skin are destroyed in first- and second-degree burns, these are sometimes termed partial-thickness burns. Further damage destroys all skin layers and results in charred, painless areas (third-degree burn) also termed full-thickness burns. Second- and third-degree burned skin swells and "leaks" large amounts of fluid, accounting for the need to provide intravenous fluids. Even further burning will damage deeper structures such as muscle, blood vessels, bone, and vital organs.

Other organ systems affected by burns include the upper airway (respiratory tract), lungs, and eyes. *Airway burns may result in rapidly life-threatening swelling and obstruction (Figure 4-4). Signs of potential airway burns are listed in Table 4-2. Stridor is a particularly ominous sign and demands immediate attention.* Lower respiratory tract (lung) burns are rare but can be caused by superheated steam. Signs include dyspnea, cough, and crackles from pulmonary edema. Eye burns can result in vision loss. Pain, conjunctival erythema ("red eye"), tearing, and blurry vision are likely signs.

TABLE 4-2

SIGNS OF POTENTIAL AIRWAY BURNS

- Stridor
- Oropharyngeal swelling
- Hoarseness
- Drooling
- Difficulty swallowing
- Carbonaceous sputum
- Singed nasal or facial hair
- Dyspnea

Body Surface Area

A key principle in determining the extent of a burn is estimating the total **body surface area** (BSA) affected by second- or third-degree burns (first- degree burns are not counted). Figure 4-5 illustrates the proportion of each body area. With practice, the tactical medic should be able to make burn estimates on a given casualty in under 1 minute. Within reason, accuracy is important since tactical treatment and triage largely depend on good estimates of the total BSA burned.

Management

The general prehospital management of burns applies to the tactical environment. Following is an outline of the tactical implications of burn care. Readers requiring a review of general burn care are encouraged to consult any one of the many good emergency-care texts available.

The first step in burn care is to stop the burning process. Immediately smother any flames with a jacket, blanket, or available material. Water is exceptionally useful since it simultaneously smothers flames and cools hot tissue (Figure 4-6). Rolling the casualty on the ground is also effective.

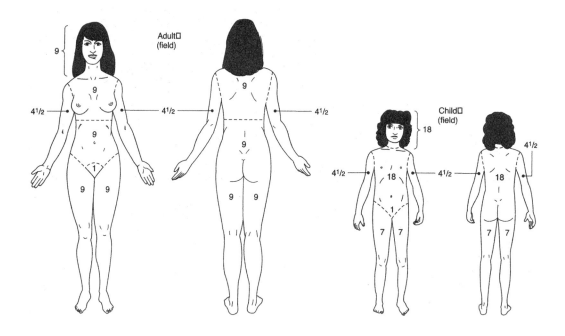

Figure 4-5 Rule of 9s to estimate body surface area.

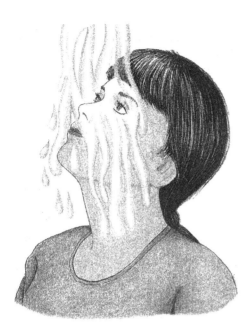

Figure 4-6 Rapid cooling of a burn can be accomplished with copious water.

Once the burning has stopped, perform an initial assessment. Concentrate on the airway since this is the most likely imminent threat from burns. Skin burns themselves are not immediately fatal and can wait until other priorities are addressed.

Remove the casualty's clothing and gear for the focused and detailed assessments. Be certain to replace protective items (body armor, kevlar helmet, NBC mask) if possible. Keep the casualty warm since burned skin is unable properly to maintain body temperature. Estimate the total BSA burned.

Cover all second- and third-degree burns with dry, sterile dressings. Do not apply ointments or creams unless directed by a physician. Initiate a large-bore saline lock (two if signs of shock are present), and administer fluid as described later. Burns can be extremely painful, and parenteral narcotic analgesia is indicated (see chapter 1, Tactical Environment of Care, and Appendix A, Medications for the Tactical Environment). Antibiotics are contraindicated.

Fluid Resuscitation

Severe burns require fluid resuscitation. The choice of fluid (normal saline, lactated ringers, colloid solutions) is the subject of ongoing discussion and research. To date, the optimal fluid for burn resuscitation is not identified. Nonetheless, normal saline can be recommended because of its effectiveness, availability, and cost. Lactated ringers is an acceptable alternative and can be substituted one-for-one with normal saline.

All burn casualties exhibiting signs of uncompensated shock should receive an immediate bolus of 1000 ml (20 ml/kg) of saline. Casualties with a BSA > 20% (10% for children) will require additional fluid, even if signs of shock are absent. However, if evacuation times are short (<2 hours), this can be safely deferred unitl the patient reaches more definitive care.

If evacuation times are long (> 2 hours), then casualties with a total BSA burned greater than 20% (10% for children) will require the additional fluid to be administered by the tactical medic. For the first 4 hours of evacuation delay, administer fluid according to the following formula:

0.5 ml Normal Saline x Patient Weight (kg) x Total BSA Burned

This amount may be repeated if the delay extends for 4 to 8 hours. For even longer delays, the amount of fluid administered (using the formula) is the same, but the timing interval increases. Thus, for a delay of 8 to 16 hours, the fluid dose may be repeated a third time, and for 16-24 hours, repeated a fourth time. In 24 hours, the casualty should receive:

2 ml Normal Saline x Patient Weight (kg) x Total BSA Burned

Ideally, the fluid should be administered as a drip. However, for the adult, it is acceptable to divide the fluid dose into 500- to 1000-ml boluses and administer them individually.

Triage

Potential or suspected airway burns should be categorized as immediate. Burns 20% to 70% total BSA are considered delayed. Burns less than 20%-unless they involve the head, hands, feet, or genital area-are considered minimal. Burns greater than 70% (50% for elderly or chronically ill patients) total BSA are likely to be lethal, and these casualties are expectant.

FLAME AND INCENDIARY WEAPONS

Flame and incendiary weapons and munitions include napalm, thermite, and white phosphorous. Although these weapons are neither new nor unconventional, they do produce injury patterns sufficiently different from conventional munitions to warrant separate discussion.

There are many types of incendiary devices. Table 4-3 lists four common types of materials used to produce the incendiary effect. Most incendiary devices are designed to be employed against equipment; however, some, especially napalm, are used against personnel.

Incendiary devices are designed to burn at very high temperatures. This burning process is the primary mechanism of injury. Magnesium burns the hottest, and it is capable of rapidly melting through steel armor. Thermite burns at slightly lower temperatures. Any individuals in the vicinity of these munitions will likely suffer severe burns.

Napalm burns at a lower temperature, but its design and employment against personnel will frequently result in many more burns than other devices. White phosphorous deserves special mention because it can spontaneously combust in air.

TABLE 4-3

TYPES OF INCENDIARY MATERIALS

TYPE	BURNING TEMPERATURE (°C)
Napalm	1000
Thermite	2000-3000
Magnesium	3000
White phosphorous	800

Medical Effects

The primary effect of incendiary and flame munitions is to cause severe burns. Contact with the superheated gases and flames from an incendiary device will result in skin burns. Airway burns are also possible, particularly if the casualty is in an enclosed space such as a bunker, ship compartment, or armored vehicle. In general, the burns caused by incendiary devices are similar to those caused by explosives and fires, only more severe.

Assessment

Tactical management of incendiary or flame munitions injury is the same as for any burn. The first priority is to stop the burning process, if necessary. Immediately smother flames by wrapping the casualty in a blanket or by rolling on the ground. If available, copious water is very effective at stopping the burning process (Figure 4-6).

Once the burning process is stopped, the focus of the initial assessment is on airway patency and adequacy of respirations. Facial burns, singed facial hair, sooty, carbonaceous sputum, or oropharyngeal swelling are all signs of possible airway burns. Tachypnea (respiratory rate > 24 in an adult or > 60 in an infant) and stridor (high-pitched "whooping" sound heard on each inspiration) are particularly ominous (Table 4-2).

Focused assessment includes an estimation of body surface area burned and the degree or depth of burns. In the detailed assessment, search for associated blast, missile, or fragment wounds that may accompany incendiary detonations.

Treatment

Incendiary and flame munitions casualties require standard burn care treatment. Initial treatment should focus on potential airway compromise from airway burns. Casualties exhibiting severe respiratory compromise will require assisted (overdrive) ventilations. Intubation is indicated for casualties exhibiting severe airway compromise, including severe dyspnea, stridor, and oropharyngeal swelling. If intubation is not feasible, manual airway maneuvers (jaw thrust, chin lift techniques, and so forth) may buy sufficient time until the casualty reaches additional care. On rare occasions, surgical airway may be life-saving in the face of severe upper airway swelling from burns (see Appendix D, Advanced Airway Procedures). Supplemental oxygen is indicated for any casualty with dyspnea.

Standard emergency care for burns includes the application of dry sterile dressings to all second- and third-degree burns. Avoid the application of ointments or other substances to burns unless expressly directed by a physician. Initiate at least one large-bore IV and connect a saline lock. Fluid resuscitation is indicated for any evidence of decompensated shock (see chapter 1, The Tactical Environment of Care). If evacuation time is short (<2 hours), no additional fluid is warranted in the field unless signs of decompensated shock are present. Prolonged evacuation may require the administration of IV fluid to maintain adequate hydration. This is especially true for second- and third-degree burns covering more than 20% of an adult. First-degree burns and second- or third-degree burns less than 20% BSA of an adult rarely require IV fluids. (see chapter 9, Evacuation Care, for additional discussion of fluids during prolonged evacuation).

Serious burns are quite painful, and morphine 2 mg IV/IM should be administered. This dose may be repeated as needed. Medication endpoints are relief of suffering (not elimination of all pain) or untoward side effects, including decreased level of consciousness, hypotension, or respiratory depression (see Appendix A, Medications for the Tactical Environment). Antibiotics are not indicated for burn injury and, in fact, may worsen the outcome.

Care for minor burns (1º < 20%, 2º/3º < 5%) includes dry, sterile dressings and elevation of the affected part (hands or feet, for example). Elevation can significantly reduce swelling and is indicated for all but the most trivial burns. Referral of the casualty to the physician is required but may be safely delayed for minor burns until the mission at hand is completed.

White phosphorous (WP) burns deserve special note because WP combusts spontaneously in air. On occasion, a casualty will be showered with WP fragments from a nearby explosion. This WP "shrapnel" can become embedded in the skin and continue to burn. Treatment includes covering the WP with water. If possible, submerge the affected body part in lukewarm (not hot or cold) water. Or use saline-soaked bandages to cover the wounds. Keep the WP covered with water until the casualty reaches definitive care.

Triage

Potential airway obstruction and dyspnea are critical markers of significant burn injury and warrant an immediate categorization. Second- and third-degree burns greater than 20% BSA (but less than 70%) of an adult ordinarily would be considered delayed. Less than 20% second- or third-degree burns would be minimal. Serious, whole-body burns greater than 70% in a young adult (50% in an older or chronically ill individual) are likely lethal, and therefore, such casualties can be classified as expectant.

DIRECTED ENERGY WEAPONS

Directed energy weapons, also called directed-beam weapons, include lasers, masers, and mass-beam devices. Additionally, nonweapon lasers and microwave power sources are common components of many weapon systems (for example, rangefinders or radar).

Injury from weapon and nonweapon energy sources is possible, and the tactical medic must be prepared to care for such casualties.

LASERS

Originally, LASER stood for Light Amplification and Stimulated Emission of Radiation. Lasers operate by charging or pumping a lasing material (such as a ruby rod) with energy, such as from a bright xenon flash tube or an electric current. Once the lasing material is sufficiently pumped, it begins to emit light in a single wavelength (color) and direction (Figure 4-7). Mirrors at each end of the lasing material reflect the beam back and forth. Each time the beam passes through the lasing material, it further pumps it, causing the light emissions to amplify by chain reaction. One of the mirrors is only partially reflective, and the light emerges as a pencil-thin, highly concentrated laser beam. The entire process takes only a fraction of a second to occur and can produce a continuous beam by constantly supplying energy to the "pump." Figure 4-8 graphically depicts a typical laser.

Beam Characteristics

Lasers produce a very thin but highly concentrated beam of light. The beam comprises a single wavelength (color) and phase, travels extremely fast, and diverges or widens very little, even over long distances. Thus, laser beams travel in a very straight line and do not deviate unless reflected by an object. Laser beams also travel at the speed of light (186,000 miles per second), which for practical, earthly uses, is instantaneous.

Reflection

Laser beams travel in a straight line toward the target. However, if the beam strikes a target or other object, part or all of the beam can be reflected. The exact angle of reflection depends on the incident angle of the beam and the geometry and characteristics of the object struck. Nonetheless, the reflected portion of the laser beam can contain substantial amounts of energy and pose a significant hazard. This reflected energy is referred to as specular hazard.

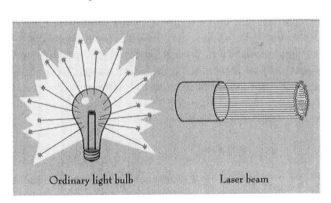

Ordinary light bulb   Laser beam

Figure 4-7 Laser light differs from ordinary light in that all energy is the same wavelength and direction.

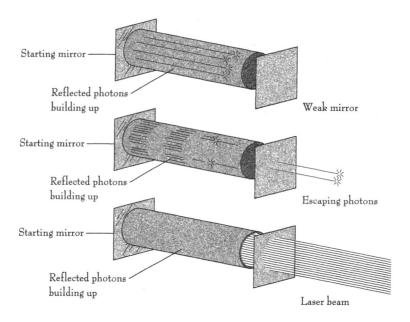

Figure 4-8 Schematic diagram of a simple laser.

Virtually all objects can reflect some laser energy although flat or shiny objects pose the greatest threat. Glass and metallic objects fall into this category. In the tactical environment, vehicle windshields, aircraft canopies, armored vehicle hulls, bodies of water (such as a puddle, pond, or ocean), and snow are all possible sources of specular hazards.

Attenuation

Laser beams can travel for many miles in clear conditions. Objects between the laser and the target, such as trees, brush, and buildings, will greatly diminish or attenuate the effects of the beam. Clouds, fog, haze, smoke, rain, and other atmospheric conditions will have variable effects on laser penetration. Low-frequency lasers operating at the near-infrared portion of the spectrum can penetrate fog and water-vapor clouds with little loss of energy. *Thus, laser damage to the target can occur even if the target itself is obscured by fog or clouds.* Of course, such laser light is below the frequency threshold of human vision and is thus invisible despite its damaging potential.

Medical Effects

Lasers exert their primary effect on biological systems by direct local heating at the site of the laser beam contact. Weapons-grade lasers operate at very high power, and the energy in the beam can raise the target spot to thousands of degrees in an instant. Obviously, this causes immediate vaporization of the target spot and severe local damage. High-powered lasers can literally "burn a hole" in flesh with resulting damage to any organ the beam passes through. Low-powered lasers common to range finders and targeting equipment do not burn or cause damage to the skin, but can damage the eyes.

Skin

The skin is vulnerable to all types of laser radiation from infrared to ultraviolet wavelengths. Mild effects include reddening (erythema) and discomfort, and are considered first-degree burns. More severe effects include blistering, charring, and tissue vaporization. This is second- and third-degree burns, respectively. The actual effects and skin damage are determined by the beam power, wavelength, and duration of exposure. In general, the greater the power, wavelength (for example, infrared), and duration of exposure, the more severe the damage.

Eye

Without doubt, the eyes are the most vulnerable organ system to lasers. Even low-powered, nonweapon lasers can cause severe eye damage under certain circumstances. Thus all lasers in tactical use must be considered potentially hazardous and handled properly.

The structure of the eye most affected by a given laser depends largely on the laser wavelength (Figure 4-9). Since the eye is an optical structure, beams of different wavelengths will penetrate the transparent eye to varying depths (Table 4-4). Thus lasers of different wavelengths can cause different types of damage, giving different signs and symptoms.

Retina

The retina is the light-sensing organ located at the posterior pole of the eye globe. Because of its function and location at the rear of a transparent, light-collecting organ, the retina is particularly vulnerable to visible and near-infrared laser beams. If the energy in the beam is low and the exposure is short, the effect on the retina can be temporary. More severe effects include retinal erythema, edema, charring, and hemorrhage. Very high energy transfers can physically disrupt the retina and destroy it. The net effect of lasers on the retina is to cause painless visual changes and blindness, either temporary or permanent.

Lens

Near UV (UVA) lasers primarily cause damage to the lens of the eye. The lens absorbs the energy and opacifies, or no longer transmits clear images. The clinical result is painless visual changes.

Cornea

The cornea is the outer covering of the globe. Besides protecting the eye structures, the cornea contributes to the optical properties of the eye. Ultraviolet (UVB & C) and far

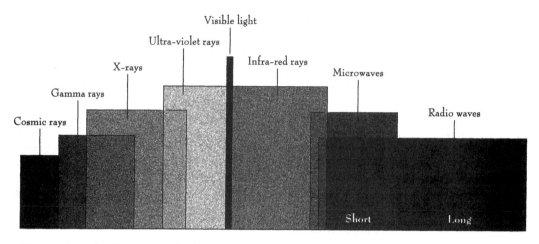

Figure 4-9 Graphic illustration of the electromagnetic spectrum.

TABLE 4-4

ABSORPTION OF LASERS BY STRUCTURES OF THE EYES

WAVELENGTH	STRUCTURE OF ABSORPTION
UVB+C (far ultraviolet)	Cornea
UVA (near ultraviolet)	Lens
Visible	Retina
IRA (near infrared)	Retina
IRB+C (far infrared)	Cornea

infrared (IRB & C) lasers tend to affect the cornea. Mild exposures result in painful inflammation resembling ultraviolet keratitis ("snow blindness"). Severe effects may opacify the cornea. The clinical results of laser injury to the cornea are painful visual changes.

Assessment

Laser casualties should be approached like any other casualty. Tactical initial assessment is unchanged and remains focused on the airway, breathing, and circulation. Focused assessment of a laser casualty will usually reveal localized, severe thermal burns in the areas hit by the laser. Varying degrees of visual loss can be expected. Eye pain may or may not be present. Even if the laser does not directly strike the eyes, specular reflections can still cause damage. Thus blindness or visual deficits may be the only symptoms present. Delayed effects are also possible, particularly with low-powered or specular hits. Delayed symptoms may appear hours later and include irritation, pain, blurring, and visual changes.

Management

The tactical emergency care for laser injuries is not different from other casualties. The focus remains on primary life-threats, regardless of cause. Second- and third-degree skin burns are immediately cooled with water, or preferably sterile saline, if necessary. If the eyes are obviously burned and still suspected to be hot, then irrigation with sterile saline or water is indicated. First-degree burns to the skin and mild injury to the eyes require no immediate treatment, and these injuries can be deferred until more serious matters are addressed.

Burns

Second- and third-degree laser burns are covered with dry, sterile dressings. Avoid applying ointments or other substances to the burn. Obvious burns to the eye are ideally treated by covering with a dry sterile dressing. *In the tactical situation, if the patient can partially see out of the affected eye and can otherwise ambulate, it is acceptable to defer dressing the eye until the casualty has evacuated himself or herself out of danger. In a similar vein, avoid covering both eyes if only one eye is injured.* This renders the casualty unable to effectively ambulate on his or her own (Figure 4-10). In some tactical situations, this burden would be unacceptable. Fortunately, leaving the uninjured eye uncovered will not worsen the injury and allows the casualty to see.

Supportive Care

If the casualty is severely injured by the laser, the usual emergency care expected in the tactical environment is indicated. Begin high-flow oxygen, initiate a large-bore saline lock, and monitor the patient closely. Laser burns are treated just like any other thermal burns. Surface area burns may be estimated using the familiar "rule of 9s." Second- or third-degree burns greater than 20% can be considered serious and deserve aggressive management. If signs or symptoms of shock are present, infuse a normal saline fluid bolus (see chapter 1, Tactical Environment of Care). Keep the casualty warm and reassured.

Body surface area burned is not the only criterion used to judge laser injuries. Lasers, by design, are penetrating weapons and can cause deep damage with only a small visible surface wound. Therefore, casualties with serious signs or symptoms and only a small laser burn should be treated accordingly.

Laser burns of the skin and cornea can be quite painful and incapacitating. Severe pain should be treated with morphine 2 mg IV or IM and may be repeated (see Appendix A, Medications for the Tactical Environment). In contrast to missile wounds, direct energy wounds and burns are not treated with prophylactic antibiotics.

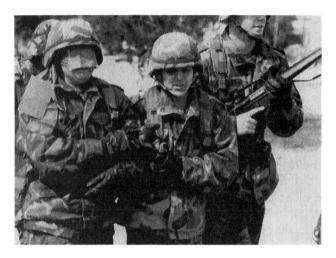

Figure 4-10 Laser burns to the eyes may cause temporary or permanent blindness.

Triage

Laser injuries require no special skills to triage. Knowledge of the medical effects of lasers, in particular on the eyes and in the depth of wounds caused, can be used to triage laser injuries accurately. Casualties suffering severe, deep, or extensive burns (for example, second or third degree > 20% BSA) can be categorized as delayed. Very extensive deep burns (for example, > 70% BSA) have little hope of recovery and may be categorized as expectant. Unless life-threatening airway compromise or exsanguinating hemorrhage is present, few isolated laser casualties will be categorized as immediate. Most isolated laser injuries to the eyes are categorized as delayed. Mild skin burns from lasers that do not represent severe threats to life or bodily function are considered minimal.

Definitive Care

Definitive care for serious laser injuries requires evacuation to units capable of specialized burn and ophthalmological care. The prospects of recovery for laser casualties depend on the nature and extent of injuries. Serious retinal burns are likely to lead to permanent blindness, as are severe thermal burns to other eye structures. With time, skin burns can heal though this may take many weeks.

Laser Protection

The basic principle of laser protection is the same as for any direct-fire weapon (for example, rifle bullet). Cover and concealment offer the best protection. Any opaque object (concealment) will attenuate a laser beam. This may reduce but not eliminate injury potential. Substantial cover such as an armored vehicle, boulder, or bunker affords more protection. However, much like exploding ordnance can scatter shrapnel in all directions, so too can specular reflections from lasers. Overhead and rear cover become important in these instances.

Body Armor

Although not specifically designed for laser protection, standard body armor and helmets afford some protection against laser strikes. A truly high-powered laser will easily defeat such personal armor. Fortunately, such weapons systems are not yet a large threat on the tactical horizon. More likely threats include medium-powered laser weapons and specular hazards from the rare high-powered laser. Personal armor can play a role in minimizing injury in these cases.

Eye Protection

Because of their exquisite sensitivity, the eyes deserve special attention when discussing laser protection. Even a low-powered, nonweapon laser can cause eye damage under certain circumstances. Therefore, proper eye protection is essential.

Certain transparent materials will block or attenuate some commonly used laser wavelengths and are useful for protective eyewear. Standard military ballistic laser protective spectacles afford modest protection against low-powered and specular laser hazards. Special multicoated lenses can protect against a broader array of wavelengths but are expensive and not widely available. Even standard (ANSI Z87) industrial-type protective eyewear affords limited protection. Nonetheless, some protection is superior to no protection, and all tactical team members should consider polycarbonate or other effective protective eyewear.

MASERS AND MICROWAVE DEVICES

Masers are direct energy devices operating in principle like a laser, but utilizing microwave or radio frequency (RF) energy instead of light (Figure 4-9). Because of the nature and properties of maser energy, it is less likely to be used as an offensive weapon. However, the weapon's potential still exists, and the tactical medic must be prepared for this possibility. Furthermore, many nonweapon devices in tactical use utilize high-energy RF (for example, radar) and can cause accidental injury similar to that of masers. This section outlines the medical effects and treatment of RF injuries to include masers, microwave emissions, and radar.

Biological Effects

RF energy effects biological systems by vibrating water molecules in the living system. The net effect is heating of the water molecules. Since humans comprise largely water, absorption of RF energy will cause heating of tissues and organs. This phenomenon is exploited, in fact, by physical therapy diathermy units and is the same principle of the common microwave oven.

Penetration

The penetration of RF energy into tissues is a function of frequency. High-frequency (gigahertz) energy penetrates very little and would be expected to produce superficial effects. Lower-frequency RF (megahertz) can penetrate deeper tissues. Damage to internal organs can be expected with this energy.

Medical Effects

Masers and high-powered RF generators such as radar cause skin and deep tissue burns. This can occur without obvious initial changes to the skin surface. Lower levels of RF energy over long periods may cause damage to the lens of the eye and the male testes. Fortunately, this is less of a tactical concern and more of a medical surveillance and preventive medicine issue.

Signs and symptoms include all the signs of superficial and deep burns. Hyperthermia and localized first-, second-, and third-degree burns are all possible. A deep, burning pain is the most likely early symptom. Late signs of exposure to high-energy RF might include hyperthermia (T > 104ºF or 40ºC) and shock.

Management

The key management principle for high-energy RF exposures is to recognize the potential for deep tissue damage in addition to any superficial effects. Burns and hyperthermia are treated in the usual fashion. Immediate cooling is indicated to stop the burning process and reverse hyperthermia. Serious burns and patients with the potential for shock should receive high-flow oxygen and have a large-bore saline lock placed. All casualties with other than trivial RF injury should be evaluated by a physician because of the possibility of occult (hidden) deep injury.

Triage

Triage of RF energy casualties is straightforward and is based on initial assessment of airway, breathing, and perfusion. Most serious RF casualties will be categorized as delayed, unless airway compromise or uncompensated shock is present. The latter casualties should be considered immediate. Minor, superficial burns can be categorized as minimal. It is difficult to judge the extent of deep RF energy injury in the tactical environment. Therefore, few such patients can easily be categorized as expectant. Examples falling into the expectant category would include casualties with absent pulse and respiration.

Protection

RF energy has variable capacity to penetrate physical barriers, depending on wavelength (frequency). In general, metallic barriers (for example, armored vehicles) provide the best protection. However, because of the long wavelength of RF energy, the beam may diffuse in and around many barriers. Thus, RF energy is not strictly dependent on line-of-site transmission. For example, crouching behind a large boulder may not afford complete protection from a nearby high-powered RF generator. Expert guidance is needed to protect tactical team members employed near high-powered RF generators such as radar sets (Figure 4-11).

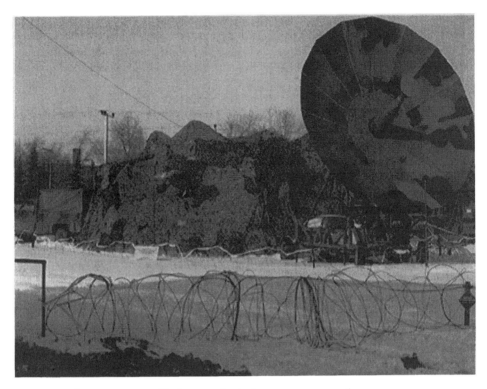

Figure 4-11 A common source of high-powered radio frequency energy is radar sets.

PARTICLE BEAM WEAPONS

Particle beam weapons use subatomic particles (protons, neutrons, and electrons) or nuclear fragments accelerated to high energies and formed into a beam. Unlike electro-magnetic beams (for example, lasers and masers), particle beams have mass (weight) and are sometimes referred to as mass beam weapons.

Particle beam generation is complex, expensive, and requires lots of power. Fortunately, these challenges have limited development and employment of these weapons, and currently, they are considered experimental. In the near term, tactical medics will be unlikely to encounter casualties caused by particle beams. Nonetheless, some knowledge of these weapons is useful.

Medical Effects

Because particle beam weapons are new and experimental, little information is known about their medical effects. What little is known is largely extrapolated from experimental models and the effects of similar weapons such as lasers.

Particle beam weapons can be expected to cause superficial and deep tissue thermal burns. Additionally, since the particles have mass, they may transfer kinetic energy to the victim, causing physical disruption to tissue somewhat akin to missile injuries. The high energy levels of particle beams may also result in ionizing radiation when the beam strikes a target. Depending on range and other factors, this ionizing radiation may cause delayed effects similar to nuclear radiation (see Chapter 7, Care of Nuclear Casualties).

Management

Treatment of particle beam casualties is similar to the care of other high-energy beams. Attention to deep and superficial burns requires standard burn care. Shock is treated as usual.

SUMMARY

Blast and burn injuries represent significant modern threats, and all tactical medics must be proficient in treating these casualties. Knowledge and understanding of the basic mechanisms of injury coupled with a recognition of key signs and symptoms is important to the successful field treatment of these patients.

FOR FURTHER READING

Technical Bulletin Medical (TB Med) 524, Occupational and Environmental Health Control of Hazards to Health from Laser Radiation, Department of the Army, Washington, DC, 1985.

Technical Bulletin Medical (TB Med) 523, Control of Hazards from Microwave and Radio Frequency Radiation and Ultrasound, Department of the Army, Washington, DC, 1980.

MOSELEY H: Non-ionising Radiation: Microwaves, Ultraviolet and Laser Radiation. Adam Hilger, Bristol, England, 1988.

Field Manual 8-50, Prevention and Medical Management of Laser Injuries, Department of the Army, Washington, DC, 1990.

Technical Guide 081, Laser Protective Eyewear, U.S. Army Environmental Hygiene Agency, Aberdeen Proving Grounds, MD, 1982.

Technical Bulletin Medical (TB Med) 506, Occupational and Environmental Health, Occupational Vision, Department of the Army, Washington, DC, 1981.

BELLAMY RF et al. (eds): Conventional Warfare: Ballistic, Blast and Burn Injuries, Department of the Army, Washington, DC, 1991.

BOWEN TE et al.: Emergency War Surgery, U.S. Government Printing Office, Washington, DC, 1988.

TRUNKEY DD et al.: Management of Battle Casualties, in Feliziano DV et al. (eds): Trauma, Appleton & Lang, Stamford, CT, 1996.

HECHT J: Beam Weapons, Plenum Press, New York, NY, 1984.

5

CARE OF CHEMICAL CASUALTIES

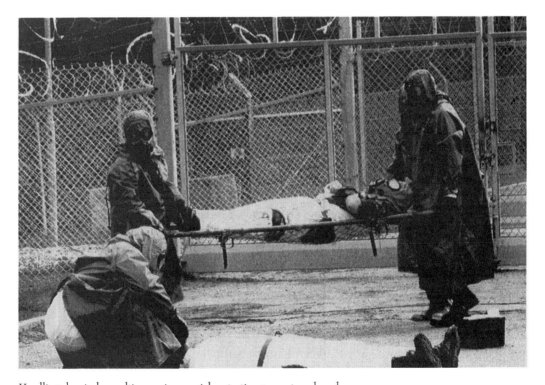

Handling chemical casualties requires special protective garments and mask.

OBJECTIVES

After reading this chapter, you will be able to:

1. Describe the nature of chemical weapons in terms of state (solid, liquid, or gas), volatility, persistence, and portal of entry.

2. List the five major types of chemical agents, and describe the general characteristics of each.

3. Understand the mechanism of toxicity of nerve agents, vesicants, cyanide, pulmonary agents, and riot control exposure.

4. List the signs and symptoms of nerve agents, vesicants, cyanide, pulmonary agents, and riot control exposure.

5. Describe the emergency treatment for nerve agents, vesicants, cyanide, pulmonary agents, and riot control exposure.

6. Outline the factors to be considered in making triage and patient disposition decisions for patients suffering from nerve agent, vesicant, cyanide, pulmonary agent, and riot control exposure.

7. Understand the steps to take and the equipment needed to ensure personal protection when working in a chemically contaminated area.

8. Describe the principles of patient decontamination from chemical agents.

CASE

You are a Navy corpsman assigned to a frigate patrolling the sea lanes in the Middle East. Over the past several weeks, the ship has experienced several "near-miss" attacks from missiles fired from the rogue nation of Crustaceae. Intelligence reports indicate Crustaceae has chemical weapons and plans to use them. In response, the ship's captain has ordered extensive drills in chemical defense, and all equipment is on hand.

While staffing the ship's sick bay, several sailors working the top deck report symptoms of blurry vision, runny nose, and chest tightness. Focused assessment reveals pinpoint pupils, diaphoresis, dyspnea, and crackles on auscultation of the lungs. Shortly thereafter, more sailors working the top deck report the same symptoms. Quickly recognizing the possible signs of nerve agent exposure, you immediately don your chemical protective ensemble and sound the alarm. You also immediately instruct your patients to do the same. To counteract the effects of the nerve agent, you instruct each of the patients to self-inject a single Mark I kit containing atropine and pralidoxime into his or her thigh. Because their symptoms were mild and treatment was rendered, the patients were returned to duty. The captain will need all hands to prepare a defense and counter the chemical attack.

INTRODUCTION

Chemical weapons can be among the most terrifying of all weapons of mass destruction. Yet with proper training and equipment, it is possible to operate in a chemically contaminated environment and perform basic patient care. This chapter reviews the medical effects of chemical weapons, emergency field treatment, and expedient decontamination of casualties. Additionally, the use of self-protective masks and garments and other equipment is reviewed.

History

Although thought of as a modern invention, chemical weapons use dates back to ancient times. In the Peloponnesian War in 423 BC, smoke was used against a fort in Athens, Greece. In this century, poison gas was used by both Germany and Britain in World War I. Although the chemical weapons were not decisive in the war, the psychological shock and blinding and choking injuries were devastating.

Chemical Weapons Ban

Following World War I, most nations were so horrified by the use of poison gas that its use was outlawed by international treaty. To date, this treaty has been successful in preventing large-scale chemical weapons use in war and peace. In 1997, a new treaty banned not only the use, but also the manufacture of chemical weapons.

Current Threat

Revelations of recent chemical weapons manufacture by Iraq and limited use by the former Soviet Union and Cambodia renewed concern among tactical medical providers that they might face chemical casualties. The specter of a terrorist attack against civilians using chemical weapons was underscored by the sarin nerve gas attack on a Tokyo subway in 1996. With the relative ease by which terrorist groups can acquire or manufacture chemical weapons, it is now imperative that all EMS providers be familiar with chemical casualty management.

NATURE OF CHEMICAL WEAPONS

To care properly for casualties of **chemical agents**, it is important to understand the nature and properties of the chemicals. With a basic knowledge of chemical agents, the medic can anticipate the type and severity of injuries expected. Furthermore, by understanding how chemical agents are deployed and used tactically, the medic can better protect against personal injury when working in a contaminated environment or on chemical-exposed patients.

Solids, Liquids, and Gases

Most chemical agents are stored in munitions (shells, rockets, and bombs) as a liquid. When the munition explodes, the liquid turns into an aerosol, or tiny droplets of liquid suspended in the air. A few riot control agents are stored as solids, but like liquid agents, become aerosols after deployment. Thus "tear gas" is not a gas at all, but aerosolized solid agent. Likewise, "mustard gas" is a liquid suspended in the air. These properties of chemical agents become important when chemical defense and decontamination is discussed later in the chapter.

Volatility and Persistence

Some agents, such as hydrogen cyanide, chlorine, and phosgene, may be gases during warm weather. Other agents, such as nerve and mustard, are liquids at these temperatures but nonetheless will evaporate just like a puddle of water. This tendency to evaporate is called volatility. A volatile liquid evaporates easily, rapidly forming a dangerous, breathable vapor. The opposite of volatility is persistence. Agents that tend not to evaporate quickly remain as concentrated, dangerous puddles and droplets on surfaces. Because of this, they may remain hazardous to touch for days or weeks after deployment. *In general, the warmer the temperatures, the greater the evaporation (and danger from breathing vapors); the colder the temperature, the greater the persistence (and danger from direct contact) of the agent.*

Portal of Entry

Chemical agents in the form of aerosolized liquids or solids, vapor, or gas can enter the body through the respiratory tract (lungs), eyes, or skin. This is the portal of entry. The lungs are by far the most important route for these agents. Although local damage to the lungs, eyes, and skin is also possible, the large absorptive area of the lungs allows large quantities of aerosols, vapors, and gases to enter the body. Thus, severe systemic effects are possible by this route.

Liquid agents tend to be absorbed primarily through the skin and eyes. Both severe local effect (chemical burns) and serious systemic effects are possible by this manner. Although infrequently encountered, accidental ingestion of chemical agents (for example, eating contaminated food) can also lead to serious local and systemic effects. The specific effects of various chemical agents are discussed in the following section.

Types of Chemical Agents

Five major types of chemical agents are discussed: (1) nerve agents, (2) vesicants, (3) cyanide, (4) pulmonary agents, and (5) riot control agents. We discuss the toxicity, signs and symptoms, emergency care, triage, and decision making for each class of agent.

NERVE AGENTS

Overview

Nerve agents are among the deadliest compounds known to man (Table 5-1). Because of this lethality, nerve agents represent the biggest threat to troops and noncombatants alike on the chemical battlefield. Because of their potency and relatively easy manufacture, they make similarly deadly weapons in the hands of terrorists. For this reason, all tactical medics and civilian EMS providers need to be familiar with these agents and their effects.

TABLE 5-1

LETHAL DOSES* OF VARIOUS NERVE AGENTS

AGENT	SKIN DOSE (mg)	VAPOR DOSE (mg-min/m³)
GA (tabun)	1000	400
GB (sarin)	1700	100
GD (soman)	50	70
GF	30	Unknown
VX	10	50

*50% fatality rate, other 50% severely incapacitated.

Nerve agents were invented by the Germans in World War II, but they were never used. The United States currently has the agents GB and VX in its inventory but is committed to destroying this stockpile over the next decade or so. The technology to manufacture, store, and deploy nerve agents is not terribly complex, and many rogue nations are felt to have this technical capability.

Nerve agents are liquid under most weather conditions. When dispersed, the more volatile ones represent both a vapor and liquid hazard. The least volatile agent GF is persistent and is mostly a liquid hazard.

Toxicity

Nerve agents exert their toxic effects by inhibiting or blocking the action of acetylcholinesterase, (AChE), a critical enzyme. AChE is found in the plasma, red blood cells, and nervous tissue. Although nerve agents will affect the enzyme in all three areas, the neurological effects are most important and are the focus of this discussion.

Acetylcholine, a neurotransmitter, functions in many sites in the body, primarily the smooth and skeletal muscles, the central nervous system, and most glands. Its action is to excite or turn "on" the muscle, gland, or nerve across the synapse, or connection (Figure 5-1). To excite the end organ (for example, skeletal muscle), the nerve ending releases acetylcholine into the synapse, and the muscle contracts. The muscle will continue to contract as long as acetylcholine is present, so to release the muscle contraction, AChE rapidly metabolizes the acetylcholine into inactive substances. This turns the muscle "off." Normally, the "on-off" process is very rapid and efficient, and allows for effective control over muscles.

A nerve agent works by blocking or inhibiting the action of AChE. This allows acetylcholine to rapidly build up in the synapse, causing it to remain in the on state. The net effect on muscles at first is uncontrolled and uncoordinated contraction of the muscle fibers. This is seen as fasciculations. Shortly afterward, the muscles fatigue and cease to work. Death usually results from respiratory muscle failure.

Nerve agents are extremely potent blockers of AChE. Only a small amount (Table 5-1) is needed to block effectively all the AChE in the body and produce serious consequences.

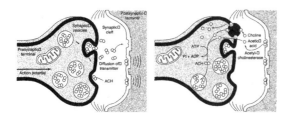

Figure 5-1 Synapse showing Acetylcholine flowing across the synapse to excite the end organ (muscle, gland, or nerve), and AChE rapidly metabolizing the Acetylcholine into inactive substances.

Fortunately, several medications exist that can break the bond between the nerve agent and AChE, thus regenerating the AChE. Unfortunately, over time (minutes to hours), the nerve agent becomes permanently attached to the AChE, preventing any regeneration of AChE. This "aging" process will markedly reduce the effectiveness of antidotal therapy. Therefore, early use of proper antidotes is critical in nerve agent poisoning.

Several compounds exist that are related to nerve agents, but are much less deadly. The most common of these are the organophosphate and carbamate insecticides and medications. These compounds cause similar symptoms to nerve agents and, in large doses, can resemble acute nerve agent poisoning. Organophosphates and carbamates do not, however, permanently bind to AChE. The principles of care outlined in this section for nerve agents also apply to organophosphate and carbamate poisonings.

Assessment

The signs and symptoms of nerve agent poisoning will depend on the dose and route of exposure. In general, larger doses and directly breathing nerve agent vapor results in quicker onset and greater severity of effects. Table 5-2 summarizes the signs and symptoms of nerve agent exposure.

The most important effects of nerve agents are on the lungs and airways, and the nervous system. *Large doses of nerve agent will wreak havoc with the brain's ability to function and result in rapid loss of consciousness, convulsions (seizures), and apnea.* Lower doses can result in difficulty concentrating, insomnia, impaired judgment, and depression. Hallucinations and confusion do not occur.

The pulmonary system is affected by two separate mechanisms that together often contribute to death. First is respiratory failure from paralysis of the respiratory muscles (diaphragm, abdominal, and thoracic muscles). The result is apnea. The second mechanism is copious airway secretions leading to obstructed larger airways and bronchoconstriction leading to obstruction of the smaller airways. The casualty may be drooling or pooling secretions in the

TABLE 5-2

Vapor	Small exposure	Miosis, rhinorrhea, mild dyspnea
	Large exposure	Sudden unconsciousness, convulsions, apnea, copious secretions, miosis
Liquid	Small exposure	Localized sweating, nausea, vomiting, fatigue, localized fasiculations
	Large exposure	Sudden unconsciousness, convulsions, apnea, paralysis, copious secretions

oropharynx. Wheezing may be prominent if air exchange is still good, or diminished if respiratory failure ensues.

Other clinical effects of nerve agents are less important but can give important clues to the cause of the poisoning. Perhaps most characteristic is pinpoint pupils or miosis. This finding, in combination with the right tactical setting and other suspicious symptoms, can lead the medic to suspect nerve agent exposure. Other, less characteristic, signs and symptoms include runny nose (rhinorrhea), copious salivation, tearing of the eyes, blurry vision, nausea and vomiting, diarrhea, sweating, and loss of bladder control. The mnemonic SLUDGE helps identify some of these findings. It stands for Salivation, Lacrimation, Urination, Defecation, and Gastric Emptying. Initially, vital signs may reflect tachypnea (rapid breathing), tachycardia or bradycardia (fast pulse or slow pulse), and normal blood pressure. Later, as effects worsen to life-threatening levels, the casualty will usually have apnea, tachycardia, and hypotension (low blood pressure).

Identification of an Attack

The early signs of a chemical attack are the same clinical signs and symptoms mentioned in the preceding paragraphs. All team members should be on the lookout for these signs, but the medic must be particularly alert in this regard. Before the nerve agent has reached incapacitating levels, most or all of the team members will experience blurry vision, runny nose, feelings of tight chest, and mild weakness or fatigue. If the medic should notice these signs in himself or herself or in the team, he or she should sound the alarm. These early effects serve as a warning signal, and all team members must don their chemical protective gear first, and then inject themselves with a single Mark I antidote kit.

Emergency Care

The first action when encountering a suspected nerve agent casualty is to protect yourself and your team from exposure (Figure 5-2). The casualty should also be protected form further exposure through decontamination. The usual measures of basic and

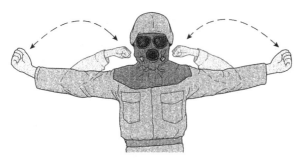

Figure 5-2 After donning your mask, sound the alarm to warn others of a chemical attack.

advanced life support apply for chemical casualties. This section highlights the key elements of treating and resuscitating casualties of chemical agents (Table 5-3).

Initial Resuscitation

Initial resuscitation should be directed at obtaining an airway and providing adequate ventilation. If able to do so, intubate the patient orally. Portable suction may be needed to clear the oropharynx of pooled secretions. If unable to intubate, an oral or nasopharyngeal airway in combination with the jaw-thrust or head-tilt, chin-lift manual method will work. Provide positive pressure ventilation at a rate of 20 breaths per minute for an adult casualty. Position the casualty in the recovery position (preferred) or supine.

Antidote

The next key step in the resuscitation is the administration of an antidote. *Currently, two drugs are available to counter the effects of nerve agents: atropine and pralidoxime (2-pam-chloride, Protopam).* Atropine, an anticholinergic, works by blocking the effect of excess acetylcholine at peripheral nervous synapses. This reduces the effects of the nerve agent. In particular, secretions will be reduced, and ventilation will be easier. For early symptoms, self-administration of atropine is indicated.

TABLE 5-3

KEY MEASURES IN RESUSCITATING NERVE AGENT CASUALTIES

- Secure airway and provide positive pressure ventilation
- Administer atropine and pralidoxime
- Administer diazepam
- Repeat atropine and pralidoxime as needed

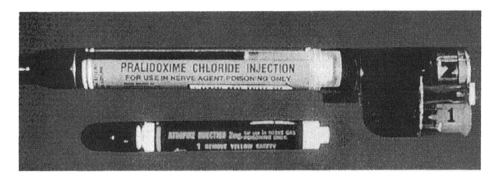

Figure 5-3 Military Mark I autoinjector kit.

Pralidoxime works by breaking the bond between the nerve agent and AChE, thus regenerating the AChE. Pralidoxime is able to work only if the bond has not "aged" and become permanent. Different nerve agents age at different rates (minutes to hours) with GD (soman) bonding permanently within 2 minutes. Pralidoxime does not work as rapidly as atropine, so it is usually administered simultaneously with each dose of atropine.

A third medication useful in the resuscitation of chemical casualties is diazepam (Valium). Diazepam does not directly counteract the nerve agent, but instead treats or reduces the likelihood of convulsions or seizures. Other benzodiazepines such as lorazepam (ativan) are equally effective and may be substituted at the appropriate doses. Unlike atropine and pralidoxime, diazepam and other benzodiazepines are never self-administered. A casualty needing diazepam would be incapacitated and unable to self-administer it.

Autoinjectors

Atropine, pralidoxime, and diazepam are all available in autoinjector form (Figure 5-3) for easy self-administration. Standard military doctrine calls for each soldier to carry three autoinjectors of atropine and pralidoxime (Mark I kits). The medic can also inject the casualty using the casualty's autoinjectors if necessary. One autoinjector of valium is also carried, but this is for use on the soldier's buddy or by a medic since any soldier needing diazepam would not be able to self-administer it.

The medic can certainly use the autoinjectors to treat casualties. Autoinjectors are a rapid method of administering antidotes (Figure 5-4). However, the intramuscular route (autoinjectors use this route) is not ideal. If time and circumstances permit, an IV should be started and atropine, pralidoxime, and diazepam administered IV. Atropine and diazepam can also be administered through the endotracheal tube, if necessary. (Some have suggested that the first dose of atropine should always be administered IM to avoid cardiac dysrhythmias. Most experts, however, feel IV/ET atropine is safe and effective in nerve agent poisoning.)

TABLE 5-4

GUIDELINES FOR INITIAL ANTIDOTE CLOSING IN CHEMICAL AGENT EXPOSURES

CONDITION	WHO ADMINISTERS	DRUG	ROUTE
Mild • Miosis, • blurry vision, • mild dyspnea, • runny nose	Self	Atropine 2 mg pralidoxime 600 mg	Autoinjector (one Mark I); repeat in 10 minutes if not improved (two Mark I's total)
Severe • above plus • generalized fasciculations, • convulsions, • unconscious	Buddy (or medic) Diazepam 10 mg	Atropine 6 mg pralidoxime 1800 mg	Autoinjector (three Mark I's) Autoinjector
Continued resuscitation	Medic every 5 minutes	Above, plus atropine 2 mg or autoinjector up to 20 mg total. Diazepam 5 mg every 5 minutes up to 20 mg total	IV, IM, ET, IV, IM, ET, or autoinjector

Additional Concerns

Injuries or wounds from conventional weapons should be treated in the usual fashion with attention to decontaminating and covering wounds to prevent further absorption of nerve agent. Keep the casualty warm, and evacuate as soon as possible.

Individuals with small exposures may develop only mild effects, such as shortness of breath, blurry vision, runny nose, tearing, and fatigue. Aggressive treatment with autoinjection is warranted, and these casualties will likely demonstrate some improvement. However, since the antidotes themselves (particularly atropine) cause uncomfortable and sometimes incapacitating effects (see Appendix A, Medications for the Tactical Environment), these casualties will likely need to be evacuated, too.

A rational approach to antidote dosing is given in Table 5-4. These guidelines were modified from military recommendations to include the capabilities of advanced-level medics and EMTs. Table 5-5 provides guidelines for the continued dosing of drugs if the casualty remains in the field or undergoes prolonged evacuation.

If the nerve agent exposure is not too large and the casualty receives prompt treatment, the chances of survival are good. Most important is early antidote administration and continued support of ventilation. If at all possible, begin antidotal therapy using autoinjectors even before decontamination is complete. The autoinjector can be used even if the casualty is wearing a full protective ensemble. The sharp steel needle will easily penetrate several layers of clothing (Figure 5-4). If resuscitation is prompt, modest improvement can

TABLE 5-5

GUIDELINES FOR CONTINUED DOSING IN CHEMICAL AGENT EXPOSURES WITH SEVERE EFFECTS (SEVERE DYSPNEA, CONVULSIONS, UNCONSCIOUSNESS)

DRUG	DOSE	INTERVAL	PREFERRED ROUTE	ENDPOINT
Atropine	2 mg	5 min	IV (or IM, ET)	Drying of secretions or 20 mg
Pralidoxime	1 gm	60 min	IV over 20 min (or IM)	Spontaneous respirations
Diazepam	10 mg	every 2-3 hr	IV (or IM, ET)	Seizure control

be expected in a few hours. The casualty will begin spontaneously breathing and will require less atropine to control secretions. The casualty's level of consciousness will improve although he or she will remain intermittently obtunded and very weak. Care at this point includes administration of supplemental oxygen, keeping the patient warm, and prompt evacuation.

Triage and Decision Making

The principles of triage for chemical casualties are the same as for conventional casualties (chapter 10, Tactical Triage). Nerve agent casualties with severe difficulty breathing, apnea, unconsciousness, or convulsions would be considered immediate. If available, treatment and securing of the airway and breathing followed by antidotal therapy should be started right away. If, however, the casualty has no pulse or blood pressure, he or she would not be expected to survive even with aggressive therapy. This casualty would be considered expectant.

A casualty with severe symptoms but conscious and breathing has an excellent chance of survival. The triage category of immediate is appropriate with initial therapy

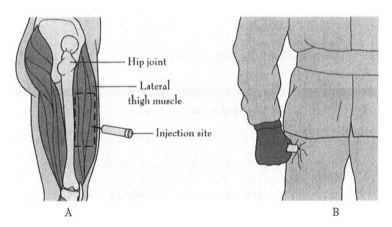

Hip joint

Lateral thigh muscle

Injection site

A   B

Figure 5-4 Self-injecting nerve agent antidote using Mark I autoinjector.

being the administration of three Mark I kits plus one valium autoinjector. This therapy is effective and requires only 1 to 2 minutes to accomplish. The casualty should, however, be watched for worsening of his or her condition.

Ambulatory or walking casualties are considered minimal. However, they should be instructed to self-administer one Mark I autoinjector (Figure 5-4) and then be observed for any changes. If symptoms do not worsen or, better yet, improve in several hours, many of these casualties can be returned to duty although their effectiveness will be diminished. In a mass casualty incident, these individuals could be expected to take a bus or truck, or perhaps walk to the hospital.

VESICANTS

Overview

Vesicants are a group of chemical agents that cause damage to exposed skin, lungs, eyes, and can also cause generalized illness if a significant amount is absorbed. Vesicants date back to World War I when sulfur mustard was first used. The current threat includes sulfur and nitrogen mustards, lewisite and phosgene oxide (Table 5-6). All these agents cause localized blistering, burning, and tissue damage on contact. The eyes, skin, and lungs are the most commonly affected organs. *The key difference between the mustard agents and the others is the onset of effects. Lewisite and phosgene oxime produce immediate pain and redness on contact. Mustard, however, causes little initial discomfort but will cause severe damage within a few hours.* All the vesicants can cause systemic or generalized illness if significant amounts are absorbed.

All the vesicants except phosgene oxime are thick, oily liquids. They have low volatility and hence tend to be persistent. In warm temperatures, all the vesicants pose a significant vapor hazard. Mustard has an odor of onions, garlic, or mustard, whereas phosgene oxime smells of newly mown grass or hay. However, the sense of smell is unreliable and should never be used for chemical agent detection.

Toxicity

Vesicant agents cause damage on contact. The agent causes local damage at the cellular level, leading to tissue destruction. Blisters commonly form, hence the old term *blister*

TABLE 5-6

CURRENT VESICANT AGENTS AND ONSET OF SYMPTOMS

HD	Sulfur mustard	Delayed
HN	Nitrogen mustard	Delayed
L	Lewisite	Immediate
CX	Phosgene oxime	Immediate

agent. Mucous membranes, particularly the eyes and respiratory tract, are very sensitive to vesicants. The net result is a chemical burn of the affected area.

Vesicants can also be absorbed into the body and blood stream and cause systemic damage. Mustard, in particular, will damage the blood-forming organs (bone marrow) and can cause life-threatening illness days or weeks after the initial skin injury. However, the body fluids of vesicant casualties do not contain hazardous levels of the agent, and no special precautions are needed beyond standard universal precautions.

Assessment

Vesicant agents cause burning, redness (erythema), blistering, and necrosis of exposed skin. Eye contact results in stinging, tearing, and development of eyesight-threatening ulcers. Inhalation of vesicant vapors causes shortness of breath, cough, wheezing, and possibly, pulmonary edema. Other nonspecific symptoms include nausea, vomiting, and fatigue. Table 5-7 summarizes the signs and symptoms of vesicant agents.

The key difference between mustard agents and other vesicants is the onset of signs and symptoms. Lewisite and phosgene oxime cause immediate burning and pain to the skin, eyes, and respiratory tract. Exposed individuals will usually exit the area or don their protective mask and garments immediately upon exposure. This usually limits the total exposure of the casualty and consequently limits injury.

In contrast, mustard agents cause no immediate symptoms on contact. Thus, individuals may not be aware of the exposure and fail to decontaminate or protect themselves from further exposure. Unfortunately, mustard exposure of only a few minutes will lead to significant pain, redness, and blistering within 2 to 24 hours. Eye damage may occur earlier, often within 1 to 2 hours after exposure.

Severely exposed individuals may develop widespread skin and mucous membrane damage. Essentially, such casualties have suffered large chemical burns. Pain, blindness, and respiratory distress will be prominent features in such casualties.

Emergency Care

The most important action when caring for a vesicant-exposed casualty is immediate removal of the agent. The window of opportunity for preventing damage is only a few minutes in duration. Immediate irrigation with water or a chemical decontamination kit is crucial. Since time is essential, this care must be provided by the casualty himself or herself or by a buddy (self-

---

TABLE 5-7

SIGNS AND SYMPTOMS OF VESICANT AGENT EXPOSURE

Skin	Burning, erythema, blistering
Eyes	Stinging, tearing, ulcer formation
Respiratory	Shortness of breath, cough, wheeze
Gastrointestinal	Nausea and vomiting
Other	Fatigue, lethargy

TABLE 5-8

EMERGENCY TREATMENT OF VESICANT CASUALTIES

Immediate	Copious irrigation and decontamination
Mild skin irritation	No special treatment
Severe skin lesions, blisters	Sterile dry dressing
Severe eye lesions	Eye patch
Severe pain	Morphine IV/IM
Severe respiratory distress	Oxygen, intubation if needed

aid or buddy aid). By the time the casualty reaches the medic, at least some damage has been done. Nonetheless, medical treatment includes continuing irrigation and decontamination. The type and amount of irrigation used will depend on the available supply of water. If available, a hose (low pressure) provides plenty of water. However, in a pinch, the small amount in a canteen is better than nothing. Saline from an IV bag is also useful and is particularly suited for eye irrigation. However, never delay irrigation of the eyes while searching for sterile saline. Use plain, uncontaminated water instead.

Once blisters or other damage occurs, emergency care is the same as for ordinary chemical burns. Dry sterile dressings are applied loosely. Severe eye injuries should be patched. Most casualties will be suffering significant pain and should receive intravenous morphine. Unlike thermal burns, most serious vesicant casualties do not require fluid resuscitation. Table 5-8 outlines the emergency treatment of casualties exposed to vesicants.

Triage and Decision Making

Most vesicant casualties with less than 50% BSA affected will be categorized as delayed. Over 50% BSA affected would usually be considered expectant. This unfortunate casualty could be saved, but only at the expense of great medical resources. Casualties with eye involvement are considered delayed. Less than 5% BSA affected are triaged minimal. Few if any vesicant casualties will be triaged as immediate, except perhaps to institute immediate irrigation. This, however, should have been instituted as part of self-aid or buddy aid prior to reaching medical care.

CYANIDE

Overview

Cyanide is a rapidly acting lethal agent that directly poisons the body's cellular metabolism. It is the representative agent of what used to be termed "blood agents." This old term is a misnomer because the site of action of cyanide is not the blood or red blood cells. Related chemicals with similar toxicities include hydrogen cyanide (AC), cyanogen chloride (CK), and cyanogen bromide. Although it is a potent poison, cyanide is 25 to 50 times less toxic by the inhalation route than the nerve agent GB (sarin). This limits its tactical usefulness. However, cyanide is relatively easy and inexpensive to produce, and hence may represent a significant terrorist threat.

Cyanide was used in large quantities by the French in World War I, but the military effectiveness was small. Japan allegedly used cyanide against China in World War II, and Iraq may have used the agent against the Kurds in the 1980s. The high volatility of cyanide means that it evaporates and disperses quickly. Thus, it is likely to affect only those individuals in the immediate area at the time of a cyanide release. An important exception might be a closed-space release, such as in a building. In this case, the enclosed space would slow the dispersion.

Cyanide exposure risk is not limited to chemical warfare and terrorist attacks. Thousands of tons of commercial cyanide and related compounds are manufactured and transported across the United States and other countries every year. Combustion of plastics, as in a structure fire, can also produce cyanide. Thus, all EMS providers must be familiar with the management of cyanide-poisoned patients.

Toxicity

Cyanide is usually absorbed by inhaling the vapor; however, poisoning can also occur by ingesting cyanide-contaminated food or water. Once in the body, cyanide acts rapidly. If a large concentration is inhaled, loss of consciousness occurs within 1 minute and death within 6 to 8 minutes. Moderate exposure will also produce unconsciousness and death, but may take many minutes to occur. It is for these latter cases that emergency care is directed because there is sufficient time in which the medic can act. Low-dose exposures can make the casualty briefly ill, but most will recover without treatment. This "all or nothing" phenomenon of cyanide has important implications for treatment and triage, as will be discussed.

Cyanide rapidly inactivates a metabolic enzyme called **cytochrome a$_3$**. This enzyme is critical to all cells in the body, and it allows the utilization of oxygen for cellular energy. When cytochrome a$_3$ is inactivated by cyanide, the cell immediately starves for oxygen and begins to die. No amount of supplemental oxygen can overcome this process (yet supplemental oxygen is still important to maximize oxygen delivery to those cells not yet poisoned by cyanide). The body can rid itself of small amounts of cyanide, and this accounts for the spontaneous recovery of casualties with minimal exposures. Larger exposures overwhelm the body's natural cyanide detoxification, and unless treatment is promptly started, the casualty will likely die.

Assessment

Cyanide works rapidly and primarily targets the brain and heart. Within a minute of inhaling a high concentration of cyanide, the victim loses consciousness and may convulse (seize). Two or three minutes later, the casualty stops breathing. Cardiac arrest occurs within 6 to 8 minutes of exposure.

Lower concentrations or ingestion of cyanide produces milder symptoms and a slower rate of onset. Anxiety, weakness, dizziness, nausea, and muscular trembling are common. Physical findings are nonspecific and may include elevated heart and respiratory rate. It is possible for symptoms to progress to loss of consciousness, apnea, and death. The

TABLE 5-9

SIGNS AND SYMPTOMS OF CYANIDE POISONING

High concentration inhaled	30-60 sec loss of consciousness, convulsions 2-3 min apnea 6-8 min cardiac arrest
Ingestion or low concentration inhaled	Tachycardia Tachypnea Dizziness Nausea Weakness May progress to LOC, apnea and death

"cherry red" color of the lips and extremities classically associated with cyanide poisoning is unreliable. The casualty may be pale, cyanotic, or normal color. Importantly, the pulse oximeter may give a false sense of reassurance in cyanide poisoning. Although the blood may be well saturated with oxygen, the cyanide causes cellular hypoxia by blocking the utilization of oxygen. Table 5-9 outlines the signs and symptoms of cyanide poisoning.

Emergency Care

To be effective, treatment of serious cyanide poisoning must be started early. Serious vapor exposures will likely result in severe respiratory distress or apnea in addition to unconsciousness. Rapid airway intervention (endotracheal intubation, if available) and ventilatory support with a bag-valve-mask is indicated as a first priority. However, a rapid shift to antidotal therapy will be required to save the patient.

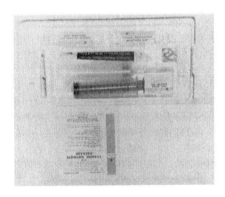

Figure 5-5 Cyanide antidote kit.

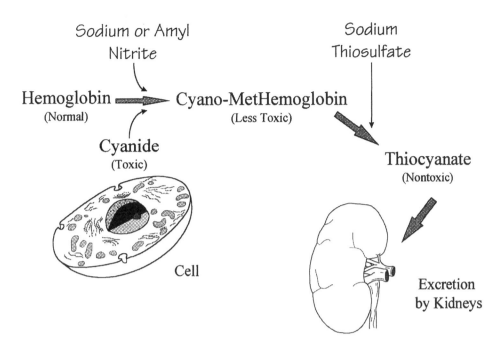

Figure 5-6 Removal of cyanide from cytochrome a3 by use of nitrite- and sulfur-containing antidotes.

The antidote for cyanide is a two-stage process using a nitrite compound followed by a sulfur-containing compound (Figure 5-5). The nitrite acts by converting the **hemoglobin** (the primary oxygen-carrying protein) in the blood to **methemoglobin**. Methemoglobin binds the cyanide, removing it from the cytochrome a$_3$. The sulfur-containing antidote then removes the cyanide by forming a nontoxic compound that is excreted in the urine. This process is depicted in Figure 5-6.

The nitrites for clinical use are sodium nitrite and amyl nitrite. If an IV is already established, administer sodium nitrite 300 mg over 2 to 4 minutes. Amyl nitrite is used only when an IV is not yet established. Crush one ampule for the patient to inhale. If the patient has spontaneous respirations, place the ampule under an oxygen mask with high-flow O$_2$ running. In patients needing ventilatory support, place it in the bag or oxygen reservoir of the bag-valve-mask. In all cases, be certain to avoid letting the ampule fall into the casualty's mouth or down the ET tube. Always follow inhaled amyl nitrate with intravenous sodium nitrite. Do not use amyl nitrite if the casualty has already received sodium nitrite.

Following administration of IV sodium nitrite, administer 12.5 gm of sodium thiosulfate. Do not use sodium thiosulfate unless the casualty has received IV sodium nitrite since it does not work by itself. Appendix A, Medications for the Tactical Environment, provides additional details on the use of cyanide antidotes. Table 5-10 outlines the dose and administration of cyanide antidotes. A highly effective and much

TABLE 5-10

DOSE AND ADMINISTRATION OF CYANIDE ANTIDOTES

ANTIDOTE	DOSE	ROUTE	COMMENTS
Oxygen	High flow	Nonrebreather, BVM	Ventilatory support may be needed
Amyl nitrite	1 ampule	Inhaled	Only if no IV access
Sodium nitrite	300 mg	IV	Primary antidote
Sodium thiosulfate	12.5 gm	IV	Use only after sodium nitrite is given

safer antidote (it is related to vitamin B_{12}) is on the horizon, but is not yet available for general use in the United States.

Triage and Decision Making

Casualties with severe or progressing symptoms should be triaged as immediate patients. Casualties who are pulseless are expectant. Those casualties with mild, non-progressing symptoms would be considered delayed or minimal depending on the severity of symptoms. Ambulatory casualties, for example, would likely be minimal. In fact, if most symptoms resolve, these casualties require no further treatment and can return to duty.

The key decision facing the medic when confronted with a potential cyanide poisoning is not triage, however. *The hardest decision is whether to initiate antidotal therapy when hard evidence of cyanide poisoning is not present. Since the window of opportunity in treating cyanide poisoning is brief, the medic must decide with whatever information is at hand.* Certainly, if intelligence reports or chemical detection equipment indicates the presence of cyanide, the medic should treat any patient with compatible signs and symptoms (Table 5-9) with antidotes.

Unfortunately, treatment with nitrites is not without side effects and risks. Hypotension and hypoxemia are possible effects. Keeping the casualty supine (lying down) and providing supplemental oxygen will minimize these adverse effects.

PULMONARY AGENTS

Overview

Pulmonary agents include phosgene (CG), other halogen compounds, and various nitrogen-oxygen compounds. These agents act primarily to cause lung injury, hence the obsolete term *choking* agents. In World War I, both Germany and Britain used phosgene, usually in combination with chlorine, another pulmonary agent. Currently, phosgene and related agents are not considered very suitable for military use. However, the widespread availability of phosgene makes it a potential weapon for terrorists.

More than one billion pounds of phosgene are produced by industry in the United States for chemical processes. Additionally, pulmonary agents can be incidentally produced during combustion of plastics (particularly Teflon, or polytetrafluoroethylene) or munitions, including smoke (HC). Thus the tactical medic or civilian EMS provider has plenty of opportunity to encounter pulmonary agents in the field.

Phosgene is the representative agent in this group, and the remainder of this section focuses on it. Phosgene is transported as a liquid, but it rapidly converts into a gas that tends to settle in low-lying locations. It has the odor of newly mown hay.

Toxicity

Phosgene works by directly attacking the airway and lung tissue (Figure 5-7). The smaller airways and alveoli are most susceptible (Figure 5-8). The damaged airways and alveoli leak fluid, which leads to pulmonary edema and inflammation (Figure 5-9). This, of course, causes dyspnea, hypoxemia, and if severe enough, respiratory failure.

Assessment

Relatively low concentrations of phosgene irritate the mucous membranes (mouth, eyes, nose, and throat), so initial symptoms will reflect tearing, runny nose, and throat irritation. If the casualty is exposed to a higher concentration, airway and lung damage may also occur. However, symptoms of pulmonary edema will take several hours. Thus a key point in dealing with phosgene casualties is realizing that initially mild symptoms may lead to a serious condition within a few hours. Table 5-11 summarizes the signs and symptoms of phosgene inhalation. Exertion can worsen symptoms.

TABLE 5-11

TREATMENT OF PHOSGENE OR PULMONARY AGENT EXPOSURE

Mild symptoms	Beta-agonist nebulized (Albuterol)
Mild dyspnea	Oxygen
Wheezing	Rest
Cough	
Severe symptoms	Above, plus
Pulmonary edema	Airway management
Severe dyspnea	Positive pressure ventilation
Stridor	
Airway obstruction	

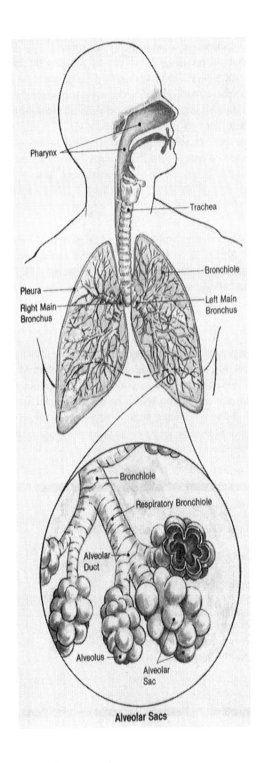

Pharynx

Trachea

Bronchiole

Pleura

Right Main
Bronchus

Left Main
Bronchus

Bronchiole

Respiratory Bronchiole

Alveolar
Duct

Alveolus

Alveolar
Sac

Alveolar Sacs

Figure 5-7 Human respiratory system consists of airways that direct inhaled air to the alveoli.

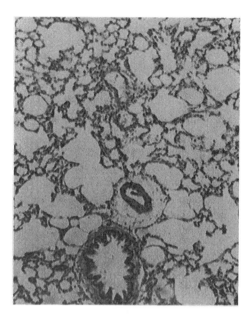

Figure 5-8 Normal alveoli and bronchiole under light microscope.

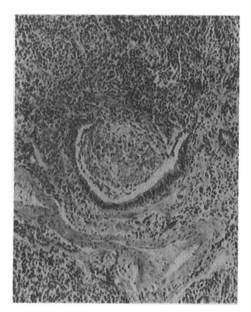

Figure 5-9 Inflamed alveoli and bronchiole under light microscope.

Emergency Care

Initial care of phosgene inhalation is the same as for other toxic inhalations. Priority is given to airway and breathing concerns. Mild to moderately symptomatic casualties are treated with high flow oxygen and rest. Severe dyspnea may require airway control to include intubation. Signs of airway compromise, including obstruction and stridor, mandate immediate intubation. In extreme cases, needle cricothyrostomy or cricothyrotomy may be lifesaving.

Rest is an important component in the field treatment of phosgene exposure. Exertion or exercise worsens the symptoms of the exposure. Therefore, all patients with moderate to severe symptoms should not be allowed to ambulate unless absolutely necessary. Additionally, the delayed effects of phosgene require that all exposed individuals undergo a period of observation for signs of worsening. Ideally, 24 hours is optimal, but even 3 to 6 hours of observation will be helpful in identifying progressing cases.

Casualties exhibiting copious secretions will require suctioning. Shortness of breath, wheezing, tachypnea, or muscular retractions should all be treated with a beta-2 agonist such as albuterol. The beta-2 agonist can be administered by inhalation using a mouthpiece, mask, or endotracheal tube. A typical regimen might be 0.5 ml of albuterol solution dissolved in 5-ml normal saline administered by nebulization. This treatment may be repeated every 20 minutes up to three times. This regimen may need to be repeated every 3 to 4 hours during long evacuations. No significant dosing or interval changes are required for pediatric patients. Appendix A, Medications for the Tactical Environment, provides additional details on the use of albuterol in phosgene exposure. Table 5-11 summarizes treatment.

Triage and Decision Making

Casualties suffering severe dyspnea, stridor, or pulmonary edema require immediate field treatment to survive and are triaged as immediate. Casualties with shortness of breath but no tachypnea, wheezing, crackles, or stridor are delayed. A casualty with a known exposure but little or no signs or symptoms can be classified as minimal. These latter two categories must be rested and should be observed and reclassified, if needed. Expectant casualties manifest with signs of severe pulmonary edema (severe dyspnea, hypoxemia, crackles, muscular retractions, altered mental status) and hypotension. Even with intensive treatment, many of these patients will not survive.

RIOT CONTROL AGENTS

Overview

Riot control agents include the common terms *tear gas* and *mace*. Specific agents include CS, CN, CA, CR, and pepper spray (oleoresin capsicum, OC). Their common effect is intense irritation of the eyes, nose, and other mucous membranes. In the concentrations employed for field use, these agents are all considered nonlethal.

Agents in use today by military and police forces are limited to CS, CN (mace), and pepper spray. Pepper spray has gained widespread acceptance as a safe agent for use in direct employment against individual suspects by civilian police. Thus all EMS providers must be familiar with these agents.

With the exception of pepper spray, all riot control agents are solids. The dispersion method aerosolizes the solid, which is seen as a white or gray cloud of "gas." Each of these agents causes pain without tissue damage. At extremely high concentrations (a closed room, for example, or very close range), it is possible, however, for these agents to have serious effects.

Assessment

Severe eye pain and tearing are characteristic of riot agents and lead to a temporary "blinding" of exposed individuals. Additionally, nose, throat, and skin irritation are also common. Cough and shortness of breath can also occur. In rare cases, wheezing and bronchospasm may occur. Riot control agents, by design, give only temporary symptoms. Once in fresh air, exposed individuals will feel relief within 15 minutes. Mild lingering effects may last for hours, however. Table 5-12 outlines the signs and symptoms of riot agents.

Emergency Care

Under most field conditions, emergency care is limited to removal of the casualty to fresh air. The effects of riot control agents are self-limited, and no further treatment is usually needed. On occasion, a casualty may experience severe shortness of breath and wheezing. This should be treated with oxygen and beta-2 agonists as described in Appendix A, Medications for the Tactical Environment. Also, it is possible that a casualty close to the dispersion or detonation of the riot control agent may get a particle stuck in the eye. Treatment in this case involves copious irrigation with saline, Ringers Lactate, or plain water. Commercial products are being marketed to treat the effects of riot control agents but are not necessary because these agents cause only self-limited effects.

Triage and Decision Making

Because most casualties will recover spontaneously, triage and emergency care are not needed. Those few casualties with severe or persistent symptoms should be triaged in accordance with their injuries.

TABLE 5-12

SIGNS AND SYMPTOMS OF RIOT AGENT EXPOSURES

Tearing and eye pain
Temporary "blindness"
Nose, throat, and skin irritation
Coughing and shortness of breath

PROTECTION FROM CHEMICAL AGENTS

Overview

This section introduces the concepts of protection from chemical agents. All the protections against chemical agents are also effective against biological agents, and provide limited protection against fallout radiation. In many ways, these principles parallel hazardous materials (hazmat) guidelines already familiar to EMS providers. Thus any EMS provider or medic who may potentially care for casualties of chemical, biological, or radiological agents must be familiar with the principles of self-protection.

Hazmat Teams

Hazardous materials teams are equipped with sophisticated barrier protection and self-contained breathing apparatus. In the military, this might be a chemical or NBC team. This equipment is very effective in chemical or biological protection. However, this equipment is expensive and requires extensive training in its use. Most medics will not have access to this equipment. Instead, medics can expect to use other forms of protection as discussed in the following paragraphs and in Appendix B, Chemical Agent Protective Measures.

It is not the intent of this section to provide a thorough discussion of the technique of chemical protection. Appendix B, Chemical Agent Protective Measures, provides additional details on the step-by-step procedures for certain protection techniques. For more detailed information, see the reading list at the end of the chapter.

Masks

Since the primary route of entry for most chemical and biological agents and radioactive fallout is the mouth, nose, lungs, and eyes, a face mask is a critical component in an NBC protection system. Masks in common use are listed in Table 5-13 and depicted in Figures 5-10 to 5-13. All provide excellent protection against all known chemical and biological agents when properly donned and worn (see Appendix B, Chemical Agent Protective Measures).

Garments

A mask alone is not sufficient protection against some agents, particularly nerve and vesicant agents. Complete protection requires a suitable garment or suit to include gloves and

---

TABLE 5-13

NBC PROTECTION MASKS IN COMMON USE

M17	Old-style military mask
M24/25	Combat vehicle/aircraft mask
M40/42	Newer style field/vehicle mask
Civilian-style	Full face piece mask
Civilian-style	Half face price mask

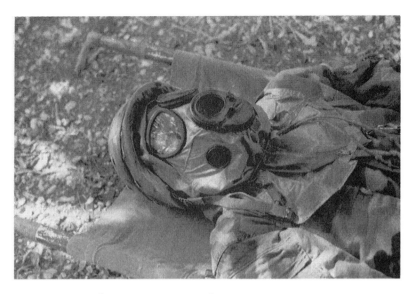

Figure 5-10 Casualty wearing an M-17 mask.

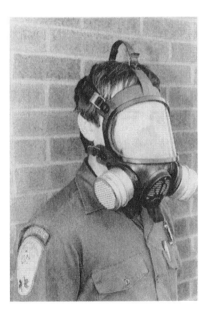
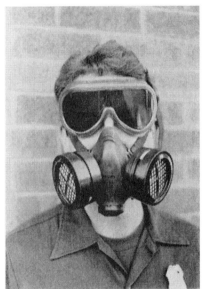

Figure 5-11 Full-face piece
civilian mask.

boots. Two main types are available: the military overgarment and civilian Tyvex suit. Both provide excellent protection against all known chemical and biological agents. The military overgarment (Figure 5-13) is a charcoal-embedded, liquid repellent material, and

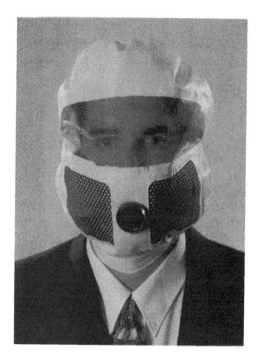

Figure 5-12 Disposable civilian full-face piece mask.

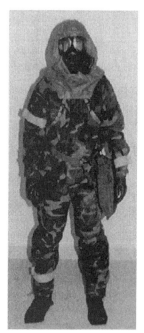

Figure 5-13 Military M40 mask and NBC overgarment with boots and gloves.

the Tyvex suit is impervious plastic (Figure 5-14). The military overgarment has the advantage of being breathable and durable, with a wear time of 30 days in an uncontaminated environment. Vinyl boots and hood and butyl rubber gloves

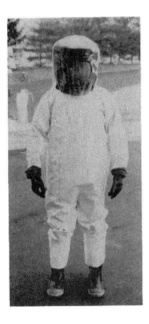

Figure 5-14 Civilian style Tyvek suit.

complete the protective ensemble. The Tyvex suit is less expensive, easier to store, and widely available in the commercial market. It is much less durable and does not breath, however. Neither type offers positive pressure (Level A and B) protection, but both do provide proven protection against known chemical and biological threats.

Working in Protective Garments

The medic in full NBC protective ensemble will quickly realize the hot, bulky, and cumbersome nature of the gear. Vision and hearing are consequently limited, and manual dexterity is markedly degraded. Heat buildup quickly becomes a problem in all but the coolest conditions. During hot weather, heat exhaustion is a real risk for personnel wearing the ensemble for longer than a few minutes. A rule of thumb is to add 5°-9°C (10°-15°F) to the ambient temperature as an estimate of the heat burden.

Despite these limitations, it is possible to work and provide adequate medical care when wearing the full protective ensemble. Intubation, starting an intravenous infusion, and assessing vital signs are all possible. Certainly, these procedures will take longer than usual to perform. However, careful palpation, auscultation, and rechecking of critical findings will improve accuracy and efficiency. Practice drills and simulated patient care are essential training tasks for all medics preparing to treat chemical or biological casualties.

Chemical Agent Prophylaxis

Prophylaxis is the use of medications to pretreat individuals not yet exposed but at risk for contact with chemical agents. Pretreatment has the goal of providing some degree of protection against potential chemical threats. The only effective prophylaxis or pretreatment against chemical agents that is currently available is pyridostigmine. This medication is effective against some types of nerve agents, particularly GD (soman). Although pyridostigmine does not offer complete protection against soman, it will improve survival of many exposed individuals. However, it may not be effective against GB (sarin) or VX. Pyridostigmine is not an antidote and should not be administered to patients already exposed to nerve agents since it can worsen symptoms.

Pyridostigmine is taken every 8 hours whenever the risk of nerve agent exposure is high (see Appendix A, Medications for the Tactical Environment). The drug causes side effects (mainly vomiting, diarrhea, and urinary frequency) in up to 50% of those taking the regimen. However, it is usually well tolerated in healthy adults, and less than 1% will need to discontinue the medication. Thousands of U.S. troops received the regimen during the Gulf War, and pyridostigmine was speculated to be a factor in the mysterious "Gulf War Syndrome." However, strong data supports the safety of the drug. If a serious risk of nerve agent exposure is imminent, the benefits of pyridostigmine pretreatment outweigh any possible risk.

Individual Decontamination

This section introduces individual decontamination techniques for chemical agents. Patient decontamination is discussed in later sections. All these discussions assume the medic and patient are fully dressed in the chemical protective ensemble.

Physical Removal

Liquid and solid agent residue on skin, clothing, and equipment is the greatest hazard. Therefore, the primary focus of chemical agent decontamination is physical removal of the offending agent. Use whatever means are available under the circumstances (Table 5-14). A field expedient method is to simply use a stick or tree branch to scrape as much of the agent off as possible. If available, copious amounts of water are extremely effective. The amount of water needed is large, such as from a low-pressure fire hose or industrial decontamination shower. (Smaller amounts of water may be used but only with great

TABLE 5-14

SOME METHODS OF PHYSICALLY REMOVING CHEMICAL
AGENT FROM SKIN AND CLOTHING

METHOD	NOTES
Removal with stick or tree branch	Field expedient method
Copious water irrigation	Large amounts needed
Fuller earth	Absorbs chemical agent
Diatomaceous earth	Substitute for Fuller earth

care. There is a risk of a counterproductive effect because it may spread contamination and not fully wash the offending agent away.) Few tactical units have the luxury of large amounts of water. Naval vessels and encampments alongside an ocean, river, or lake may be able to take advantage of this method. Care must be exercised to control the waste water and avoid environmental contamination.

Another method to physically remove chemical agent is to absorb it into highly absorbant Fuller earth (a clay-based, highly absorbant quarry product) and then dispose of the Fuller earth. A big handful of Fuller earth is rubbed briskly over outer garments or skin. This process is repeated until all surfaces are covered. Diatomaceous earth is a similar substance and is an acceptable alternative. Both are widely available from commercial sources and are inexpensive.

Military Decontamination

The current portable mainstay of individual decontamination is two kits available from the military, M291 and M258 (Figure 5-15). Both kits contain wipes designed to remove and neutralize chemical agents from the skin and protective equipment. M258, the older of the two kits, is being phased out. The active ingredients are caustic and work by alkaline hydrolysis. M291 is newer and contains highly adsorbent activated charcoal and chemical agent-destroying resin. Both kits are effective for a wide variety of liquid agents and are

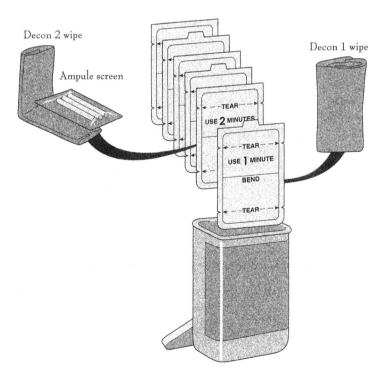

Figure 5-15 M258 Individual decontamination kit.

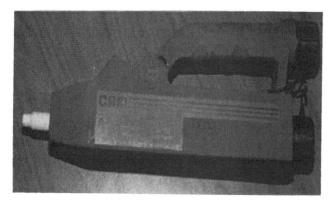

Figure 5-16 Chemical Agent Monitor (CAM).

safe for use on skin or equipment. Caution must be used, however, to avoid contacting the eyes or mouth with decontamination material. Appendix B, Chemical Agent Protective Measures, provides additional details on the proper use of individual decontamination kits.

Civilian Decontamination

Most civilian decontamination plans call for the use of commercially available decontamination showers and tubs. Casualties are sprayed down with warm, soapy water and the runoff is captured in tanks. Less sophisticated approaches may employ plastic children's wading pools, tarps, and other basins to wash and decontaminate casualties. In all cases, a well-rehearsed plan is essential to successfully employing a decontamination operation in a contingency.

Nuclear, Biologic, and Chemical Detection Equipment

A wide variety of detection equipment (such as the Chemical Agent Monitor, CAM, depicted in Figure 5-16) and supplies are available and being developed, primarily by the military. Use and maintenance of this equipment is beyond the scope of this textbook. Interested readers are referred to the sources listed at the end of this chapter. Needless to say, proper training and experience is essential for reliable use of this equipment. All medics and EMS personnel who may need to treat NBC casualties must be familiar with the equipment they will use. Chapter 7, Care of Nuclear Casualties, provides a brief discussion of radiation detection equipment.

Caring for Casualties in a Contaminated Environment

Undoubtedly, caring for casualties in a contaminated environment will be a challenge. Not only must the medic be protected by a cumbersome protective ensemble, so too must the casualty. This will naturally limit the degree and sophistication of care provided. Nonetheless, life-saving care can occur in this circumstance. Three special pieces of equipment are available to aid the medic in caring for patients in contaminated environments: (1) patient protective wrap, (2) decontaminable litter, and (3) resuscitation device individual chemical (RDIC).

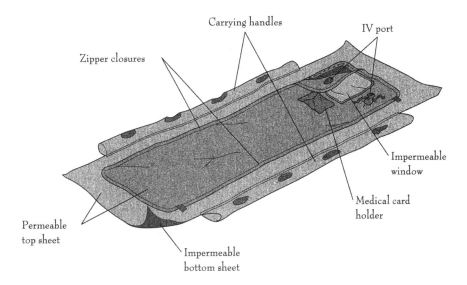

Figure 5-17 Patient protective wrap.

The patient protective wrap (Figure 5-17) is a disposable wrap designed to be placed around a casualty once he or she is stripped of his or her overgarments and underclothes. The wrap is permeable to oxygen and carbon dioxide to allow the casualty to breath. It is designed to be used on a litter but can be used as a field-expedient litter by itself if necessary. Patients can spend up to 6 hours in the wrap.

The decontaminable litter resembles an ordinary military folding litter but is specially designed to allow thorough patient and litter decontamination. The RDIC is essentially a bag-valve-mask filled with a chemical/biologic filter to allow positive pressure ventilation of intubated casualties. It is used in the same way as a standard bag-valve-mask device.

PATIENT DECONTAMINATION

Overview

Casualties exposed to chemical, biological, or radiologic agents will need to be decontaminated before being allowed to enter the evacuation or transport system. Failure to decontaminate the patient properly will result in dangerous agents being carried into areas where personnel may not be wearing protective ensembles. This, of course, places the medical team and others at risk. Furthermore, failing to decontaminate the casualty adequately allows greater potential exposure of the casualty to hazardous agents. Thus thorough and rapid decontamination is a critical medical skill for all EMS providers and medics. Fortunately, the principles of NBC decontamination are parallel to routine hazmat principles practiced by all emergency services.

TABLE 5-15

Wind direction and site selection
Security and control of the side
Litter patient decontamination
Ambulatory patient decontamination

This section focuses on the decontamination provided in the field. Only a general outline provided in this section. Readers interested in further details of patient decontamination are referred to the references at the end of the chapter or Appendix B, Chemical Agent Protective Measures. The key points to consider in patient decontamination are listed in Table 5-15.

Wind Direction and Site Selections

Choose a site on relatively high ground that slopes toward the contaminated zone. Also place the site upwind of the zone of contamination. These measures will reduce the spread of hazardous materials from the contaminated zone (hot or dirty side) to the uncontaminated zone (cold or clean side). If available, establish waste-water collection procedures to reduce environmental contamination and spread of the agent.

Security and Control of the Site

Security and control of the site is needed to avoid personnel from inadvertently tracking contamination across to the uncontaminated side. Establish a "hot line" boundary between the dirty (contaminated) and clean (decontaminated) sides (Figure 5-18). All personnel on the dirty side must be in full protective ensemble. Personnel on the clean side but close to the hot line should be in protective ensemble, too.

Garment Removal

An important first step in patient decontamination is removal of gross contamination followed by careful removal of all garments (protective and underclothes) except mask. Care must be taken to avoid touching the outer portions of clothing to the casualty's skin. Appendix B, Chemical Agent Protective Measures, outlines the details of garment removal.

Physical Removal

If possible, use copious amounts of water to thoroughly wash all body surfaces of the patient. A low-pressure fire hose or low-pressure power cleaner is ideal since it is able to deliver many gallons of water per minute. However, most tactical operations will

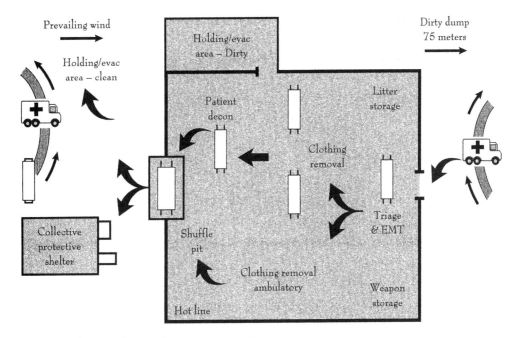

Figure 5-18 Schematic of patient decontamination station.

not have the luxury of a large water supply. An alternative is Fuller or Diatomaceous earth (Table 5-14). However, when water or other methods of physical removal are not available, the medic must rely on decontamination solutions to neutralize any agent residue.

Decontamination Solutions

A highly effective decontamination solution is readily available in a hypochlorite solution (Table 5-16). The 0.5% solution is used on all patient skin surfaces and the protective mask. The 5% solution is used on all garments and equipment (except mask). Avoid getting either solution in the eyes. Copious normal saline is the decontamination solution of choice for the eyes. Lactated Ringer solution or plain water is an acceptable substitute if saline is unavailable. The hypochlorite decontamination solutions are effective for all chemical and biologic agents. However, several minutes of contact are needed for the hypochlorite to adequately to neutralize chemical agents. If available, copious water (for example, garden hose) can be used to rinse the casualty after using the hypochlorite solutions. Civilian experience has shown that low-pressure power cleaners are very effective in decontamination procedures and should be employed when available to supplement the hypochlorite rinses.

TABLE 5-16

MAKING A HYPOCHLORITE DECONTAMINATION SOLUTION

5%	Add eight 6-ounce containers of calcium hypochlorite (HTH) to 5-gal water or Household bleach straight from bottle
0.5%	Add one 6-ounce container of HTH to 5-gal water or Add 64 fluid oz (half gal) of bleach to 5-gal water

Litter Patient Decontamination

Once brought to the decontamination station, litter patients should be transferred to a decontaminable litter. Then, following the procedures outlined in Appendix B, Chemical Agent Protective Measures, the patient is decontaminated. Care is taken not to break the mask seal during the process.

Ambulatory Patient Decontamination

Patients able to walk are segregated to a separate decontamination line. They, too, are systematically decontaminated; however, the sequence is slightly different from that for litter patients (see Appendix B, Chemical Agent Protective Measures).

SUMMARY

Chemical agents pose a serious threat to military medics and civilian EMS providers alike. However, with proper training and equipment, it is possible to provide advanced-level emergency care to casualties of chemical agents. Knowledge of symptoms and signs and specific management and antidote treatments is critical for optimal chemical casualty care. Finally, familiarization with protective equipment will enable the medic to provide emergency care in contaminated environments with less risk to himself or herself.

FOR FURTHER READING

Medical Management of Chemical Casualties, 2d ed. U.S. Army Medical Research Institute of Chemical Defense, Aberdeen Proving Grounds, MD, 1995.

Field Manual 3-5 NBC Decontamination. Department of the Army, Washington, DC, 1993.

Field Manual 3-4 NBC Protection. Department of the Army, Washington, DC, 1992.

Field Manual 8-285, Treatment of Chemical Agent Casualties and Conventional Military Chemical Casualties. Department of the Army, Washington, DC, 1995.

Field Manual 8-9, NATO Handbook on Medical Aspects of NBC Defensive Operations. Department of the Army, Washington, DC, 1996.

Emergency Response to Terrorism: Basic Concepts Student Manual. US Fire Administration, National Fire Academy. Emmitsburg, MD, 1997.

McCAUGHEY BG et al.: Combat Casualties in Conventional and Chemical Warfare Environment. Military Medicine, 1988; 153: 227-229.

DANON YL et al. (eds): Chemical Warfare Medicine. Gefen Publishing House, Ltd. Jerusalem, 1994.

SPIERS EM: Chemical and Biological Weapons. St. Martin's Press. New York, 1984.

ZAJTCHUK R et al. (eds): Medical Aspects of Chemical and Biological Warfare. Department of the Army, Office of the Surgeon General, Washington, DC, 1997.

BORAK J ET AL.: Hazardous Materials Exposure. Brady, Englewood Cliffs, NJ, 1991.

6

CARE OF BIOLOGICAL CASUALTIES

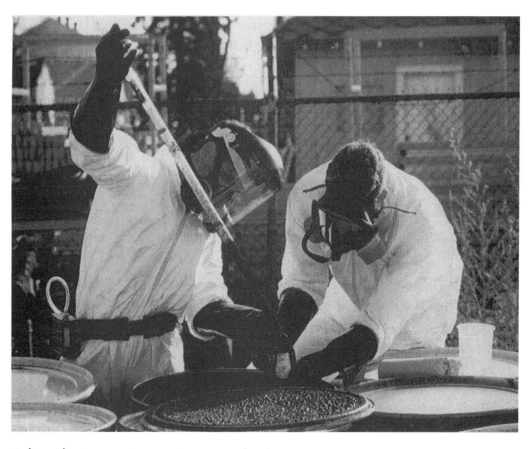

Working with toxic agents using protective garment and mask.

OBJECTIVES

After reading this chapter, you will be able to:

1. Describe the nature of biological agents to include the delivery, route of exposure, disease states, and lethality of the agents.

2. List the eight main categories of biological agents: pneumonialike, encephalitislike, cholera, viral hemorrhagic fevers, botulinum, SEB, ricin, and T2 mycotoxin.

3. Outline the principles of how to recognize a biological agent attack.

4. List the chief signs and symptoms of the each of the eight main categories of biological agents.

5. Know the principles of emergency care for biological agents to include recognition and identification, isolation, supportive care, and antibiotic/antitoxin therapy.

6. Describe the role of the medic in the emergency care for biological casualties.

7. Outline the principles of triage and patient disposition decision making for biological casualties.

8. Know the principles of biological agent protection and decontamination.

CASE

You are a National Guard medic deployed to Asia on a humanitarian mission to feed starving refugees. The refugees have been driven out of their homeland by warring factions trying to gain control of the country. Recently, reports have come in alleging the use of biologic warfare on the border towns near your encampment. The commander has ordered your unit to investigate.

On arrival, the town is littered with dead bodies. There are no obvious marks or evidence of trauma on the bodies. As a precaution, your unit leader had already ordered the donning of the full NBC protective ensemble. Suddenly, two news reporters who had been in the town for several days appear, seeking an interview. As they step closer, however, they begin to complain of weakness, double vision, difficulty swallowing, and shortness of breath. Several hours later, they stumble to the ground, unable to talk or breathe.

You recognize the symptoms as possible botulinum poisoning. After a rapid scene size-up, your initial assessment confirms the casualties are flaccid (completely paralyzed with no muscle tone) and apneic. You open the airway of the first patient and begin artificial ventilation with a bag-valve-mask. You then prepare for intubation, realizing the casualty has an excellent chance of survival if ventilation can be maintained. Your partner does the same for the second victim. Since the resources are available, all efforts are made to resuscitate the casualties, and a preparation is made to evacuate the patients.

INTRODUCTION

Overview

Biological agents are living organisms (or the toxins produced by living organisms) that are deliberately used to cause disease in the target population. Biological weapons are no different from naturally occurring disease except they are concentrated and delivered with the intent to cause harm.

Because a small amount of agent can cause widespread casualties, biological weapons are potential weapons of mass destruction. Furthermore, because they cause disease that is identical to naturally occurring disease, it can be difficult (at least initially) to detect and identify the attack. Also, the potential spread or contagiousness of many biological agents adds a new dimension to the threat and fear associated with weapons of mass destruction.

This chapter reviews the principles of biological weapons and discusses a few example types of agents. Identification and treatment priorities are highlighted, along with the protective measures needed to safely care for casualties of biological agents.

History

Crude forms of biological warfare date as far back as the 14th to 18th centuries when attackers were known to hurl the corpses of bubonic plague victims over the walls of besieged cities. In the 1750s, the English "donated" smallpox-laden blankets to Indians loyal to the French in the French and Indian War. This caused many casualties among the native Americans defending alongside the French.

In World War II, the Japanese in particular had an active biological weapons program. After the war and until 1972, the United States manufactured and stockpiled a number of biological agents. Since 1972, international treaty has banned the development or use of biological weapons. Unfortunately, several nations, including Iraq and several republics of the former Soviet Union, are still felt to posses offensive biological agents.

Current Threat

Today, the threat of biological attack is felt to be higher than in the past. Several countries with terrorist tendencies continue to experiment with these agents. Because of the difficulty in tracing an attack, terrorist groups may find biological agents useful tools to carry out their deadly work. For this reason, all prehospital providers must be knowledgeable and skilled in dealing with its potential threat.

NATURE OF BIOLOGICAL AGENTS

Biological agents for warfare or terrorism are simply disease-causing organisms (or the products of organisms) that are collected, processed, and delivered for maximal effect, usually death. Any of the disease-forming groups such as viruses, bacteria, or fungus are potential candidates as biologic agents. Fortunately, weapons makers have only a few good candidates to choose from because the agent must be effective, efficient, easily delivered, and easy to manufacture. This limits the list of potential agents to a small number. The tactical medic can easily prepare and train to care for this limited number of likely biological agents.

Delivery

To be effective, the biological agent must get to its target. This is usually accomplished by spraying a liquid containing the agent through a nozzle. Such a nozzle attached to an airplane could deliver the agent over a wide area. A particle size of 1 to 5 microns is optimal because it has the greatest chance of dispersing and also of reaching deep into the respiratory tract, the most effective portal of entry. Obviously, wind, speed, direction, rain, and sunlight can have great effect on delivery. High winds will tend to disperse the agent but also can carry it great distances. Rain and sunshine usually work to diminish the agent's effectiveness. Ideal conditions for the release of biological agents usually occur at night and very early morning.

Route of Exposure

By far, the respiratory tract is the most common and efficient portal of entry for most biological agents. Particle size is important (Figure 6-1). If the particle is too big (> 5 microns), it will impact in the upper respiratory tract and be less effective. If it is too small (< 1 micron), it will not impact in the lungs but will merely be exhaled back out. Lesser portals include the mouth, nose, and eye mucous membranes. Ingestion of the biological agent is a serious consideration if the attacker contaminates the food or water supply.

Disease States

Most biological warfare agents are intended to kill their victims. Anthrax, botulinum toxin, and tularemia are examples of lethal agents. Other agents tend to incapacitate,

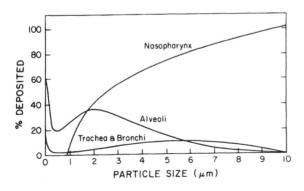

Figure 6-1 Particle size is important to deposition in the respiratory tract.

TABLE 6-1

TOXICITY OF SOME BIOLOGICAL AGENTS AND OTHER POISONS

AGENT	LETHAL DOSE ug/kg	LETHAL DOSE 70 kg ADULT
Botulinum toxin	0.001	0.07 ug
Ricin	3.0	210 ug
VX nerve agent	15.0	1 mg
SEB	27.0	2 mg
Sarin (GB)	100	7 mg
T_2 mycotoxin	1210	85 mg

Adapted from Medical Management of Biological Casualties, 2d ed., U.S. Army
Research Institute of Infectious Diseases, Ft Detrick, MD, 1996.

such as Q fever and Staphylococcal enterotoxin B. The actual disease state varies with each agent. Plague and Q fever cause a pneumonia-like picture of cough, fever, and shortness of breath. Cholera, on the other hand, produces vomiting and diarrhea.

Lethality

Biological agents can be extremely potent weapons. Some of the most toxic substances known to man are potential biological weapons. Table 6-1 lists the toxicity of several biological agents as compared to other poisons. For example, 50 kg of anthrax dispersed upwind of a large city could kill up to 220,000 people. Thus, the potential power of biological weapons should not be underestimated.

SPECIFIC AGENTS

A dozen biological agents are sufficiently threatening to deserve discussion. They can be roughly divided into four groups: (1) pneumonia-like agents, (2) encephalitis-like agents, (3) biological toxins, and (4) other agents. Although these groupings are artificial, they are useful to the medic who must recognize and treat biological casualties without the benefit of extensive experience in exotic infectious diagnosis and sophisticated laboratory support.

Recognition of Attack

Key to distinguishing a biological attack from an isolated case of ordinary (or perhaps exotic) disease is the number and timing of cases. Isolated disease strikes one or at most a few persons. If cases are contagious (like the common cold), more may become infected, but only over time. Biological attacks, in contrast, usually strike a large number of individuals at virtually the same time. Symptoms all develop within hours or, at most, days of each other. This situation is easily distinguishable from isolated cases.

A little more challenging is differentiating a biological attack from ordinary mass food-poisoning, or perhaps epidemic meningitis. The key here is to recognize the common bond shared by all the ill patients-a shared meal, water source, or living quarters. Biological attacks usually strike victims across large areas and without regard to job, residence, or similar factors.

Pneumonia-Like Agents

This group (Table 6-2) includes anthrax, tularemia, plague, and Q fever. Common symptoms include cough, dyspnea, fever, and malaise. Anthrax is by far the most lethal, infecting and killing up to half the exposed persons. Q fever, on the other hand, is an incapacitating agent and rarely causes death. In general, these are the agents most likely to be used in a biological weapon.

Anthrax

Anthrax is caused by the bacterium *Bacillus anthracis* and, in nature, usually infects cattle, sheep, and horses. The handling of meat, bone meal, and hides of these animals can pass the disease to humans, usually through direct contact. The bacteria can also form spores, which are highly resistant to heat and drying and can be easily aerosolized. The spore is the usual infective form in biological weapons.

Several nations, including the United States, the republics of the former Soviet Union, and Iraq are believed to have been, or to be, capable of making anthrax. Relatively speaking, it is easy to manufacture and store anthrax. Delivery, particularly over wide areas, is more difficult, but could be accomplished by aerosolization of the spores from aircraft or by detonating small bombs encased by anthrax spores.

Anthrax has a very high fatality rate; that is, 90% or more of those who contract the disease from inhaling the organism will die. After an incubation period of 1 to 6 days, a nonspecific illness of fever, malaise, nonproductive cough, and chest discomfort will occur. In theory, persons aggressively treated at this stage may recover. Untreated, however, anthrax progresses to a brief (hours to days) period of improvement followed by

TABLE 6-2

BIOLOGICAL AGENTS CAUSING PNEUMONIA-LIKE ILLNESS

AGENT	COMMON SYMPTOMS	SPECIFIC FINDINGS
Anthrax	Cough, shortness of breath, fever, malaise, headache, hemoptysis	Severe dyspnea, shock, death within 24-36 hours
Plague		Severe dyspnea, death
Q fever		Resolves 2-14 days
Tularemia		Respirophasic chest pain, headache

the rapid appearance of respiratory distress and diaphoresis. The lesions and scabs characteristic of skin exposure may not occur from inhalational anthrax. Shock and death ensue within 1 to 2 days.

Treatment of anthrax requires aggressive respiratory and cardiovascular support. Oxygen and intubation will be required in many cases. Most casualties will require intravenous fluids to counteract septic shock. Intravenous ciprofloxacin 400 mg q 8-12 hours or doxycycline 100 mg q 12 hours are the antibiotics of choice. Despite aggressive therapy, many patients with pulmonary anthrax will die.

Prophylaxis is possible with a licensed vaccine that requires six initial doses over a year followed by yearly boosters. Vaccination may not entirely prevent disease but can provide reasonable protection. In the face of an imminent anthrax attack, ciprofloxacin 500 mg po bid or doxycycline 1000 mg po bid may offer some protection. Contact isolation is required for infected patients.

Plague

Plague is caused by the bacterium *Yersinia pestis* that naturally infects rodents such as mice, rats, and squirrels in some parts of the world. Fleas that live on the rodents can occasionally pass the disease to humans. Crowded and unsanitary conditions can allow the disease to spread and account for the millions killed by plague in the European Dark Ages. Yersinia is quite hardy and can tolerate drying, freezing, and heat well.

The most likely form of plague from a biological attack is pneumonic plague. This is usually caused by the inhalation of organisms although it can occasionally occur from systemic spread through the blood. After an incubation period of 2 to 3 days, the victim develops high fever, chills, cough with hemoptysis (bloody sputum), headache, and malaise. The pneumonia progresses rapidly, and the patient soon develops cyanosis and shock. Death is from respiratory failure and septic shock. The black, necrotic skin lesions of cutaneous or bubonic plague are not usually seen in primary pneumonic plaque. All patients with pneumonic plague will die without treatment.

Treatment focuses on the respiratory and cardiovascular systems. Oxygen, intubation, mechanical ventilation, and aggressive fluid resuscitation may all be required. If treatment with antibiotics is provided early in the course of the disease, recovery is possible. Intravenous doxycycline 100 mg q 12 hours or intramuscular streptomycin 30 mg/kg/day bid are the drugs of choice.

A licensed vaccine is available, but it requires biannual boosters. Doxycycline 100 mg po bid is potentially effective in the face of imminent attack. Contact and respiratory isolation is required for pneumonic plague patients.

Tularemia

Tularemia is caused by the bacterium *Francisella tularensis* and naturally infects rabbits. Humans can acquire the disease through handling infected materials, or by the bites of deerflies, mosquitos, and ticks. The bacterium is highly resistant to freezing but is susceptible to high heat. As few as 10 to 50 organisms can cause infection if inhaled.

Tularemia can appear in several forms in humans, depending on the route of exposure. Biological weapons will usually employ the aerosol route and cause typhoidal disease or pneumonia. Typical symptoms include fever, substernal chest discomfort, and nonproductive cough. Treatment includes respiratory and fluid support as needed, and either streptomycin (1 gm q 12 hours IM) or gentamycin (3-5 mg/kg/day IV). A vaccine is under development. Contact isolation is required for infected patients.

Q Fever

Q fever is caused by the rickettsial organism *Coxiella burnetii*. In nature, it infects sheep, cattle, and goats. Humans may acquire the disease through aerosolization of infected urine, feces, or milk. The organism is extremely potent: only a single inhaled organism may cause disease. Fortunately, Q fever is rarely fatal, and would thus be classified as an incapacitating agent.

Incubation lasts from 10 to 20 days, and then victims develop symptoms lasting 2 days to 2 weeks. The usual symptoms are fever, myalgias (body aches), headache, and malaise. Cough and respirophasic (pleuritic) chest pain can occur in about one-fourth of cases. Complications can occur but are uncommon.

Treatment with oral tetracycline 500 mg qid or doxycycline 100 mg bid may shorten the course of the disease. A vaccine is under development, but is not yet available. Prophylactic administration of oral tetracycline or doxycycline can prevent or delay the onset of disease.

Encephalitis-Like Agents

Table 6-3 lists two agents that cause symptoms vaguely resembling influenza or the flu, including fever, headache, and malaise. However, these diseases are many times more lethal than the flu. Their predilection for affecting the brain and central nervous system accounts for their rough classification as encephalitis agents. In this group, both the smallpox and Venezuelan equine encephalitis viruses have very high attack rates, affecting more than 90% of those exposed. Both groups of agents can cause fatalities, with smallpox being the most deadly.

TABLE 6-3

BIOLOGICAL AGENTS CAUSING ENCEPHALITIS-LIKE ILLNESS

AGENT	COMMON SYMPTOMS	SPECIFIC FINDINGS
Small Pox	Headache Fever Malaise	Characteristic rash develops in 2-3 days
Venezuelan Equine Encephalitis		Photophobia Severe headache

Smallpox

Smallpox is caused by the variola virus. Smallpox is believed to be eradicated from nature; however, laboratory repositories remain in the United States and Russia. It is possible that other nations have secretly kept smallpox stocks. Upwards of 30% of infected victims may die of the disease. Even vaccinated individuals may contract smallpox, and up to 3% will die.

Incubation lasts about 12 days, after which the patient develops abrupt fever, malaise, rigors, headache, backache, and vomiting. About 15% will develop mental status changes (delirium). Two or three days later, the characteristic rash appears on the face, hands, and forearms. Later, the rash spreads to the lower extremities and finally begins to scab and heal in 8 to 14 days.

Treatment is supportive since antibiotics are ineffective against viruses. Respiratory and contact isolation is needed for infected patients. All contacts with an infected person should be quarantined for 17 days. A licensed vaccine is available.

Venezuelan Equine Encephalitis

Venezuelan equine encephalitis (VEE) is caused by an alphavirus and is endemic to parts of Central and South America and Florida. As its name implies, horses, donkeys, and mules are the natural reservoir. It is transmitted to humans by mosquitos. The attack rate of the disease is very high, approaching 90%. Fortunately, most recover, and only 1% will die.

After a 1 to 5 day incubation period, the victim develops abrupt fever, chills, severe headache, photophobia, and myalgias. Nausea, vomiting, and sore throat may also occur. The disease peaks for 2 to 3 days, then subsides; however, malaise may last for 1 to 2 weeks. Complications include neurologic problems, including brain damage. Children appear more susceptible to complications.

Treatment for VEE is supportive only. An experimental vaccine is under development. Infected patients require blood and body fluid precautions.

Miscellaneous Agents

Three agents—cholera, brucellosis, and viral hemorrhagic fevers—give signs and symptoms different from each other and from the other agents discussed so far (Table 6-4). Viral hemorrhagic fevers include the infamous Ebola virus and the agents of dengue and yellow fever. These agents are lethal, causing death in 5% to 50% of infected individuals. Cholera is interesting because it regularly causes natural outbreaks and epidemics in developing nations. The watery diarrhea can be profuse and can easily dehydrate and kill a small child in less than one day or an adult in 2 or 3 days.

Cholera

Cholera is caused by the *Vibrio cholerae* bacterium and naturally occurs in man. Transmission is by the "fecal-oral" route, that is, by eating or drinking contaminated food and water. The organism is very susceptible to drying, heat, and water chlorination. It can live for days in untreated water, however.

TABLE 6-4

AGENT	SYMPTOMS AND FINDINGS
Cholera	Vomiting, abdominal distension, profuse watery diarrhea, severe dehydration possible
Viral hemorrhagic fevers	Malaise, body aches, headache, vomiting, early easy bleeding, hypotension, shock late
Brucellosis	Fever, malaise, body aches, joint pain, headache, cough

Following an incubation period of 12 to 72 hours, victims experience sudden and uncomfortable abdominal cramping and a profuse, watery diarrhea. Vomiting and malaise may accompany the diarrhea. The diarrhea can result in the loss of 5 to 10 liters of water per day and can easily lead to dehydration and hypovolemic shock. Death results from electrolyte imbalance and hypovolemia. Up to 50% of untreated victims will die. With adequate treatment, however, survival is excellent.

Treatment is aimed at preventing and correcting hypovolemic shock. Oral hydration with "World Health Organization oral rehydration solution" (contains water, sodium chloride, potassium chloride, sodium bicarbonate, and glucose) is frequently successful in adults and some children. Field expedient substitutes include juices and "sports drinks" such as Gatorade and the drink packets of Meals, ready to eat (MREs). Intravenous normal saline (preferably with bicarbonate and potassium added) can be lifesaving for seriously ill individuals. Children are much more susceptible to serious dehydration from cholera than are adults. Antibiotic treatment with tetracycline 500 mg qid or doxycycline 100 mg bid is frequently helpful. Resistant strains of cholera may require treatment with ciprofloxacin 500 mg bid or erythromycin 500 mg qid. Children should be treated with tetracycline 50 mg/kg/day qid for 3 days, erythromycin 40 mg/kg/day qid or trimethoprim-sulfamethoxazole 40 mg/kg/day bid, all for 3 days duration.

A vaccine is available but is only about 50% effective in preventing disease, and requires a booster every 6 months. Since biological attacks must reach their victims through ingestion of the organism, the major mode of prevention is good sanitation (see Chapter 11, Tactical Environmental and Preventive Medicine). Careful selection of food and water sources, proper storage of foodstuffs, adequate water chlorination, and good handwashing technique will go a long way to prevent disease. Infected individuals require enteric precautions, and all persons in contact should practice effective handwashing.

Brucellosis

Brucellosis is caused by the organism of the genus *Brucella*. This bacteria naturally infects sheep, pigs, goats, dogs, and other mammals. Disease occurs in man from contact with infected animals or their milk. Brucella is highly infectious and can gain entry to the body through breaks in the skin, the mucous membranes, the lungs, and the gastrointestinal tract. The most likely route for a biological attack would be by inhalation.

The signs and symptoms of brucellosis are nonspecific and can vary form person to person. The incubation period lasts from 3 days to 3 weeks. Fever, malaise, myalgias (body aches), sweats, and arthralgias (joint pain) are the most common symptoms. Cough and headache are also common, but these symptoms do not predominate. Untreated, the symptoms can last for weeks or months. Common complications include debilitating bone and joint disease. A rare complication is involvement of the heart called endocarditis, and this complication accounts for 80% of deaths from brucellosis.

Treatment is aimed at preventing and treating shock and cardiovascular collapse. Intravenous fluids will be necessary in severe cases. Endocarditis is a particularly feared complication since treatment of heart-valve damage is difficult. Treatment with oral doxycycline 200 mg/day for 6 weeks combined with streptomycin 1 gm/day IM for 2 to 3 weeks is effective therapy. Endocarditis or other serious complications may require triple antibiotic coverage for 6 weeks or longer.

Doxycycline and rifampin may be taken orally in combination for prophylaxis, but the effectiveness of this regimen is untested. No vaccine is available. Infected patients require standard universal precautions.

Viral Hemorrhagic Fevers

Viral hemorrhagic fevers (VHFs) include the deadly Ebola and Marburg virus (*Filoviridae*), Lassa fever, Argentine hemorrhagic fever (*Arenaviridae*), Hantavirus (*Bunyaviridae*), Rift Valley fever (*Phleboviridae*), and yellow and dengue fever (*Flaviviridae*). These viral diseases all have similar clinical features and are therefore considered together. Some, such as Ebola and Marburg, occur naturally in primates, including man. Argentine hemorrhagic fever occurs naturally in rodents and is spread by fecal matter. Yellow and dengue fever are spread by mosquitos. All the VHFs (except dengue virus) are infectious as aerosols and through direct contact with infectious material. Therefore, each has some potential as a biological weapon.

The incubation period for the VHFs is variable, but generally lasts a few days to a week. Early symptoms include fever and malaise, and early signs include conjunctival injection and petechia (tiny patches of bleeding in the skin). Full-blown disease involves widespread damage to the capillary beds with easy bleeding, petechia, hypotension, and liver disease. Mortality can be in the range of 5% to 20%, with Ebola, in particular, causing death in 50% to 90% of those infected.

Treatment is supportive and includes judicious use of intravenous fluids. Overhydration is to be avoided, owing to the leaky capillary beds that may lead to pulmonary edema. Antibiotics are not helpful. However, the antiviral drug ribavirin has shown promise in treating some VHFs.

A yellow fever vaccine is available now, and other VHF vaccines are under development. Barrier isolation (mask, gown, and gloves) is required for all infected patients. VHF viruses can be present in high concentrations in the blood of infected patients, so careful handling of specimens and sharps is required.

Biological Toxins

Biological toxins are perhaps the most significant threat of all the biological agents. Unlike anthrax, tularemia, and the other previously discussed agents, toxins are not living organisms. Instead, they are the products of living organisms. Therefore, toxins cannot be transmitted from one affected individual to another. This does not diminish the toxin threat, however, since biologic toxins are among the most dangerous compounds known to man. By way of example, botulinum toxin is 15,000 times as potent as VX, the most deadly of all nerve agents.

There are dozens of potential biological toxins. Fortunately, only four are of significance: botulinum, ricin, staphylococcus enterotoxin 13 (SEB), and trichothecene mycotoxins (T_2) give varied and different effects (Table 6-5). Of importance is recognition of the paralysis and double vision (with normal mental status) of botulinum toxin and the skin lesions of T_2.

Botulinum

Botulinum toxin is produced by the bacterium *Clostridium botulinum* and is the most toxic substance known to man. As little as 1 nanogram (1 billionth of a gram) per kilogram of botulinum will kill a man. The route of exposure can be either inhalation or

TABLE 6-5

CLINICAL EFFECTS OF BIOLOGICAL TOXINS

AGENT	EFFECTS
Botulinum	Generalized weakness and paralysis; droopy eyelids; double vision; difficulty speaking, swallowing, and breathing; respiratory failure and death
SEB	Fever, chills, headache, body aches, cough, shock and death at high exposures
Ricin	Weakness, fever, cough, hypotension and death
T_2	Pain, itching, redness and lesions on exposed skin, nose and throat pain, runny nose and sneezing, shock and death at high exposures

ingestion. A few sporadic cases of botulinum poisoning occur in the United States each year, mostly from improperly canned food. Botulinum toxin is very stable and resists heat and freezing. Hypochlorite solution (see chapter 5, Care of Chemical Casualties) effectively inactivates the toxin. Because of its incredible potency and relative ease of manufacture, botulinum is considered a likely biological weapon threat.

Botulinum toxin acts by permanently binding to the presynaptic terminal of the neuromuscular junction (Figure 6-2). This inhibits nerve transmission and results in widespread muscular weakness and paralysis. Essentially, the nerve cannot release the neurotransmitter acetylcholine (ACh), and thus cannot stimulate the muscle. This may be thought of as the opposite effect of nerve agents poisoning, which causes an excess of ACh. The net effect of botulinum toxicity is complete paralysis, including the respiratory muscles, yet preservation of cardiac and higher mental functions. Untreated, foodborne botulism kills 60% of victims. Weaponized botulinum may kill an even higher percentage of exposed victims.

As soon as 24 to 36 hours after ingestion or inhalation, victims experience blurred vision, dry mouth, and difficulty talking and swallowing. A characteristic symptom is double vision (diplopia), and a useful sign is dilated pupils (mydriasis). A short time later, muscular weakness and paralysis sets in, which may eventually lead to respiratory arrest. Fever is absent, and mental status is preserved (unless the patient is hypoxic from respiratory failure). It is important to distinguish botulinum toxicity from nerve agent poisoning and atropine overdose (Table 6-6).

Treatment focuses on respiratory support. Oxygen, intubation, and mechanical ventilation can be lifesaving. Complete recovery from even severe botulinum toxicity is possible if respiratory support is initiated and continued until recovery (which can take weeks). Unfortunately, this aggressive approach is not practical in a mass casualty situation, but is completely reasonable if only a few casualties are encountered. Antitoxin therapy is an important adjunct to airway and breathing support. The antitoxin will neutralize any circulating botulinum toxin in the blood, but it cannot reverse any toxin already bound to the nerve endings; 10 ml is administered intravenously over 20 minutes. Because the antitoxin can cause life-threatening anaphylaxis as well as other serious side effects, it may require skin testing and should be administered only by medical professionals familiar with its use.

An experimental vaccine is being developed against botulinum toxin. Unfortunately, it often causes uncomfortable local reactions and requires boosters each year. Intoxicated patients are not able to transmit the disease, and no special isolation measures (beyond universal precautions) are required.

Staphylococcal Enterotoxin B

Staphylococcal enterotoxin B (SEB) is produced by the common bacterium *Staphylococcus aureus*. This is one of the toxins that can cause ordinary food poisoning after eating improperly handled foods. SEB can enter the body through the inhalational or oral route, and produces differing clinical pictures depending on which route. The toxin is resistant to heat, and only tiny quantities are needed to produce symptoms. Under most circumstances, SEB is not lethal, but it can effectively incapacitate at least 50% of those exposed.

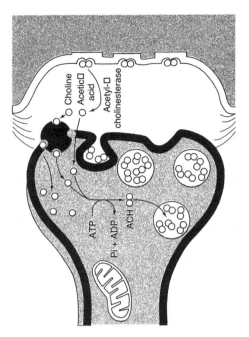

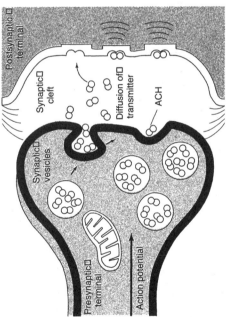

Figure 6-2 Presynaptic nerve ending at the neuromuscular junction. Normally, Acetylcholine is released and stimulates the muscle. Botulinum blocks this release and prevents stimulation.

TABLE 6-6

DIFFERENTIATING NERVE AGENT, BOTULINUM, AND ATROPINE POISONING

FACTOR	NERVE AGENT	BOTULINUM	ATROPINE OVERDOSE
Time of onset	Minutes	Hours	Minutes
Mental status	Normal initially Unconscious late	Normal	Altered (delirium)
Pupils	Miosis (constricted)	Mydriasis (dilated)	Mydriasis (dilated)
Vision	Blurred	Often double (diplopia)	Blurred
Heart rate	Decreased (bradycardia)	Normal	Increased (tachycardia)
Skin	Moist	Dry	Dry
Muscle tone	Fasciculations early Seizures late	Progressive Flaccid paralysis	Normal
Secretions	Copious	Normal	Dry
Small airways	Bronchoconstriction	Normal	Bronchodilation

Approximately 3 to 12 hours after inhalation, SEB causes fever, chills, body aches, and nonproductive cough. Shortness of breath and chest pain are possible. The fever may last for 5 days, and the cough for up to a month. Ingested SEB produces severe nausea and vomiting, and occasionally diarrhea. It is possible to have patients with overlapping symptoms since some aerosolized SEB may land on the hands or on food and be inadvertently swallowed by the victim.

Treatment is supportive since there is no known antidote or effective treatment. Patients with dyspnea should receive oxygen, and hypotension and dehydration should be treated with intravenous saline fluid boluses. Except in cases of overwhelming toxicity, recovery is the rule. There is no known prophylaxis. Hypochlorite solution effectively inactivates the toxin when applied to most nonporous surfaces.

Ricin

Ricin is derived from the beans of the castor plant *(Ricinus Communis)*, which is grown worldwide. Ricin is a natural byproduct of castor oil production, making the acquisition of large quantities of the toxin relatively easy. The toxin may be either inhaled or ingested. It is a protein complex and thus susceptible to heat and weak hypochlorite solutions.

Ricin exerts its toxicity directly on cells by inhibiting protein synthesis. This causes cellular death and tissue necrosis. The aerosol route causes primary lung damage, pulmonary edema, respiratory distress, and hypoxia. Ingested ricin causes severe vomiting, diarrhea, abdominal cramping, and shock. Complications of ricin poisoning include multiple organ failure and disseminated intravascular coagulation.

After a latent period of about 8 hours, aerosol-exposed individuals experience dyspnea, chest tightness, cough, fever, malaise, and body aches (myalgias). Death occurs within 36 to 72 hours from pulmonary edema and respiratory failure.

Treatment is supportive since there is no known antitoxin. Respiratory failure is treated with oxygen and, if needed, intubation and mechanical ventilation. Hypotension and shock will require intravenous fluids. There is currently no vaccine available. Ricin-intoxicated individuals require no special isolation or precautions once they have had effective skin decontamination.

Trichothecene Mycotoxins

Trichothecene mycotoxins (T_2) are the products of fungus molds Fusarium, Trichoderma, Myrotecium, Stachybotrys, and others. These are the alleged toxins of "Yellow Rain" in Laos, Kampuchea, and Afghanistan. Given its appearance in several global locations over time, T_2 should be considered a potential biological weapon.

T_2 acts directly on cellular growth by inhibiting protein and nucleic acid synthesis. Rapidly dividing cells are most affected and account for the symptoms referable to the skin, mucous membranes, gastrointestinal tract, and bone marrow. In a biological attack, exposure is possible through inhalation, contact, and oral routes. This will produce a broad array of effects on the victim. The toxin is very stable even under high heat and prolonged sunlight.

T_2 acts almost immediately, causing symptoms within minutes to hours of exposure. Burning skin, redness, pain, blistering, and bleeding at exposed skin sites occurs. Contact with the upper respiratory tract causes nose and throat pain, rhinorrhea (nasal discharge), and nosebleed (epistaxis). Lower respiratory symptoms include dyspnea, wheezing, and hemoptysis (bloody sputum). Eye exposure causes redness, pain, tearing, and blurry vision. Gastrointestinal exposure results in nausea, vomiting, bloody diarrhea, and abdominal cramping. Significant exposure can result in dizziness, loss of balance and coordination, hypotension, and death.

T_2 exposure can be difficult to differentiate from mustard agent poisoning (see chapter 5, Care of Chemical Casualties). However, mustard agents have a characteristic odor and are readily detected by field tests. Mustard usually has a slower onset of action, taking several hours to produce symptoms.

There is no specific therapy for T_2 mycotoxins. Medical management should focus on thorough decontamination (hypochlorite solution is effective). Saline should be used to decontaminate the eyes. Respiratory distress should be treated with oxygen, aerosolized beta-agonists (albuterol), and if necessary, intubation and mechanical ventilation. Skin lesions should be dressed with dry gauze. Hypotension and shock is treated with intravenous fluids such as saline. No vaccine or prophylaxis is available. Decontaminated patients require no special isolation or precautions.

EMERGENCY CARE

Recognition and Identification

A number of principles are important to recognize when faced with a biological casualty (Table 6-7). Recognition is crucial to the successful management of biological casualties.

TABLE 6-7

PRINCIPLES OF EMERGENCY CARE FOR BIOLOGICAL AGENT CASUALTIES

Recognition and identification
Isolation in selected cases
Respiratory and fluid support as needed
Arrange antibiotic or antitoxin therapy

A key discriminator between chemical and biological weapons is that most biological weapons take hours or days to cause effects. Chemical agents cause effects in minutes to at most a few hours. By the very nature of biological attacks, many casualties can be expected, and the medic will need to call additional resources as early as possible. A top priority is self-protection. Physicians (or physician assistants) will be needed to prescribe the proper antibiotic coverage and antitoxin treatment that is so crucial in treating biological agents. Infectious disease and biological agent experts and laboratory support will also be needed to help positively identify the agent and recommend further treatment.

Isolation

Fortunately, only a few biological agents are highly contagious from one infected individual to another. In particular, smallpox, plague, and Ebola are highly transmissible. As much as practical in the field, isolate biological casualties from unaffected individuals. Enforce the protective measures outlined in this chapter. Once the agent is identified as nontransmissible, overt protection can be discontinued. Of course, in all situations of patient care, observe body substance isolation if contact with body fluids is likely.

Supportive Care

The usual principles of emergency care apply to the care of biological casualties. Priority goes to securing and maintaining an airway and ensuring adequate ventilation. Provide high-flow oxygen by nonrebreather mask to all patients in moderate to severe respiratory distress. Respiratory failure or apnea will necessitate orotracheal intubation or positive pressure ventilation with a bag-valve-mask. Respiratory support is particularly crucial in botulinum poisoning. The cause of death in botulinum poisoning is respiratory failure. If ventilation can be maintained for the casualty, the chance of survival is good. Unfortunately, ventilation may need to be continued in the hospital for weeks or months.

Intravenous lifelines or saline locks should be initiated on all nonambulatory biological casualties. Many agents will cause dehydration, hypotension, or septic shock, and thus early IV access is important. Adult casualties with signs of compensated shock should receive 1000 ml of normal saline as a bolus. Children should receive 20 ml/kg. Uncompensated shock (for example, hypotension or signs of inadequate perfusion) should receive repeat boluses up to 3000 ml for adults or 60 ml/kg for children. During prolonged evacuation, casualties may receive up to 1000 ml (20 ml/kg) every 2 hours as a bolus if signs of shock persist.

Antibiotic and Antitoxin Therapy

A mainstay of treatment for many biological agents is treatment with specific antibiotics or antitoxins. These treatments, however, require the expertise of a physician or PA to select the right drug, dose, and route. It is beyond the scope of practice and beyond the expectations of tactical medics to initiate this therapy. However, the medic plays a crucial role in summoning the assistance of a physician when necessary, and can assist the physician's treatment of biological casualties with antibiotics or antitoxins. For the purposes of familiarity, some antibiotics and antitoxins are mentioned in this chapter; however, selection and use of these medications are best left to a physician familiar with the management of biological agent illness.

TRIAGE AND DECISION MAKING

Triage for biological casualties is no different from triage of any other patient (chapter 10, Tactical Triage). By the very nature of biological attacks, the medic will likely face mass casualties (Figure 6-3). In general, ambulatory patients will be classified as minimal, whereas those with moderate to severe symptoms (severe headache, cough, malaise,

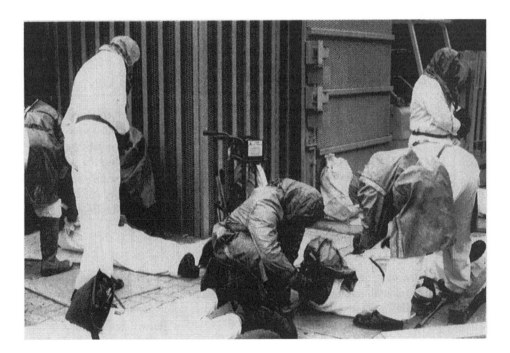

Figure 6-3 Mass casualties are a likely possibility in biological attacks.

TABLE 6-8

GENERAL TRIAGE CATEGORIES FOR BIOLOGICAL CASUALTIES

Minimal	All ambulatory patients
Delayed	Moderate to severe symptoms
Immediate	Respiratory failure and decompensated shock
Expectant	Pulseless and persistent decompensated shock despite adequate IV fluids

vomiting, and so on) and those unable to walk would be considered delayed. Casualties requiring immediate respiratory support with positive pressure ventilation and those in uncompensated shock are immediate. Pulseless casualties and those with persistent uncompensated shock despite initial IV fluid boluses are generally considered expectant. Table 6-8 summarizes the triage decision making of biological mass casualty incidents.

As in all triage, it is essential continually to reassess casualties and retriage casualties as appropriate. Most biological casualties will progress over time, much as natural disease does. Unlike chemical casualties, most biologic casualties will take hours, rather than minutes, to worsen. This affords the medic the opportunity to summon the required help to treat and evacuate the casualties.

BIOLOGICAL AGENT PROTECTION AND DECONTAMINATION

Self-protection against biological agents is achievable, and all medics and prehospital care providers should be familiar with these measures. Fortunately, all the techniques used to protect workers from chemical agents are also very effective for biological agents. Thus, the medic need only be familiar with one set of techniques for both biological and chemical agents. Chapter 5, Care of Chemical Casualties, and Appendix B, Chemical Agent Protective Measures, describe in detail the self-protection devices and equipment used for chemical and biological defense. The following paragraphs amplify important points.

Protective Mask

Because most biological agents enter the body through the mouth, nose, and lungs, a properly fitted and maintained protective mask is a crucial element in self-protection. If a standard NBC mask is not available and the agent is known to be biological, then a medical high-efficiency particulate air (HEPA, OSHA N95) filter will afford modest protection. Of course, many of these masks do not protect the eyes, nor the rest of the body. The best protection, however, is a self-contained breathing apparatus and full hazardous materials

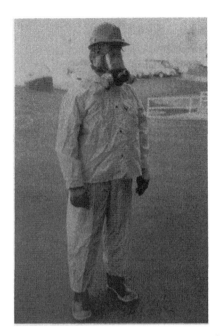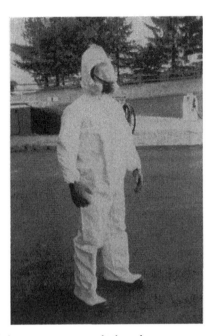

Figure 6-4 Full mask and overgarment ensemble for protection against biological agents.

ensemble (OSHA level A ensemble, Figure 6-4). Unfortunately, this equipment is expensive and available only in very limited quantities. Furthermore, it is very bulky and heavy, and without replacement of the air cylinders, will afford protection for at most a few hours. In contrast, the military chemical protective overgarment and mask is widely available and can be worn for several days while still maintaining effectiveness.

Protective Overgarment

Intact skin affords good barrier protection against most biological agents. Nonetheless, a protective overgarment is essential until safety can be assured. This includes the use of hood, gloves, and boots. Chapter 5, Care of Chemical Casualties, and Appendix B, Chemical Agent Protective Measures, provide details on the wear and use of protective equipment.

Immunization and Prophylaxis

Perhaps the best protection against biological weapons is prevention. A key tool to prevent any disease is immunization or prophylaxis. Immunization involves taking substances related to the biological agent (but nontoxic or non-infectious) to develop resistance or antibodies in the body. Immunizations are available against many biological agent threats. Prophylaxis is the taking of antibiotics prior to exposure. It, too, can be effective. Of course, good intelligence reports are needed to pinpoint the agent and timing of an attack

TABLE 6-9

IMMUNIZATION AND ANTIBIOTIC PROPHYLAXIS STRATEGIES AVAILABLE FOR SOME POTENTIAL BIOLOGICAL AGENTS

AGENT	STRATEGY
Anthrax	Vaccine, or ciprofloxacin/doxycycline prophylaxis
Plague	Vaccine, or doxycycline prophylaxis
Q fever	Vaccine (experimental) or tetracycline prophylaxis
Brucellosis	Doxycycline and rifampin prophylaxis
Tularemia	Vaccine (experimental) or tetracycline prophylaxis
Smallpox	Vaccine
Venezuelan equine encephalitis	Vaccine (experimental)
Viral hemorrhagic fevers	Vaccine (experimental)
Botulinum	Vaccine

to make this strategy useful. Several effective immunizations and prophylaxis strategies are available. The most notable is the anthrax vaccine, which may be up to 95% effective and is relatively free of side effects. Other immunizations and prophylactic antibiotics are administered only when the threat is high. Table 6-9 lists several common preventive strategies against biological agents.

Decontamination

Self-decontamination and decontamination of patients is accomplished as outlined for chemical agents (chapter 5, Care of Chemical Casualties, and Appendix B, Chemical Agent Protective Measures). Sodium hypochlorite solution (5% for overgarment and equipment, 0.5% for skin and mask) is the decontamination fluid of choice. Contact with the solution for 15 minutes will kill or inactivate all known biological agents. Decontaminating the eyes and wounds requires normal saline, Ringers Lactate, or plain water instead of hypochlorite solution.

SUMMARY

Biological weapons represent serious potential threats both on and off the battlefield. However, by recognizing that only a few agents are likely threats, the medic can prepare for this possiblilty. Biological agents can give varied symptoms, and it is important to focus on common and characteristic presentations. Field care for biological agents is largely supportive, but the medic plays an important role in assisting with and facilitating antibiotic and antitoxin therapy.

FURTHER READING

Medical Management of Biological Casualties. U.S. Army Research Institute of Infectious Diseases, 2d ed., Ft Detrick, MD, 1996.

Emergency Response to Terrorism: Basic Concepts Student Manual. U.S. Fire Administration, National Fire Academy. Emmitsburg, MD, 1997.

FRANZ DR et al.: Clinical Recognition and Management of Patients Exposed to Biological Warfare Agents. JAMA, 1997, 278: 399-411.

HOLLOWAY HC et al.: The Threat of Biological Weapons. JAMA, 1997, 278: 425-427.

CHRISTOPHER GW et al.: Biological Warfare: A Historical Perspective. JAMA, 1997, 278: 412-417.

SPIERS EM: Chemical and Biological Weapons. St. Martin's Press, New York, 1984.

ZAJTCHUK R et al. (eds): Medical Aspects of Chemical and Biological Warfare. Department of the Army, Office of the Surgeon General, Washington, DC, 1997.

BORAK J et al.: Hazardous Materials Exposure. Brady, Englewood Cliffs, NJ, 1991.

7

CARE OF NUCLEAR CASUALTIES

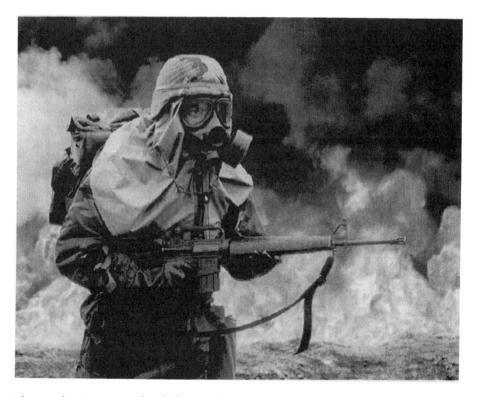

The tactical environment can be a frightening place.

OBJECTIVES

After reading this chapter, you will be able to:

1. Explain the process by which nuclear reactions develop their energy.
2. Relate the differences between fusion and fission and the relative energies they develop.
3. Describe the three major mechanisms of injury associated with a nuclear explosion.
4. Discuss how increasing acute radiation exposures affect the human body.
5. Identify the nature and severity of nonradiation-induced injury associated with nuclear detonation.
6. Describe the triage considerations when dealing with nuclear detonation and the associated injuries.
7. Define the equipment and techniques used to detect and measure nuclear radiation.
8. Explain the personal precautions taken to protect against radiation exposure and fallout.
9. Describe the decontamination procedures for a patient contaminated with radioactive fallout.
10. Describe the triage, assessment, and care for casualties associated with nuclear detonation and radiation accidents.
11. Given several preprogrammed and simulated nuclear casualties, provide the appropriate scene size-up; triage; initial, focused, and ongoing assessment; and then the appropriate care.

CASE

Your battalion is ordered to provide scene security at the crash site of a long-range bomber. It has impacted just inside a rural village of several hundred civilians. As your medical unit arrives at the site, word comes in that the craft may have been carrying nuclear weapons. There has been no detonation, though the craft wreckage is strewn about a few thousand square meters. All personnel are directed to don NBC gear and dosimeters, and geiger counters are passed out to all field medics.

As you approach the crash debris, you close the detection chamber of your geiger counter to detect only gamma radiation. There appear to be several small locations where the radioactivity is high, but most of the scene is not hot. As per command direction, you place red flags at locations of radioactivity and move back from the area, scanning for further contamination. There are clearly no survivors, and spectators are beginning to gather. Security personnel begin to evacuate the civilians from the village. Half your medical unit establishes an aid station while the other half continues to search the crash site and village for signs of radioactive contamination.

At the aid station, you provide care for several minor injuries, mostly related to falls or contact with sharp debris. However, one soldier arrives with hand injuries. Close examination reveals erythema and a complaint of a warm and burning sensation. Questioning of the casualty reveals he picked up a small cylinder of metal and handled it for a while before setting it down. Recognizing that this is likely the result of acute, local radiation exposure, you alert the battalion surgeon and arrange for immediate evacuation from the scene. The casualty is scanned for radiation but found to be clean. The battalion commander is alerted, and all personnel are advised not to handle any debris. The mission continues without incident until you and your battalion are relieved by a crash investigation and radiological teams.

INTRODUCTION

The extensive U.S. effort to develop a nuclear bomb in the 1940s set the stage for both warfare and power generation utilizing the atom's awesome power. The wartime detonations over Nagasaki and Hiroshima, Japan, and the accident at Chernobyl, USSR, demonstrate the potential for both warfare and peacetime casualty generation. Serious injury and death can also be associated with nuclear fuel or weapon transportation accidents or terrorist acts. The injuries produced by nuclear detonation and accidents can occur from several mechanisms and challenge the assessment and care skills of the medic. To better respond to this challenge, let us look at the nuclear explosion, how it produces energy, and ultimately, how it produces casualties.

THE NUCLEAR EXPLOSION

Conventional munitions gain their explosive power by breaking or changing the chemical bonds within the ordnance molecules. The result is kinetic energy, generally expressed as heat. (Heat is the measurement of molecule movement in a substance.) Nuclear energy is generated as the bonds inside the atom, and specifically the center of the atom (the **nucleus**), are broken and rearranged. *Nuclear bonds are much stronger than chemical bonds, hence, release much more energy when broken.*

NUCLEAR FUSION/FISSION

There are two types of nuclear reactions, fusion and fission. **Fission** breaks apart a large and unstable nucleus into multiple, smaller, and somewhat more stable nuclei. To create a reaction, forms (**isotopes**) of uranium and plutonium are pushed into high concentrations, interreact, release energy and particles, and ultimately, form more stable atoms. This reaction is controlled to generate power and was used in the nuclear weapons of World War II.

Fusion takes small atoms and fuses them into heavier ones. The reaction uses isotopes of hydrogen to form helium and other heavier elements. This process generates much more energy than fission but takes tremendous heat before a chain reaction can occur. The sun is an example of the fusion process. Science is not yet able to create a controlled fusion reaction because it is difficult to control the tremendous heat required to initiate and continue the reaction. For warfare, the necessary heat is generated by detonating a fission bomb within a concentration of fusion materials.

THE CHAIN REACTION

In fission, an unstable nucleus divides (decays), forming more stable atoms, releasing heat and high energy rays and particles. This occurs over time and is the radioactivity we associate with unstable isotopes. To create a chain reaction, however, the concentration of radioactive material must be greatly enhanced. Then, when an isotope decays and releases high energy particles, they collide with other unstable isotopes, causing them to decay and release more high energy particles, and so on. If there is enough reactive material (a critical mass), the reaction rate grows dramatically, and an explosion occurs. This process occurs in but a few thousandths of a second, creates great quantities of heat and electromagnetic energy, and vaporizes and blows the bomb apart. Only about 20% of the bomb's active nuclear material is responsible for the reaction and explosion (Figure 7-1).

As a chain reaction occurs, the heat energy and outflow of radiation become extreme. The great heat vaporizes the surrounding bomb casing and unspent nuclear fuel, and creates the first flash of nuclear ignition. The reaction releases extremely concentrated X-ray, gamma, and neutron radiation that superheats the surrounding air. This forms the powerful second flash and fireball associated with the nuclear blast. The rapidly expanding, vaporized, and superheated material creates a shockwave and begins to rise

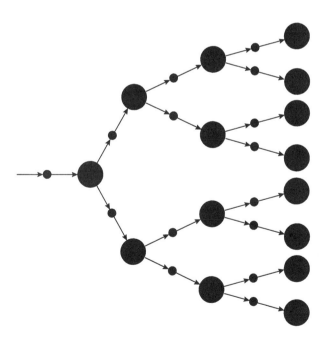

Figure 7-1 Nuclear chain reaction.

from the ignition point (called ground zero). The superheated surrounding air rises rapidly and draws air, and possibly debris, in from underneath the explosion. This material too is vaporized, bombarded with radiation, and becomes unstable (**radioactive**). It rises, cools, and condenses with the residual materials from the bomb (the characteristic mushroom cloud) forming small, radioactive particles that fall to earth as **fallout**. These events are responsible for the injury mechanisms associated with a nuclear detonation.

Fusion reactions create the same injury mechanisms as a fission detonation; however, they are generally much more powerful and also create a burst of electricity (called an electromagnetic pulse). Free electrons released from the reaction transmit an electrical surge outward. This current flow is extremely intense, and though it does not affect humans, it can have devastating effects on electrical equipment. Computers, medical diagnostic devices, communications equipment, and in many cases, vehicles may be rendered inoperative. This may impact communications and your ability to arrange for evacuation, request supplies and assistance, and report your status to higher echelons of care.

The energy expended by nuclear ignition differs greatly from a conventional explosion. The smallest of nuclear weapons (a tactical fission weapon—about 100 kg) delivers the conventional explosive energy equivalent of 500 tons (1/2 kiloton) of TNT. More modern fusion weapons deliver multimegatons (1 million tons of TNT equivalent) of energy upon detonation. This energy is distributed between the blast wave, heat energy, and radiation. Fifty percent of the bomb's energy is in the blast wave (converted from initial thermal energy), whereas 35% is released as direct thermal energy. The remaining 15% is released as initial radiation (5%) and radioactive debris (fallout; 10%). Some bombs are designed to distribute more initial radiation (approaching 30% of total output) and less physical destruction and fallout (Figures 7-2 and 7-3). These radiation-enhanced or "dirty" bombs are in the smaller range of nuclear arms and injure more personnel and fewer structures with detonation.

Nuclear Explosion Energy

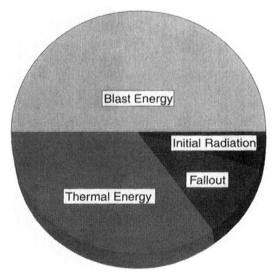

Figure 7-2 Energy distribution of a standard nuclear weapon.

Nuclear Explosion Energy

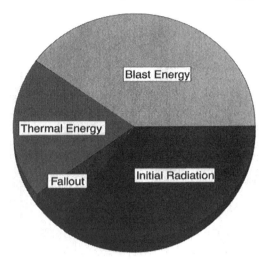

Figure 7-3 Energy distribution of a
radiation enhanced nuclear weapon.

NUCLEAR INJURY MECHANISMS

The result of nuclear detonation yields injury or death through three mechanisms: radiation, the blast, and thermal burns.

RADIATION

When an unstable (radioactive) molecule breaks apart, it releases energy in the form of rays and particles traveling at high speeds (nuclear radiation). This nuclear or ionizing radiation differs from other types of radiation (light, heat, and sound) because it can change the structure of atoms it passes. By this process, these rays and particles damage the cells of the human body. These cells then either die, repair themselves, or go on to produce damaged cells.

We are constantly bombarded by ionizing radiation from natural sources (the stars, the sun, and the earth) with little if any ill effects. However, the concentration of radiation from the nuclear chain reaction or fallout is much more intense and life endangering. X-ray, gamma, neutron, beta, and alpha radiation are the most common radiations associated with fusion, fission, and fallout (Figure 7-4).

X-Rays and Gamma Radiation

X-rays and gamma radiation are the same type of radiation though they are created by different processes. This powerful radiation is the most penetrating and occurs as unstable nuclei release energy and become more stable. The radiation is capable of traveling through 1000-2000 meters of air, penetrating deeply into all but the densest of materials, and damaging body cells in its path. X-ray and gamma radiation is generated in the reactor, bomb, and through the decay of radioactive particles, as in fallout. It is also given off when molecules are bombarded with high-speed electrons, as in the X-ray machine.

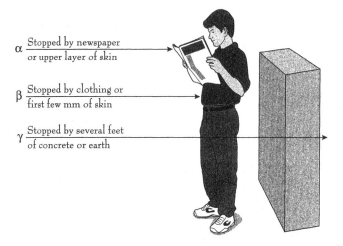

α $\frac{\text{Stopped by newspaper}}{\text{or upper layer of skin}}$

β $\frac{\text{Stopped by clothing or}}{\text{first few mm of skin}}$

γ $\frac{\text{Stopped by several feet}}{\text{of concrete or earth}}$

Figure 7-4 Radiation penetration gamma, alpha, beta, neutron.

Gamma radiation is the major external, and to a lesser extent, an internal, hazard associated with the nuclear detonation or reactor accident.

Neutron Radiation

Neutron radiation is released as the fission chain reaction occurs. It is a powerful and very damaging energy particle that penetrates several hundred meters of air and easily passes through the body. Since it occurs infrequently outside the nuclear chain reaction, its greatest threat to life occurs in proximity to an active nuclear reactor or bomb ignition. For simplicity's sake, neutron radiation, which does not penetrate as well as gamma radiation and X-rays, is considered along with this, other, more penetrating, radiation.

Beta Radiation

Beta radiation is a low-speed, low-energy particle that is easily stopped by 6-10 feet of air, clothing, or the first few millimeters (or in some cases of high energy beta radiation, the first centimeter) of skin. It is a common byproduct of fallout decay and is a serious internal hazard from ingestion of contaminated food or inhalation of airborne, contaminated particles. Although beta radiation is easily stopped by a few millimeters of soft tissue, it will cause significant ionization of those tissues.

Alpha Radiation

Alpha radiation is a very heavy and slow-moving particle that travels only inches in air and is easily shielded by clothing or the outer layer of skin. It is a very serious internal contaminant because it causes a great amount of damage along its short course of travel. Like beta radiation, alpha's greatest hazard is inhalation or ingestion of the source (radioactive) material.

RADIATION EXPOSURE

Two types of radiation exposure are associated with the nuclear explosion. They are the primary exposure associated with the intense nuclear reaction and, then, fallout.

Primary Radiation Exposure

Serious primary radiation injury during and shortly after a nuclear detonation is rather limited. The rising fireball draws the radioactive materials upward and away from the ground very quickly, with exposure occurring for only the first minute immediately after detonation. Neutron and gamma radiation also travels only around 1000-2000 meters through air, so exposure is limited to the blast proximity. Hence, *for most nuclear weapons, the mortality caused by primary radiation is overshadowed by blast and thermal injuries.* The only exception is the small, radiation-enhanced, tactical weapon where radiation doses may be sufficient to kill while the blast strength and thermal injury may not.

When exposure to radioactive energy occurs due to a nondetonation experience, like a power or research reactor or transportation accident, gamma radiation is the most serious life threat. Although these exposures are not as intense as the radiation exposure associated with an uncontrolled chain reaction, they can result in severe and life-threatening injury near the source of radiation. Here the radioactive source strength, the exposure duration, any shielding, and the distance from the source directly affect the exposures seriousness and the potential for injury and death.

Fallout

The second form of radiation exposure is fallout. Fallout is radioactive dust and particles that may present serious and life-threatening hazards not only near the blast epicenter but at some distance away. As the superheated products of nuclear detonation and surrounding debris are drawn up and into the atmosphere, they are bombarded with nuclear reaction byproducts, energized, and then distributed by winds aloft (and not always in the same direction as surface winds). If the nuclear detonation occurs at or close to the ground, the updraft of debris is increased, as is the amount of fallout.

The radioactive material may be scattered anywhere from a few miles surrounding ground zero to around the world. However, *the most immediately dangerous radiation falls shortly after (within 48 hours), in proximity to the blast, and in the form of larger, heavier particles.* This fallout is the most hazardous because it is concentrated over a relatively small geographic area and is an intense ionizing radiation source because it has not had much time to decay (Figure 7-5).

A similar condition to fallout occurring during a reactor accident is the release of radioactive particles, or gasses. The area of coverage and radiation intensity are not as great as with a bomb, but the health risk is still serious.

BLAST

The rapid heating of air surrounding the nuclear ignition creates an explosively expanding gas cloud. As the cloud's outward movement reaches the speed of sound, it creates a shockwave and a following blast of wind. The shockwave and blast wind produce the

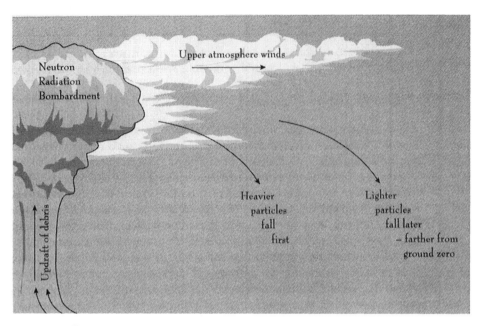

Figure 7-5 Fallout process.

same injuries associated with conventional explosives though the intensity close to, and the range of injury outward from, ground zero are much, much greater (see chapter 4, Care of Blast and Burn Casualties). The blast winds can reach more than 160 miles per hour and may displace personnel and topple structures, resulting in further trauma and death. However, like radiation, the shockwave and blast wind effects rapidly diminish the farther they travel from ground zero.

THERMAL BURNS

The mechanism resulting in most injury and death associated with nuclear detonation is the thermal burn. The nuclear reaction releases tremendous thermal energy that, unlike radiation and blast energy, travels unimpeded through air to its target. There the energy is absorbed by the contact surface, creating burns or igniting combustibles. Though the heating is of very short duration, it is extremely intense. Anything in proximity to the detonation is incinerated. *A 10-megaton bomb will result in 50% mortality due to burns 14 kilometers (10 miles) from ground zero.*

Even though thermal injury is the most prevalent injury for nuclear weapons, it is the easiest injury against which to shield. Any opaque object between the fireball and victim captures the energy. Any white or light colored clothing reflects much of the heat energy. The burn also involves only the surface facing the detonation. However, the heat energy may ignite clothing or building materials, resulting in a flame burn.

Farther out from the blast epicenter, thermal burns, caused by the short-duration flash, appear very serious and possibly charred in nature. However, they may involve only the epidermis and upper layers of dermis because of the short duration heat exposure and the skin's resistance to thermal injury. The prognosis for complete healing is very good, even with limited care, unless the burn is extensive or complicated by radiation exposure and/or trauma. Thermal burns caused by secondary mechanisms, such as clothing ignition, carry the same degree of seriousness as normal first-, second-, and third-degree thermal burns (see chapter 4, Care of Blast and Burn Casualties).

One event sometimes associated with nuclear ignition, especially when the detonation area contains substantial combustibles, is a **firestorm**. The blast and extreme heat ignite the flammable materials while the ensuing fire is fanned by air drawn into the rising mushroom cloud. The result is an extreme region of intense heat and fire. Burns associated with this event are extremely deadly.

Eye burn injuries may be associated with the brilliant light flash of nuclear detonation. The extremely intense light may cause momentary blindness as the flash stuns the retina. Much like the effects of a flash bulb in a dark room, the casualty is blinded for a few seconds or minutes, or possibly as long as 30 minutes when the flash occurs during the night. These effects completely disappear with time though they can severely impair the casualty's ability to fight and protect himself or herself. If the casualty looks directly at the detonation and focuses on the flash, the intense light may physically burn and permanently damage the retina. The injury destroys light sensitivity where the image focuses, but the casualty retains peripheral vision over the remainder of the retina.

Concentric Circles of Injury and Destruction

The explosive energy of a nuclear detonation distributes outward from ground zero. As the energy travels away from the blast center, it quickly dissipates. There is an innermost circle of complete destruction with flattened and burned buildings and foliage, and no personnel found alive. The next concentric circle contains much destruction to all but the stoutest of structures. Most personnel suffer mortal injuries from radiation, the blast wave, and burns. Some casualties may survive if they are shielded from the heat by objects between them and the blast though many die from collapsing structures. The next circle has greater survival with patients exposed to the flash suffering severe burns. The shockwave and radiation may induce serious injury, but thermal burns are the greatest cause of death. As the reaction energy moves farther from ground zero, the primary radiation exposure drops off rapidly, and pressure injuries diminish quickly. Burns remain the major cause of injury or death in these more distant circles. The more powerful the bomb, the larger the respective circles of destruction, injury, and death.

RADIATION EXPOSURE INJURY

Radiation exposure results in injury through different mechanisms than either thermal burns or injuries produced by the overpressure of the blast. These injuries also manifest in ways different from conventional-type wounds.

Ionizing radiation travels through body tissue and may alter some cell structures. Most commonly, radiation damages the **DNA** or causes chemical changes that, in turn, damage the DNA. *Since DNA is a cell's blueprint for reproduction, cells that reproduce quickly* *have the least time to affect DNA repairs and suffer most from radiation exposure.* The cells, in descending order of sensitivity, are those of the bone marrow and blood, bowel, skin, and nervous and cardiovascular systems.

Bone Marrow and Blood Cells

Moderate doses of gamma and neutron radiation penetrate the body and damage red bone marrow and blood cells. The marrow generates blood cells that carry oxygen and those that help with immunity and clotting. A reduction in the blood's oxygen-carrying capacity results in slight nausea, fatigue, and a general ill feeling (malaise). Later on, reduced platelet production induces clotting disorders and, possibly, uncontrollable hemorrhage. White blood cell destruction reduces the body's ability to rid itself of infection. The early signs and symptoms of bone marrow and blood cell injury usually take anywhere from 4 to 36 hours to become evident.

The radiation dosage necessary to damage the bone marrow and blood cells is generally survivable if not complicated by other injuries. However, when this early radiation syndrome is present, it is very important to reduce the casualty's exposure to infection. Any serious infection attacking the body when the white blood cell production is reduced may be severe and fatal.

Bowel

As the acute dosage increases, radiation penetrating the body begins to damage cells reproducing the bowel lining. This causes serious nausea, loss of appetite (anorexia), possible vomiting, diarrhea, fluid loss, and malaise. In later stages, dehydration and malnutrition, and possible bowel hemorrhage and perforation may occur. The early evidence of this syndrome appears a couple of hours after exposure and before those associated with bone marrow and blood cell damage. This syndrome may also result from the ingestion of food contaminated with emitters of alpha and beta particles, fallout. Internal contamination will take a longer time before it produces signs and symptoms. Bowel damage and the resulting signs and symptoms usually suggest a lethal dose of primary radiation. However, with extensive supportive care, and if not compounded by other injury, these patients can survive.

Skin

The upper layers of the dermis rapidly replace the dying skin cells of the body's surface. This rapid cell production makes the skin sensitive to ionizing radiation. The acute dosages creating gastrointestinal signs and symptoms often affect the skin. Cell damage causes a generalized skin reddening, called erythema. Although this injury does not significantly threaten the casualty's life, it may reflect his or her exposure to significant doses of beta, gamma, and neutron radiation. Nonuniform erythema may suggest partial shielding from the radiation. However, a weapon's thermal flash may also redden or burn the skin and confound this sign's value for assessment.

Fallout may cover unprotected skin and, with time, subject it to alpha and beta radiation. Here the skin may redden or receive a sunburnlike injury. If exposure persists and the area is subjected to extremely high radiation dosages, more serious burns may occur.

Nervous and Cardiovascular Systems

With more acute radiation exposure, blood vessel and nerve cells are affected. The result is a rapid onset of incapacitation, cardiovascular collapse, confusion, and with very extreme doses, a burning or "on fire" sensation throughout the body. Dosages sufficient to cause nervous and vascular damage, and the associated signs and symptoms, are generally very severe and do not permit survival even with very intensive, resource-consuming support efforts, especially if the casualty has sustained any thermal burn or blast injury.

Evaluating Exposure

As the radiation dosage increases, the signs and symptoms of exposure appear earlier and become more severe. The first signs of serious exposure are slight nausea and fatigue occurring within 4 to 24 hours after exposure. As the radiation dose moves into the lethal range, nausea severity increases and is joined by anorexia (lack of appetite), vomiting, diarrhea, and malaise. Erythema of the skin may be present, and fatigue becomes more intense. These signs appear within 2 to 6 hours. With increasingly fatal doses, the casualty displays all the signs of radiation exposure almost immediately, joined later by confusion, watery diarrhea, and physical collapse (Table 7-1).

With all the syndromes of radiation exposure, from the least to most serious, the casualty will display initial illness signs and symptoms, then may seem to get better, then gets worse. This occurs because the body attempts to repair itself after the initial damage. However, once the damaged cells fail to reproduce or produce damaged cells, a period of frank illness sets in. These phases of radiation sickness each span several days or weeks for the lesser doses, and hours for extremely lethal radiation exposures. It should also be noted that *there is a great individual sensitivity to radiation exposure.*

Cancer

Cancer is a flawed cell reproduction that becomes evident only many years after serious radiation exposure and only in a small portion of those exposed. Since it is impossible to determine who this problem will effect and there is no care either to prevent or to limit its development, you will not address this radiation exposure consequence.

TABLE 7-1 SIGNS AND SYMPTOMS OF INCREASING RADIATION DOSAGE

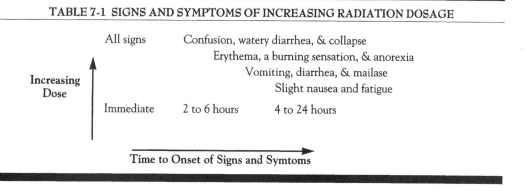

NUCLEAR CASUALTY ASSESSMENT

Both the nuclear detonation and accident drastically change your role as an emergency care provider. Your major responsibilities will probably involve triage, evacuation or sheltering, search and rescue, radioactive monitoring, decontamination, and limited casualty care. Your mission objectives and command authority are further altered between the civilian and military theaters. Let us examine the various nuclear scenarios and your respective scene size-up and initial responsibilities. These scenarios include the detonation (strategic, terrorist, and tactical) and the accident (reactor, fuel generation or transportation).

NUCLEAR DETONATION

Detonation is most likely to be a strategic weapon explosion, as part of a major offensive action, a single terrorist event, or a tactical event on the battlefield. Each type of explosion is very different in the magnitude of energy release, the command authority, the effect it has on casualties and the care provision system, and on your responsibilities as a medic.

Strategic Detonation

Strategic nuclear detonations will involve large urban or militarily useful locations and deliver multimegatons of explosive energy. There will probably be numerous detonations, and the ability to obtain significant additional medical and evacuation support will be severely limited. Because the weapon is likely a fusion bomb with a significant electrical surge, available radio communications will be compromised, as will be most vehicle operation. You will probably be brought into the area as a mass effort to provide search and rescue, triage, evacuation, radiological monitoring, decontamination, and some limited care. Military command will likely direct your actions, and it is assumed that there is no immediate danger of hostile enemy action.

Your initial assignment at a strategic nuclear detonation will be primarily search and rescue, followed by staging in anticipation of evacuation. Size-up the scene to determine the degree of radiation hazard, both on the ground and from fallout. Assure that your team and you yourself are protected from the effects of any radioactive fallout by donning NBC suits and personal **dosimeters** (see Appendix B, Chemical Agent Protective Measures). Take a quick resource inventory of your care supplies, methods of transportation, and personnel to assist with patient movement. Also determine what additional resources, supplies, personnel, and transportation, if any, might be available.

Find a suitable location to stage patients in anticipation of evacuation. Ideally, choose a location other than downwind from ground zero. This will minimize fallout accumulation. If you anticipate a delay between staging and transportation and there is a serious risk of fallout, select a large structure with a protected interior. The greater the distance between the casualties and the accumulating radioactive fallout, the less risk from continuing exposure. The center of the basement of a larger, stable, multifloor structure is ideal.

Search and rescue starts at the outer perimeter of injury and destruction and works inward, clearing routes of travel along the way. Egress to casualties may be the greatest obstacle to the entire response effort as trees, collapsed buildings, disabled vehicles, and other debris litter the disaster scene. As you find casualties, extricate them from debris and arrange for assisted movement to the staging area (if the casualties are nonambulatory). *As you move closer to ground zero, the severity and incidence of burn injuries increase and start to mix with pressure injuries to the ears, lungs, and bowel.* Close to ground zero, the burn and pressure injuries become critical and join with moderate, then serious radiation exposure.

If medical personnel are in short supply, staff the staging area to provide triage and limited supportive care. As more medical personnel become available, direct them to work with the search and rescue teams. They will provide triage and immediate life-saving care only. Because of the fallout hazard, all immediate, minimal, delayed, and ambulatory expectant casualties are sent to the staging area, then evacuated to fallout secure locations.

Since the ability to obtain outside help for one of the many strategic detonation areas is limited, some other resources will be critical for casualty survival. The devastation caused by the blast will destroy most sources of potable water, food, power, clothing, heat, and shelter. During your search-and-rescue activities and whenever outside the fallout zone, look for resources that may help meet these needs as the disaster grows older. Protect food and water sources from contamination. Assure adequate shelter from the environment and begin to acquire medical supplies (like clean fabric and makeshift splints). Locate lighting and power sources such as flashlights and operating vehicles.

Assure proper sanitary facilities (see chapter 11, Tactical Environmental and Preventive Medicine). In the disaster environment, infection quickly becomes a major concern owing to poor sanitation and the decreased infection-fighting capability of casualties. Isolate the water supply and sanitation, assure that food is well cooked and eating utensils are clean, and boil water if necessary to assure its quality. Also assure that the injured are isolated from the dead and any other source of infection.

Terrorist Detonation

Terrorist nuclear detonation will probably be limited to one small (1 to several-kiloton) detonation in a highly populated area. It is likely that international resources will rapidly be brought to the scene, and massive evacuation and extensive care is possible during the days thereafter. However, during the first few hours of the disaster, resources are severely limited, and the damage, both to structures and personnel, is great. You are likely to be brought into the scene to assist with the search and rescue, monitor radiation levels, evacuate casualties, or at a remote location, provide supportive care. Your actions will probably be directed by civilian incident command (Table 7-2).

After a terrorist nuclear detonation, your role may be similar to that associated with the strategic detonation. However, the available resources are much greater and the structural damage and number of casualties much reduced. Evacuation and shelter are given high priority owing to the radioactive fallout hazard. Intensive scene and hospital care is offered to all patients who need it, though immediate category patients will receive it first. Here, you will most likely function under the civilian incident command system. The civilian incident command will designate medical sectors such as extrication (search and rescue), triage, treatment, and transport (evacuation). Because of the incident size, several sectors may be established geographically for each designation.

TABLE 7-2 NUCLEAR WEAPON CHARACTERISITCS

	STRATEGIC WEAPON	TERROIST WEAPON	TACTICAL WEAPON
Location	Military/urban	Urban	Battlefield
Nature/Size	Fusion/Megaton	Fission/Kiloton	Fission/Kiloton
Nature			Radiation Enhanced
Incidence	Multi-sites	Isolated	Battlefield
Casualties	Millions	Thousands	Hundreds
Resources Available	Regional	National	Limited
Prioirty	Evacuation & Shelter	Evacuation & Shelter	Maintain Fighting Force

Tactical Detonation

Tactical nuclear detonation occurs on the battlefield with the purpose of destroying the enemy's will and ability to fight. The tactical nuclear weapon is of limited yield and possibly radiation enhanced. You are likely to be in the vicinity of detonation and will provide immediate advice to command regarding the detonation's effects on the combat effectiveness of the troops. You will also provide search and rescue, triage, evacuation, radiologic monitoring, decontamination, and supportive care, as needed.

Prevention from an imminent nuclear explosion depends on the amount of warning given. If possible, seek shelter in a deep or well-fortified bunker. If shelter is unavailable, seek protection in or behind an armored vehicle or other large, substantial object. Trenches or foxholes also provide moderate protection. If you are caught in the open, drop to the ground, face down, with your feet pointing toward ground zero. Avoid looking at the flash to reduce your risk of temporary blindness.

The scene size-up of a tactical nuclear detonation places a great responsibility on you. The nature and degree of destruction can be unimaginable; however, you must gather your senses and begin to organize a response. The initial radiation hazard has lifted by the time you realize what has happened. The fireball has drawn the radioactivity up and away from the battlefield and is expected to return it as fallout in about an hour. Anticipate the fallout contamination by donning your NBC suit and dosimeter and by assuring other personnell do the same, then continue your scene size-up.

Try to determine your location regarding ground zero and how intense the blast was. Although you will not calculate the bomb's nuclear output, this information may help you determine the size of the concentric circles of destruction and the potential for casualties. Also note how close the ignition was to the ground. Ground blasts draw in much more debris and create much more fallout than do the higher air bursts. Also, look at which direction the head of the nuclear cloud moves. This may suggest the direction most fallout will be carried by the winds aloft. Try to stay out from under the moving radiation cloud, if possible.

Tactical nuclear weapons may be used in conjunction with chemical or biologic weapons. Try to rule out this possibility as you evaluate the initial casualties. Chemical weapons may cause nausea and vomiting, confounding the triage of lethal radiation exposures. However, the immediate protective measures for biologic and chemical weapons are the same as for radioactive fallout, donning the NBC suit (Figure 7-6).

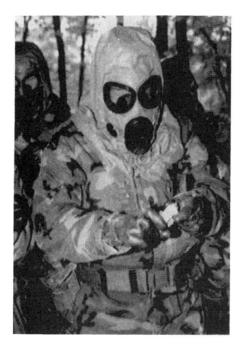

Figure 7-6 Soldier in camou-
flaged NBC protective gear.

With any tactical nuclear detonation, presume, for at least the first day or so, your casualties will far outstrip care resources at hand. Those casualties surviving the initial blast may be responsible to carry out the military mission. And the blast may be a prelude to aggressive enemy action. Many casualties sustaining lethal radiation doses may still be combat effective. It may be a day or two before they become severely incapacitated by their exposure.

NUCLEAR ACCIDENTS

Nuclear accidents are usually isolated incidents affecting only those personnel in proximity to the reactor or leak. However, on rare occasions, the accident may be a major incident contaminating many square miles and endangering thousands, or possibly, hundreds of thousands of people. The nuclear accident's ability to cause property damage or personnel injury is much, much less than even the smallest of nuclear weapons. The vast majority of accidents present serious radiation exposures to but a few personnel and very limited radiation exposures to few if any of the population. Nuclear accidents are most likely reactor or fuel-processing, or transportation accidents.

Reactor or Fuel-Processing Accident

Reactor accidents can be serious because there is a relatively large quantity of nuclear material present, and there is also a chain reaction taking place. Though the potential for a nuclear explosion is not physically possible, great heat or pressure may damage the reactor and its containment vessel. The result may be a release of radioactive steam, or vapor and the danger of contamination. There may also be internal accidents involving the handling of radioactive materials. These accidents subject a very small number of personnel to radiation danger though their injuries may be severe.

Fuel-processing accidents occur during nuclear fuel enrichment for use in power or research reactors or in weapons. It is unlikely that a critical mass is present and that an explosion will occur. However, the reaction may become uncontrolled, creating great amounts of heat, and releasing radioactive steam, smoke, or vapor into the atmosphere, or injuring plant personnel. Personnel may also be seriously or mortally injured if the shielding is compromised.

Expect reactor or plant personnel, under the direction of the health physicists, to provide any initial firefighting, radiation containment, and cleanup services. Your role as a medic will likely be to evacuate or shelter civilians, monitor radioactivity, or provide decontamination services. These services are guided by reactor or plant personnel. Your services may be most needed in very large incidents where large population evacuations are necessary.

Transportation Accidents

Transportation accidents can occur whenever radioactive materials are moved. The material can be for medical treatment or diagnosis, reactor fuels, industrial testing agents, radioactive waste, or weapons. Radioactive material is shipped in only very small quantities or in crash-proof containers. Leaks or spills affect only a small and immediate area, unless combustion, from other agents, aerosolizes the material. Owing to the limited potential for release and exposure to the populace, transportation accidents rarely require military assistance.

An exception occurs when nuclear weapons are damaged through air travel and high-velocity crashes. Although nuclear weapons are safeguarded against nuclear ignition, the conventional explosives, used to induce the nuclear detonation, may explode on impact. Weapon-grade nuclear material is then scattered around the crash site and poses a hazard within the debris perimeter. Further, any combustion, such as with jet fuel, may introduce the radiation into the atmosphere.

In the transportation accident, you may be called to monitor radioactivity or assist with evacuation and, rarely, decontamination. Since casualties are unlikely, and radiation exposure is limited, you will probably not provide much medical care. The exception might be a military aircraft crash into a populated area where you may render care for trauma and burn injuries not associated with radiation exposure.

ASSESSMENT

When assessing nuclear detonation casualties, remember this is a disaster, and assessment and triage must occur quickly (see chapter 10, Tactical Triage). Visually sweep each casualty for any signs of serious injury, most likely burns or blunt trauma. Check quickly for signs and symptoms of pressure injuries, especially any lung injury, difficulty breathing, or small strokelike symptoms (air emboli). Note the distance from the explosion center and any early complaints of radiation exposure, such as nausea or fatigue.

During a mass casualty incident, such as a detonation or serious accident, document your casualty assessment and care well. Assure you record the casualty's initial location, and narratively describe each serious injury and complaint. Identify the time after exposure that the casualty complains of any radiation-related signs and symptoms. This information will help to determine the radiation dosage and the ultimate triage category assigned the casualty.

TRIAGE

Triage is a difficult responsibility for anyone involved with a nuclear event, especially the detonation. The signs and symptoms of serious radiation exposure may not occur for several hours and do not suggest imminent death; sensitivity to radiation exposure varies greatly from individual to individual, and *sublethal radiation exposure, when mixed with other serious injuries, greatly increases mortality*. With these considerations in mind, let us look at triage approaches to evaluate nuclear detonation, then nuclear accident, casualties.

Nuclear Explosion Triage

Before employing a triage system at the nuclear explosion, carefully evaluate the resources you have at hand or that will be available shortly. When resources (medical personnel, supplies, and transportation) are adequate or will arrive soon, limit the expectant category to those who will die despite intensive care. In the strategic or tactical weapon deployment, you may be forced to triage patients as expectant who could otherwise survive with only moderate care. To act differently reduces the chances for survival of others who need less extensive care.

It is best to begin the triage process from the outer ring of destruction (Figure 7-7). Here the primary mechanism of injury is burns. Although these burns may look severe

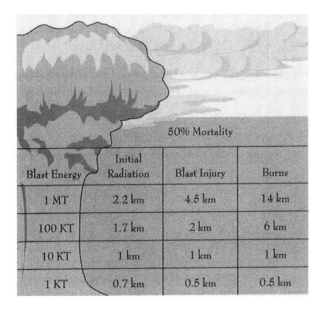

Blast Energy	Initial Radiation	Blast Injury	Burns
1 MT	2.2 km	4.5 km	14 km
100 KT	1.7 km	2 km	6 km
10 KT	1 km	1 km	1 km
1 KT	0.7 km	0.5 km	0.5 km

50% Mortality

Figure 7-7 Rings of nuclear destruction.

and, in some cases, charred, the quick delivery of the blast's thermal energy reduces the burn depth. Check for the absence of pain, indicating full thickness burns, and use the rule of 9s to approximate burn surface area (see chapter 4, Care of Blast and Burn Casualties). Remember, each adult body region-each arm, the head, the anterior chest, the posterior chest, the anterior abdomen, the posterior abdomen, each anterior leg, and each posterior leg-approximates 9% of the total surface area.

Categorize any 70% or greater full-thickness burn as expectant. Classify any burns greater than 20% full thickness as delayed. Any serious burn involving a joint area or circumferentially covering a limb or the trunk is increased in severity by one position, as are those affecting the very young or old or anyone with a preexisting or concurrent disease or serious injury. If the burn is complicated by any signs of respiratory burn injury, also move the patient's triage category one closer to immediate.

As you move closer to ground zero, the depth and severity of burns increase, and this mechanism of injury is joined by pressure injuries. Designate casualties with serious signs of lung injuries as expectant, moderate or minor lung injury signs as immediate, bowel injury signs as delayed, and ear injury signs as minimal. This concentric destruction and injury ring may also produce blunt trauma from blast wind projectiles, casualty displacement, or collapsing structures. Move any serious mixed injuries (any two or more of burn, pressure, or blunt trauma) one triage class toward expectant.

The next closest ring of destruction introduces radiation injuries along with increasingly severe burn, pressure, and blunt trauma. Here burns, pressure injuries, and radiation each account for a mortality greater than 50%. It is unlikely that many casualties will be found alive, and those that are, are likely to die, regardless of the care you provide. Place only those casualties with limited injuries and no early signs of radiation exposure, in the immediate category. All others are expectant.

Sorting casualties for radiation exposure is difficult because the signs are delayed and are often intermingled with other, more apparent injuries. Signs suggestive of moderate radiation exposure include mild to moderate nausea, vomiting, possible diarrhea, and fever. In severe radiation exposure, the casualty will display severe nausea, vomiting, and mild to severe diarrhea and fever. The severely irradiated casualty may also display erythema, hypotension, and CNS dysfunction. Remember, as the primary radiation dose increases, the signs become more severe and appear sooner. *During your early triage (the first few hours), casualties presenting with signs and symptoms of radiation injury are most likely to have the most serious exposure.*

Triaging casualties into the expectant category is a difficult task in any nuclear detonation. Patients who receive lethal radiation doses appear sick but certainly not mortally injured. You must simply comfort them without providing extensive care because those with a chance for survival need your services and supplies. You may also note that many radiation casualties seem to improve with time. Owing to the nature of radiation injury, this improvement is transient, will be followed by more serious signs and symptoms, and does not indicate that the casualty will survive.

Nuclear Accident Triage

The nuclear accident is a much easier situation to triage. The emergency medical service system is intact, and supplies, personnel, and transportation are or will be available in adequate quantities. The accident is also likely to produce fewer, and much less, serious radiation exposures and few, if any, thermal burns or pressure injuries. In the nuclear accident, it is unlikely that you will employ disaster triage.

The major injuries associated with a radiation accident will be radiation exposure and, possibly, radiation burns. Upon arrival at the scene, locate the health physics staff, and function under their direction. In their absence, place yourself at a distance from the site and with some large mass of steel, concrete, or earth between you and the radiation source. Identify the location and number of victims and, if possible, the level of radiation. If there is a hazard of fallout or radioactive smoke, steam, or other contamination, don a NBC suit. Attempt a casualty rescue if the expected total rescuer exposure will be 25 rem or less. Have the rescuers don dosimeters, and assure they move quickly toward the casualty and then away from the source. Decontaminate the casualty as necessary, then transport.

Radiation exposure injuries, most commonly skin burns, do not occur for hours, unless the exposure is from extremely strong gamma radiation or is a result of prolonged surface contamination with alpha- and beta-emitting particles. Simply provide decontamination as needed, and care for the associated burns as you would for thermal burns.

RADIOLOGICAL MONITORING

An important service you may provide at the nuclear accident or detonation is radioactive monitoring. Fallout, smoke, vapor, or steam may deposit nuclear material over a moderate to large geographic area. The accumulation is gradual, then its radioactive strength diminishes as the unstable material decays. *This decay reduces the radiation by 90% 7 hours after a detonation (10% the original strength), by another 90% after 2 days (to 1%), and by another 90% (to 0.1%) after 2 weeks.* To determine where the material has fallen and its changing strength, careful and continuous monitoring must take place (Figure 7-8).

Since you cannot feel, hear, smell, or see nuclear radiation, you must use a special monitor. This device, called a geiger counter, measures electrical discharges as ionizing radiation passes through the detection chamber. *(The chamber cover blocks all but gamma radiation; removing it will evaluate the alpha and beta dose).* The geiger counter's electronics then register a radiation exposure level, converted to a dosage per hour rate. This radiologic monitoring will help you define the hazard boundary, determine exposure levels, and suggest where special actions such as rescue, evacuation, sheltering, or decontamination are necessary (Figure 7-9).

Radiation exposure rates vary greatly. The detonation sends several hundreds or thousands of **gray** (a standardized radiation energy unit) out over the first minute within 1000-2000 meters from ground zero. A rapid dose of 300 gray will ultimately result in 50% mortality of those irradiated and produce the nausea, fatigue, and possible vomiting associated with serious radiation exposure. The radiation released from fallout arrives much more slowly and requires twice the dosage to cause the same damage. However, any radiation exposure is accumulative (dosage rate per hour times the hours of exposure).

For civilian operations, the evacuation threshold occurs whenever the expected cumulative dose will reach 1 **rem**. Elective life-saving or rescue actions may expose care providers to as much as 25 rem. In the military operation, these limits are higher to accomplish the mission; however, the objective is to minimize the radiation exposure while maintaining the fighting force.

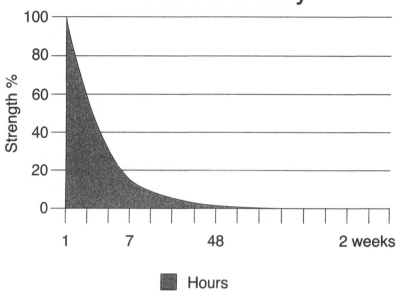

Fallout Decay

Figure 7-8 Fallout strength decay graph.

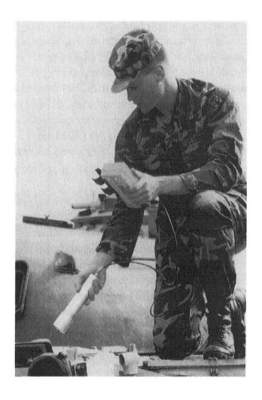

Figure 7-9 Geiger counter.

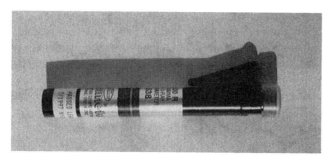

Figure 7-10 Dosimeter.

In addition to geiger counter monitoring, all personnel on the potential nuclear battlefield or assisting at a detonation or incident should wear personal dosimeters. These "penlike" devices record the accumulation of radiation and can be read optically. The device further provides a measure of the victim's exposure and may suggest when he or she should be evacuated or moved to shelter. Although dosimeters do not record the rate of exposure, their information, especially when combined with that of several casualties, can be very valuable in determining the overall exposure from the incident or detonation. It is important to assure these devices are read frequently when combatants may be exposed to radiation (Figure 7-10).

NUCLEAR INJURY CARE

The scene size-up and assessment determines whether radiation exposure is due to a nuclear detonation, fallout at some distance from the conflagration, or is an isolated noncritical mass incident. Each of these mechanisms of injury and exposure calls for you to perform different activities as a medic. These activities are common to the scenarios mentioned earlier and include search and rescue, evacuation and sheltering, decontamination, and supportive medical care.

SEARCH AND RESCUE

After donning the NBC garment, the next step is to locate casualties. Search and rescue is an essential part of the nuclear detonation response since patients may be trapped or isolated from care by debris. In most nuclear detonations, as you get closer to the area of extreme destruction, travel becomes more and more difficult. Once a casualty is found, there may be difficulties in accessing them and then removing them from the scene and to the staging area. Usually the responsibility for search and rescue will be left to nonmedical personnel since the medic's knowledge and skills are needed either at the staging area for triage and limited on-scene care or at a remote location for decontamination and supportive care.

When removing casualties from a radiation accident, *reduce rescuer exposure by minimizing exposure time, maintaining the greatest distance possible from the radioactive source, and using natural and artificial shielding.* Armored vehicles, for example, provide limited protection against fallout and radiation sources. Have rescuers move to the casualty and bring them out of the area as quickly as possible. Radioactive exposure is a cumulative danger, so shorter exposures are less damaging. Evacuate casualties to a distant location. Radiation strength falls off very quickly with increasing distance from the source. Also use any natural shielding like earthen berms, ditches, or heavy building walls between you and the source to reduce exposure. Lastly, since cancer is a significant but very delayed effect of radiation exposure, utilize older rescuers to perform actions that will garner the greatest radiation doses. Their shorter remaining life span reduces the chance of cancer developing, and if it does, it will likely occur at a greater age.

EVACUATION AND SHELTERING

Evacuation removes casualties from the danger associated with radioactive fallout. You will generally move the casualties perpendicular to the wind direction. This moves the casualties most quickly to a safe zone. However, wind direction changes frequently, so watch for wind shifts and assure the evacuation moves the casualties to safety. Radiologic monitoring will help guide evacuation and, while waiting, or in the absence of transportation, help you seek shelter from exposure.

If medical support personnel are in adequate supply, you may travel with casualties during evacuation. During this time, care for the patients triaged to immediate, delayed, and minimal categories, and provide comfort (psychological support and empathy) to the expectant. You will most likely treat thermal burns, pressure injuries, and blunt trauma.

If evacuation is not possible, shelter personnel from fallout and radioactive contamination. Sheltering is best accomplished by placing as much distance and substance between you and the accumulating radioactive material. Two inches of steel, 6 of concrete, 8 of earth, and 22 of wood, will each reduce radiation gamma exposure by 50%. If fallout is, or you expect it to become, a significant exposure threat, locate or construct a shelter (Figure 7-11).

DECONTAMINATION

Decontaminate casualties once you are remote from the scene and away from further radioactive fallout exposure. Bring the contaminated casualty to the decontamination site, and remove, bag, and set aside the clothing for proper cleaning or disposal. This simple act removes about 90% 95% of external contamination. Then gently wash the exposed areas such as the face and hands with soap and water, or if in short supply, wipe them clean (Figure 7-12). Irrigate any contaminated wounds or burns with sterile saline or water, if available. Finally, wash and/or clip the hair to remove any remaining contamination. Then scan the casualty for any further contamination with a geiger counter. *Once properly decontaminated, the casualty presents no further hazard to care personnel.*

During the decontamination process, do not vigorously scrub the casualty. This may abrade the skin and open a route for infection. Because radiation exposure injures the body's immune system, this injury may become seriously infected or permit infectious agents to invade the body. During the decontamination process, use stretchers that are easily cleaned and assure the casualty and the decontamination process does not move contamination into the patient-care area. Also contain any wash water and other contaminated material, then dispose of it safely.

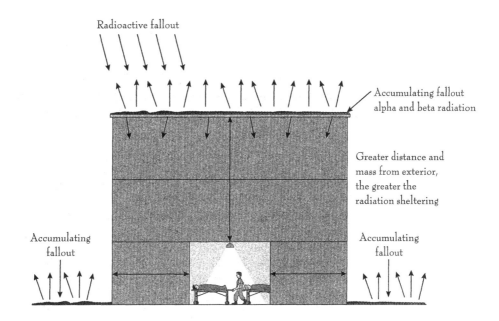

Figure 7-11 Sheltering.

Radioactive fallout

Accumulating fallout
alpha and beta radiation

Greater distance and
mass from exterior,
the greater the
radiation sheltering

Accumulating
fallout

Accumulating
fallout

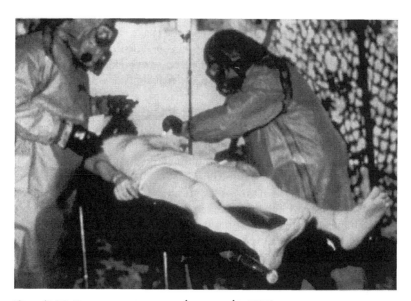

Figure 7-12 Decontamination area with personnel in NBC gear.

Emergency medical care at the nuclear incident, be it the detonation or accident, is limited. *Because of the detonation's nature, a restrictive triage must be employed to salvage the greatest number of casualties.* On the other hand, the radiation accident, even with high personal exposures, does not produce wounds that need immediate care. The only injuries requiring your attention are conventional burns and blunt or pressure injuries. However, there are helpful guidelines regarding the typical injuries associated with the nuclear incident.

Conventional (Thermal) Burn Care

Thermal burns associated with the tremendous heat of a nuclear detonation can be severe. However, care for them as you would any burn while paying special attention to reduce potential infection. If radiation exposure suppresses the immune system, the body will not be able to combat the serious infections often associated with full thickness burns.

Since burns induced by nuclear explosion heat cover a large portion of the body's surface, care for them by covering the area with clean dressings. Sterile burn sheets are ideal, but in an area of mass destruction, freshly laundered sheets are a reasonable substitute. If adjacent skin surfaces are seriously burned, such as the hands or feet, place non-adherent dressings between the digits. This keeps the injury surfaces from adhering one to another. If the body was well shielded and burns affect only small surfaces, cover them with smaller sterile dressings.

Serious burns can quickly cause serious dehydration. Third-degree burns break down the skin and dimish its function as a container for the human body. Fluid seeps through the wound and then evaporates. The result is rapid dehydration and possible hypothermia. First- and second-degree burns also increase the likelihood of hypothermia because they dilate the surface blood vessels, permitting a rapid loss of heat to the environment. Maintain the body temperature of any casualty with extensive first-, second-, and third-degree burns.

Consider fluid administration if IV solutions are in adequate supply. Administer a bolus of 1000 milliliters of normal saline in the first hour after a serious, third-degree burn affecting more than 20% of the body surface area. Administer additional fluid just as for conventionally caused burns (see chapter 4, Care of Blast and Burn Casualties). Pain medication may also be helpful for the serious or extensive burn patient. Administer morphine sulfate in 2-mg increments until pain relief, a reduced level of consciousness, or a total of 10 mg has been administered (see Appendix A, Medications for the Tactical Environment). Repeat the dosing as needed for pain. In general, antibiotics are contraindicated in the tactical phase of burn care.

Injuries to the eyes caused by the detonation blast will require little specific care. The flash blindness lasts only a few minutes during daylight and as long as 30 minutes at night. Assure the casualty that his or her eyesight will return shortly, and have a buddy remain with him or her until it does. With retinal burns, the blindness is more permanent though the casualty will have peripheral vision and be able to move about and protect himself or herself after a short period of adjustment. No tactical medical care is needed for either condition.

Blunt Trauma Care

Trauma associated with a nuclear detonation will be blunt in nature and anywhere from mild to extremely serious. Injuries occur from debris placed in motion by the blast wind, casualties thrown by the wind, and structural collapse. Fractured limbs, possible spinal injury, head and torso blunt trauma, and penetrating trauma caused by flying glass and other sharp debris are common. Care for these wounds in accordance with standard emergency care principles.

Fallout danger may require rapid evacuation of casualties before you can completely stabilize their wounds. Secure their arms to the torso, tie their legs together, and move them to the stretcher along the long axis of the body. Protect the head as you move the patient. Care for specific injuries will likely occur after triage and evacuation (see chapter 8, Tactical Evacuation).

Pressure Trauma Care

Pressure injuries needing your greatest concern and care are those affecting the lungs. The damage and tearing of the alveoli causes swelling, fluid accumulation, and possibly, pulmonary emboli. Progressive swelling and fluid accumulation makes breathing more difficult and less efficient with time. Oxygen has a more difficult time getting into the blood stream, and the patient becomes hypoxic. If any lung pressure injury signs are present, administer 100% oxygen. Use positive pressure ventilation only when necessary and then only to obtain moderate chest rise and air movement. Lung tissue damage may allow air to enter the blood stream directly and seriously threaten life. If you suspect pulmonary emboli, place the patient in a head-down position on his or her left side. This will slow the movement of air bubbles into the systemic circulation. Also monitor respirations and watch for developing dyspnea and possible tension pneumothorax. If you suspect tension pneumothorax, consider pleural decompression (see chapter 4, Care of Blast and Burn Casualties).

Ear and bowel injury caused by the blast pressure wave require only supportive care. Bowel injury presents with abdominal pain and needs no immediate field treatment other than making the casualty as comfortable as possible. If there is ear pain and/or hearing loss, keep the ear (auditory) canal clean, make the patient as comfortable as is possible, and suspect possible lung damage. Remember, casualties with diminished hearing cannot recognize danger. Their duty should be limited accordingly.

Radiation Exposure Considerations

The effects of radiation exposure, if they are indeed survivable, present after a few hours. Furthermore, the damage is diffuse throughout the body and the only helpful care is antibiotic therapy and rehydration. Unless you are with the patient for a prolonged time and resources are adequate to care for large numbers of patients, little can be offered for the radiation-exposed casualty.

When radiation exposure is combined with other trauma, pay special attention to keeping the wounds clean and reducing the chances of infection. Radiation exposure will limit the body's ability to fight off infection, and the introduction of infectious agents through any wound will seriously threaten the casualty's life. Consider irrigating

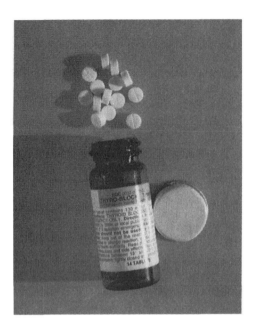

Figure 7-13 Sodium iodine.

any wound with potential contamination and applying sterile dressings and, later in care, antibiotic therapy under the supervision of a physician.

In areas of increased exposure to radiation due to detonation fallout, you may be called to help with the oral administration of sodium iodine to the population. A detonation byproduct, radioactive iodine, enters the food chain, then concentrates in the thyroid. Thyroid cell damage caused by this concentration and radioactive decay may lead to an increased incidence of cancer. Administration of nonradioactive iodine saturates the organ, reduces any radiation concentration, and hence reduces the risk of thyroid cancer. Unit (single) dose tablets of the sodium iodine are taken orally, once per day. The risk from radioactive iodine lasts for a few weeks, during which you may be asked to distribute or administer the tablets (Figure 7-13; see Appendix A, Medications for the Tactical Environment).

In rare cases, you may treat a casualty with a localized and severe radiation exposure. This is likely to occur during the handling of gamma-emitting radioactive material. Here the damage is limited to a small portion of the body, and the injury area is well defined. The patient will suffer severe burns, manifest by an intense local burning sensation, and will develop weeping wounds within a few hours. These wounds are best covered with sterile dressings and attended by a physician trained in radiation injury care.

SUMMARY

Nuclear detonation energy is released as light and thermal energy, a shockwave and blast of wind, and direct radiation, then fallout. Injury can be associated with light injury to the eye and burns to the skin, blast (pressure) injury and injury associated with being hit by objects propelled by the wind or by being thrown by it, or radiation from the bomb ignition or, later on, by falling radioactive particles. These injury mechanisms often combine during nuclear detonation, providing an assessment and care challenge for you. Understanding the injury process associated with nuclear detonation helps you in anticipating, assessing, triaging, and caring for casualties.

Your role at a nuclear disaster or accident is very different from normal emergency care. In the disaster, triage shifts to placing many casualties into the expectant category because of limited resources and the massive damage caused by the nuclear detonation. Most casualties are burned though some may suffer pressure or blunt trauma. A few may have serious radiation exposure, will show few and limited signs, yet may die without intensive supportive care. Your role at the disaster is to provide search and rescue, triage, radioactivity monitoring, evacuation, decontamination, and limited emergency care.

In the accident, assessment and care are more conventional and probably guided by civilian or health physics personnel. Your role is to monitor radiation levels, and support evacuation and decontamination. Injuries and radiation exposure is limited, as is the extent of emergency care you provide.

FOR FURTHER READING

Textbook of Military Medicine (Part 1, Volume 2) Medical Consequences of Nuclear Warfare. Office of the Surgeon General, Washington, DC, 1990.

MEYER E: Chemistry of Hazardous Materials, 2nd ed. Prentice Hall, Englewood Cliffs, NJ, 1989.

Manual of Protective Action Guidelines and Protective Action for Nuclear Incidents: Environmental Protection Agency, Washington, DC, 1992.

CASARETT A: Radiation Biology: Prentice Hall, Englewood Cliffs, NJ, 1968.

GRACE C: Nuclear Weapons: Principles, Effects and Survivability, Brassey's Limited, London, UK, 1995.

CHRISTEN H, Maniscalco P: The EMS Incident Management System: EMS Operations for Mass Casualty and High Impact Incidents. Brady, Upper Saddle River, NJ, 1998.

AUF DER HEIDE E: Disaster Response: Principles of Preparation and Coordination. C. V. Mosby Company, St. Louis, MO, 1989.

8

TACTICAL EVACUATION

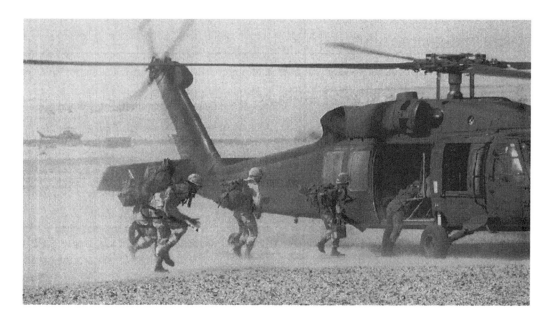

Helicopters are important tools in tactical operations.

OBJECTIVES

After reading this chapter, you will be able to:
1. Identify the general concepts and elements of tactical evacuation.
2. Evaluate the combat area to determine the best approach and techniques for casualty extraction, evacuation, or transport.
3. Explain the prioritizing of casualties and the preparation for their evacuation.

4. Describe the lifts and carries used to move combat casualties, and list the advantages and disadvantages of each.

5. Identify the various litter types, and demonstrate carries used for casualty evacuation.

6. Describe the types of ground, water, and air evacuation vehicles, their capacities for both casualties and en route care.

7. Discuss the process and considerations for requesting ground, water, or air casualty evacuation or transport.

8. Describe the setup of a proper helicopter landing zone for casualty evacuation.

CASE

Your detachment is deployed to a third-world country and assigned to search for hostile activity in a remote rural village. While marching to the village, small arms fire sounds from the front of your lines. Everyone heads for cover, draws their weapons, and waits for word on what is happening. A sergeant comes down the trail and directs you toward the firefight area. You both find cover behind a fallen tree and survey the combat zone.

The enemy fire comes from a ridge directed downward toward the lead elements of your detachment. Several soldiers are pinned down, and three appear to be wounded. The closest has a head wound and does not appear to be moving. You watch his chest with binoculars and note no motion. The second wounded combatant has a thigh wound with moderate hemorrhage. He is not moving, but is waving his hand from time to time, a prearranged signal that he's alive. You motion him to cover behind another fallen tree, and he drags himself there. The third casualty is about 40 meters away. Your current position does not permit you to determine what his injuries are. Enemy fire continues while personnel from the rear begin to move forward and flank the hostile force.

Your survey determines a route to the second casualty with limited exposure to enemy fire, and your sergeant directs you to the casualty while a few soldiers provide covering fire. There you quickly apply direct pressure to the thigh wound and maintain it with a bulky dressing, secured with the casualty's belt. The bleeding stops, and he seems, otherwise, all right. Closer to the third casualty, you can see a small amount of blood on the chest and some respiratory movement. The casualty is exposed to enemy fire though there is a ditch close by. You try to direct him to cover, but he does not respond. Again your sergeant coordinates covering fire while you crawl to the casualty and grab him by the collar and drag him a few meters to the ditch. There you assess and find him unresponsive with shallow respirations and a good pulse. You position his airway and dress his chest wound. His respirations do not improve noticeably.

With increasing friendly fire, the enemy retreats while pursued by some of your detatchment. You lift the casualty with the chest wound and transport him using a fireman's carry to the trail where you direct two litter bearers quickly to transport him to a predesignated landing zone. You quickly return to the head-injured soldier and find him unresponsive, pulseless, and apneic. With your advice, command requests helicopter evacuation for the other two live casualties, using the information associated with the standard evacuation request. You direct two other litter bearers to transport the thigh-injured casualty to the landing zone while you accompany the chest injury. The head-injured casualty is also moved to the "LZ" and will be evacuated when space is available.

At the designated landing zone, you set out four bright green panels to mark the zone and attach a cravat to a large pole to identify wind direction. When you hear the helicopter rotors, you have the radio operator identify the compass direction the sound comes from and the markings of the "LZ" using a secure radio channel. Under the direction of the flight crew, you load the casualties and give a brief patient report for each.

INTRODUCTION

Casualty evacuation from the battlefield or tactical engagement is a major responsibility of the medic and has significant impact on the mortality and morbidity of the casualty. It is also an activity that is guided by the danger associated with the operation, the seriousness of casualty injuries, the number and training of support personnel, available medical equipment and supplies, and the terrain. By carefully examining these elements of tactical evacuation, you can safely move the casualty with his or her best interest and the mission in mind.

There are several important elements of tactical evacuation. They include a general overview of evacuation considerations, stages of evacuation, principles of lifting and casualty movement, special evacuation concerns, requests for evacuation, and vehicle evacuation. These elements of tactical evacuation are discussed in the remaining pages of this chapter.

EVACUATION CONSIDERATIONS

One of your roles as a medic is to help maintain the fighting force by providing assessment, medical care, and evacuation during a conflict. You may be responsible for extracting casualties from the battlefield; evacuating casualties from the fire zone to a patient collection point; or arranging for and accomplishing evacuation from the patient collection point to an aid station, field or combat support hospital, by providing medical support services during casualty movement. This process is tactical evacuation.

The actual medical evacuation process consists of several steps that take the casualty from the time and point of injury to definitive care offered at the general hospital. Once injured, the casualty may either remain where he or she is until the battlefield is secured by friendly forces or be extracted to concealment or cover. After assessment and care, the casualty is evacuated from the fire zone to prearranged patient collection points or aid stations. From the aid stations, the casualty is then evacuated to a medical company clearing station and then evacuated further to a combat support hospital. Eventually, the casualty is evacuated outside the theater of operation. If during this process, the casualty becomes fit for service, he or she is immediately returned to duty.

Tactical evacuation is casualty movement with care provided by medically trained personnel. By contrast, transportation is casualty movement by persons without medical training and without the availability of medical care during movement. Though transportation is undesirable it may be necessary during conflict or mass casualty situations where the need for care outstrips the available personnel resources. Here it may be better to use trained medical personnel for triage and field stabilization and at patient collection points, field hospitals, and surgical hospitals.

Stages of Evacuation

Evacuation is a multiphase process that moves the casualty farther from the conflict and toward increasingly intense medical care until he or she can be stabilized and, ultimately, returned to the effective fighting force. The level of care necessary to return a casualty to the fighting force may be minor dressing and bandaging under safe cover or concealment on the battlefield, stabilization at a battalion aid station, surgical stabilization at a combat support hospital, or transport to a hospital very remote from the battlefield where intensive care and rehabilitation may take place.

As a medic, your role may be to direct a minor casualty to safe cover where you can dress superficial wounds and return him or her to the firefight. You might also direct your patient, as an ambulatory casualty, to an aid station or casualty collecting point. Or you might extract the seriously wounded casualty while under fire, provide emergent care, move him or her to cover where you provide more stabilization, and then arrange for litter transport to an aid station for further care. You might also establish a casualty collection point or helicopter landing zone, and arrange for transport to an aid station, field hospital, or surgical hospital for further, more definitive care.

In some circumstances, you might provide care in the ground ambulance, amphibious landing craft, or helicopter for numerous casualties during evacuation from a patient collection point or aid station to a field hospital or from the field hospital to hospital ship or air medical staging location. And lastly, you might provide care under the direction of a physician or physician's assistant of a medical treatment facility (aid station, field hospital, ship board medical facility, or hospital ship).

Evacuation Concepts and Elements

Two types of evacuation are associated with the tactical operation: tactical evacuation and theater evacuation. Tactical evacuation is really a continuum of movement from eminent danger of the battlefield to the safety of the rear echelon and a continuum of care from very limited stabilization while under fire to the sophisticated care of a field surgical hospital. Tactical field evacuation is further divided into to subcategories: evacuation under fire (battlefield **extraction**) and rearward evacuation. As a medic, you are responsible to determine the most appropriate field care and movement under the risk of the battlefield or combat zone environment.

Theater evacuation is a more elective and controlled casualty movement completely away from enemy threat and to the definitive level of assessment and care. When used in this context, the term *medical evacuation* (**medevac**) is usually reserved for theater evacuation. During this action, and usually under the direction of a physician, you may establish patient transfer points, move casualties to and from large transport vehicles, and provide for further, and ongoing, assessment and medical care. You may also assign the priority for evacuation and the mode to use, be it ground, air, or water.

The elements of tactical evacuation consist of identifying tactical risks, casualty evaluation, and assessment; determining priorities for care; selecting movement techniques; and arranging patient responsibility transfer. Evacuation also requires you to set the precedence for casualty transport and assure those with the most emergent need arrive at the next echelon of care first. And, in some cases, you will employ some tactical search and rescue operations.

Identify Tactical Risks

Modern warfare creates an exceptionally deadly battlefield. The advent of new highly accurate and lethal weapons such as long-range artillery, tank and antitank weapons, and air cover by rotor and fixed wing aircraft can make the intensity of injury extreme. Night vision, infrared, and computerized targeting equipment permit exceptional accuracy. And weapon design to increase its lethal nature leaves the modern battlefield a very dangerous place. The modern battlefield is also a dynamic place. With the aggressive nature of battle, the increasing range of weapons, the efficiency and speed of mechanized vehicles, and flexibility of air cover, the modern combat zone can quickly penetrate miles into enemy lines, lengthening supply and evacuation lines and leaving pockets of residual combatants. All these aspects of battle are compounded by the age-old environmental contributors such as extremes of temperature, humidity, wind, and visibility, and the variability of the terrain, foliage, and structures or debris. The result is a very dangerous and ever-changing area where you apply your skills.

Your first responsibility in the tactical environment is to survey the battlefield to identify the areas of greatest risk. Determine the source or sources of possible enemy fire or injury threat. Remember that all hazards are not small-arms fire. There may be land mines, booby traps, heavy machine guns, artillery, airborne weaponry, or chemical or biological dangers. Then assess the battleground. Look carefully for areas subject to enemy fire, areas with concealment by brush or other objects obscuring the sight of the enemy, and safe cover behind solid objects or terrain contour. Map these areas in your mind, and consider them as you plan egress to the casualty, any on-site assessment, and then extraction. Using your battleground assessment, evaluate the relative hostile fire risks of moving to and extracting the casualty from the fire ground (MET-T assessment: mission, enemy, terrain and time, Figure 8-1).

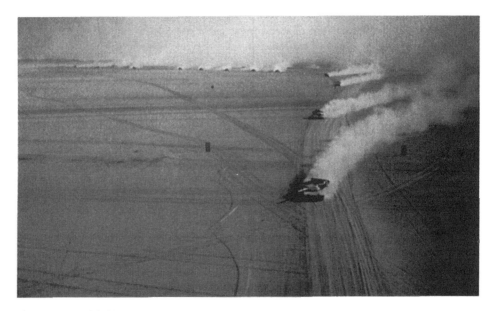

Figure 8-1 Battlefield assesment includes analyzing the mission, enemy, terrain and time.

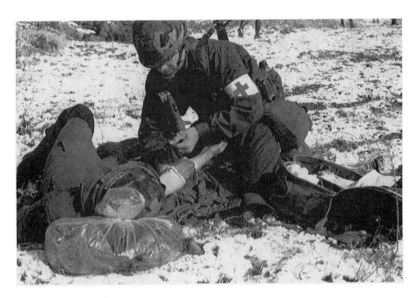

Figure 8-2 Assess the risks before attempting a rescue.

It is also necessary to evaluate the casualty's condition before considering extraction. If a soldier has sustained mortal wounds, do not endanger your life or others in moving the casualty until the battleground is secure. On the other hand, if the casualty can be instructed to self-extract from the battlefield, you can greatly reduce the hazards of rescue. Frequently, the risks of egress to or extraction of the casualty are too great for any action. However, if the casualty is seriously injured and in danger of taking more enemy fire, and you can rescue quickly with limited exposure, there might be merit to an attempt (Figure 8-2).

Chemical, biologic, and nuclear agents can also present tactical risks. If it is possible that these hazards exist, consult with command and assure the battleground is safe. If not, have the troops employ NBC protection, and observe these precautions during any rescue, assessment, and care. Remember, the NBC suit is awkward to work in, increases rescuer's fatigue, and may lead to dehydration and heat exhaustion. Be sure that you alert the rear echelons to the hazard and they consider establishing decontamination areas, clean zones, and patient collection points (see chapter 5, Care of Chemical Casualties, chapter 6, Care of Biologic Casualties, and chapter 7, Care of Nuclear Casualties).

Once remote from the danger of the battlefield, consider the hazards to evacuation vehicles such as water craft, helicopters, and ground vehicles. Their movement can draw enemy fire, so select patient collection points to minimize risk. Once outside the fire zone and at the field or combat support hospital, assessment and care carries very limited tactical risk.

Casualty Evaluation and Assessment

The tactical environment requires you to modify your approach to patient assessment. In evaluating the casualty who has fallen on the battlefield, *observe from safe cover and determine* as much about the nature of the injuries and the casualty's condition as you can from a distance. Observe the casualty carefully, possibly through binoculars or night vision goggles, and look for signs of injury and extensive hemorrhage. Look at the casualty's body position and watch carefully for signs of life and, especially, respiration. Normal respiration results in limited chest movement that may be visible only with careful observation. Count the respirations over a minute to determine the rate, and watch the mouth and nose for associated movement or air condensation with exhalation. You may also prearrange subtle signals to alert rescuers that the casualty is all right, such as having him or her blink or move a specific finger (on the side away from the enemy).

The danger from enemy fire limits the assessment you can make until you move the casualty to safe cover or he or she is remote from the battlefield. You may also risk discovery and enemy fire if you do not observe the appropriate light and noise discipline. Under these circumstances, limit the initial assessment you make at the casualty's side to a quick visual sweep to locate significant hemorrhage or other signs of severe injury. Once you move the casualty to cover or concealment, perform a more extensive evaluation for more signs and symptoms of injury while delaying a complete head-to-toe survey until the casualty is remote from the firefight.

Determine Priorities for Care

The priorities you establish for the tactical casualty's care are the same as for the civilian trauma patient. Determine the level of consciousness, assure the ABCs, and stabilize the spine if you suspect any injury. Check the patient's response to questioning and stimuli, and categorize them using the AVPU system. Quickly determine if the casualty is breathing, and assure that the airway is unobstructed. Watch chest excursion for symmetrical movement and an adequate volume of air moving with each breath. Check the pulse for a relative rate and strength and time capillary refill. Quickly view the entire body for signs of hemorrhage and significant injury. Remember that internal bleeding can account for blood loss as rapidly as external hemorrhage.

Care for any suspected airway problem with positioning, removal of fluids, or as needed, endotracheal intubation. If breathing is inadequate, ventilate the casualty with mouth to mask or bag-valve-mask ventilation. Realize that this commits one combat medic to this casualty during the entire evacuation and may not be justified or possible in an active firefight or multicasualty situation. If the pulse is rapid and weak, suspect shock and consider intravenous fluid administration. Stop any significant external hemorrhage with direct pressure and dressings. Any casualty with an uncorrected problem with the ABCs is a candidate for immediate care and urgent evacuation.

Once you assess the ABCs and find them to be stable, do a quick head-to-toe survey to locate any further injuries. Carefully examine any additional injuries, and determine the contribution they may make to shock and the stability of the ABCs. Consider any casualty you find with an injury that risks the airway, breathing, or contributes significantly to shock, including internal or external uncontrolled hemorrhage, as requiring immediate evacuation. Also consider any patient with penetrating trauma to the head, neck, chest, or abdomen as urgent. Less urgent but serious injuries include fracture of the femur or pelvis, or any casualty with a seriously altered level of consciousness.

Under tactical conditions, it may be essential to do what you can to return minor and, sometimes, serious casualties to the fight, at least until the tactical situation is stable and more elective evacuation is possible. Very minor injuries may require only quick bandaging and dressing to permit the casualty again to be a useful member of the fighting force. More seriously injured casualties may need hemorrhage control and temporary splinting but may still be able to carry a weapon and defend themselves on the battleground. Do what you can while the firefight rages to assure the fighting force. As the intensity of combat subsides, begin your in-depth assessment, care, and evacuation.

Movement Techniques

As a tactical medic, and in contrast to your civilian counterpart, you must use many different movement techniques to effect casualty extraction, then evacuation. Under danger of enemy fire, moves must be quick and expose you and the casualty to as limited fire as possible. Choose moves that will limit injury aggravation and ones you can provide alone or with another rescuer. Such moves might be the cloths, sling or neck drags, or the fireman's, pack-strap, or saddleback carries. These moves are effective in transporting the casualty short distances from danger to safe cover or concealment.

Once you stabilize the casualty and prepare him for transport from the battlefield, you can use more elective movement techniques. Here multipersonnel stretcher carries help expedite transport. However, terrain and debris may make some of the one-person carries more practical. Consider the two-, four-, and six-man stretcher carry, as well as the fireman's, supporting, arms, saddleback, and hand-seat carries. You may also find specialized stretchers techniques such as the stokes basket, long spine board, SKED, and others very useful (see Appendix E, Manual Carry and Lift Procedures, for further discussion of movement techniques).

Ongoing Assessment and Care

Another difference between civilian and military or tactical engagements is that you may be left with a casualty for a prolonged period. This necessitates a constant monitoring of the casualty's status through periodic ongoing assessments and continuing care. Use these serial assessments, in conjunction with the results of your initial and focused assessments, to determine if your casualty's condition is improving, deteriorating, or remaining the same. Ongoing assessments also may tell you quickly if interventions are helpful or if any change you notice in a casualty's signs or symptoms equates to a real change in his or her condition. The ongoing assessment results may then guide sustaining care while you await an opportunity to evacuate the wounded. To assure a continuing and current knowledge of the casualty's condition, employ frequent ongoing assessments.

Use ongoing evaluations quickly to examine the casualty's vital signs: blood pressure, pulse rate and strength, respiratory rate and volume, and level of consciousness, including orientation. Employ the ongoing assessment also to evaluate prior interventions like dressing application, splinting, spinal immobilization, hemorrhage control, and airway care. Check the pulses, temperature, capillary refill, and sensation distal to any of the casualty's bandaged wounds or splinted fractures. *Perform ongoing assessment every 5 minutes in the very seriously or critically wounded casualty.* Assess the stable casualty about every 15 minutes or so. Repeat ongoing assessment shortly after employing any significant intervention or noting any change in the patient's condition. Assess ambulatory patients less frequently, and consider pairing them with a buddy who watches for any signs of changing condition.

Use the results of the ongoing assessments to guide care and the casualty's need for supportive services. In civilian emergency care, the time spent with a patient is generally limited from a few minutes to up to an hour. In the tactical engagement, however, you may be at a casualty's side for many hours or days. Personal needs such as nutrition, hydration, maintenance of body temperature, and bladder and bowel function become very important (see chapter 9, Evacuation Care).

Casualty Responsibility Transfer

As the casualty moves from the battlefield through various evacuation stages to definitive care, the person responsible for medical care changes frequently. To assure a continuity of care, each provider in the process must clearly identify the results of the initial, focused, and detailed assessments, those of frequent ongoing assessments, and those of any significant intervention. This assurance of care continuity occurs with both the written documentation you complete and send with the casualty and in the verbal report you give as you pass care responsibilities on to the next provider. Include in your reports a complete narrative wound site description as well as the time of injury and interventions taken to care for the casualty.

Only record information gained during casualty field assessment after you move the casualty to safe cover and when your services are no longer needed by other casualties. Once you can focus your attention to a single or just a few casualties, begin more in-depth assessment, and record those results in written form. Be especially precise about vital signs, level of consciousness, and the description of signs and symptoms. Subsequent providers will use these factors to determine the patient's progress and guide their casualty care during the evacuation. It is also important that you carefully record casualty data because verbal communication may be limited because of the number of casualties received by the aid station or field hospital or because of the danger of conversation drawing enemy fire. If you must limit communication, relate only important assessment findings and vital signs outside the normal or expected range. The field medical card (FMC) is an expedient document that allows you to record brief notes about your assessment findings and casualty care (Figure 8-3).

Assure a smooth transition of patient care responsibilities. Do not surrender the care of a patient unless you are confident that the receiving personnel recognize the casualty's condition and are able to continue the necessary care. If they cannot provided this care, remain with your patient until they can.

Precedence

The tactical operation producing significant casualties may require both triaging for emergency care attention and determining **precedence** for evacuation. Although both categorize the casualty for their respective purposes, they differ in response to services available and the needs of the injured. Triage strictly identifies who needs medical care and in what order. Precedence identifies the priorities for transport. Some casualties will be easily stabilized medically at the scene, and their precedence for transport then becomes lower. Other casualties then become a higher precedence for transport. In essence, *the sorting of casualties for evacuation is precedence while the sorting for care is triage*.

In heavy combat or multi- or mass-casualty incidents, the resources for evacuation may outstrip the availability of medical vehicles and transport personnel. This situation necessitates a different approach to prioritizing for evacuation. Here casualties are sorted into four precedence categories: precedence I, urgent; precedence II, priority; precedence III, routine; and precedence IV, convenient. **Urgent casualties** are those that will probably deteriorate without significant intervention that can be offered quickly. These casualties need evacuation within 2 hours if survival is to be expected. Examples might be personnel with airway problems or serious hemorrhage. Urgent casualties are subdivided into a special category in need of surgery. These casualties are then directed to the surgical hospital. **Priority casualties** are those with serious injuries who need care but are not

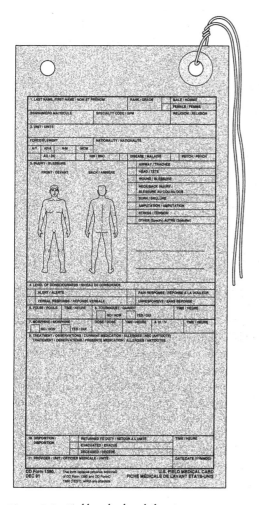

Figure 8-3a Field medical card (front).

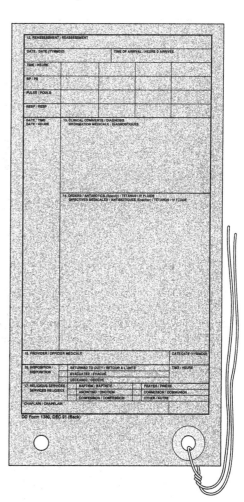

Figure 8-3b Field medical card (back).

likely to deteriorate within the next 4 hours. Such casualties might be those with lower extremity fractures or abdominal wounds without serious hemorrhage. **Routine casualties** are those personnel that are not likely to deteriorate within the next 24 hours. Examples of this category might include upper extremity fractures, minor soft tissue injuries, or limited burns. **Convenient casualties** are those casualties that have minor problems. This category also includes casualties who are dead, have sustained mortal wounds, or serious and life-threatening injury that cannot be corrected without an unreasonable commitment of resources and personnel. If you provide evacuation space to these casualties, other casualties may die or be seriously disabled because of delayed evacuation.

Tactical Search and Rescue

One of the greatest challenges to emergency tactical care is that a soldier may be injured without the knowledge of his or her platoon. The soldier may remain unaccounted for until the engagement is over or the battlefield is well defined. Then the obligation of the medical contingent is to seek out and locate the casualty. Work with and under the direction of unit leaders to determine if any personnel are missing, and then coordinate a search. This process can be both difficult and dangerous. Any search first assures that areas behind the fire zone are surveyed. Then accomplish a search of areas visible from cover and concealment. After the fire-ground is secure, complete a search for possible casualties there.

STAGES OF EVACUATION

There are three stages of evacuation, each being farther removed from danger and involving greater consideration for the casualty's injuries and condition. You will likely participate in tactical extraction, rearward evacuation, and vehicle evacuation via ground ambulance, helicopter, boat, or ship. Let us examine these evacuation stages and the role the you may play during each.

Tactical Extraction

Extraction refers to moving the casualty from the engagement area to safe cover where you can fully assess him or her, give immediate care, and prepare him or her for movement to a patient collection point or an aid station. You must provide extraction with the utmost of care and with the approval and direction of the unit command. In some cases, it may be necessary for you to leave the wounded soldier until it is safe to remove him or her, the mission is accomplished, or the engagement is better controlled by friendly forces.

Your decision to perform battlefield extraction must weigh the risks to personnel against the benefits of moving the casualty. First, assure the casualty is alive and his or her wounds are not such that you will place him or her in the expectant triage category. To risk further casualties in the rescue of a mortally wounded soldier is counterproductive. If the casualty is conscious and ambulatory, direct him or her in self-extraction, describing the way to concealment or safe cover. Otherwise, evaluate the possible injury resulting from your rapid extraction and the dangers of drawing enemy fire by your movement in and out of the fire zone. Also identify the danger caused by lack of care or enemy fire if you do not extract him or her. Finally, determine the distance, terrain, casualty weight, and other dangers caused by the extraction. If the benefits outweigh the risks, consider battlefield extraction.

Once the decision is made to extract the casualty from enemy fire, assess the terrain to identify routes of evacuation that provide some cover and limited obstacles to casualty movement. Coordinate the move with command and obtain supporting fire, smoke to conceal your actions, or other distraction to reduce the risk of effective enemy fire. Approximate the casualty's weight and your ability to move him or her. Also consider the distance to be traversed, the exposure to enemy fire, and the nature of the casualty's injuries. Then select a movement technique. Battlefield extraction, when under the danger of enemy fire, must be effected quickly.

If the risk of direct fire is high, use the low-crawl techniques to approach the casualty. Otherwise the high crawl is faster. Use whatever cover and concealment is available to protect yourself as you approach the casualty. If the casualty is not protected by effective cover, direct him or her to move toward cover by motioning, whispering, or using hand signals. If this is not possible, approach the casualty keeping a low profile and keeping the casualty between you and the enemy to cover your movements.

At this point, direct your assessment toward detecting life-threatening hemorrhage. Control only spurting or rapidly flowing blood loss. Use whatever technique is most expedient, be it direct pressure, pressure dressing, or tourniquet. Once you control bleeding, rapidly extract the casualty using the cloths, sling or neck drag, or rapid carry. Attempt to drag the casualty along the body's axis, head first.

Rearward Evacuation

Once you move the casualty to a point safe from enemy fire, your approach to assessment, care, and movement changes drastically. Your assessment is more detailed, and care focuses on stabilization in preparation for further movement. Assure that airway and breathing are secure and adequate. Quickly survey for any serious hemorrhage and use direct pressure, assumed by dressings and bandages, to control any further blood loss. Determine the casualty's level of consciousness-alert, responsive to verbal or painful stimuli, or unconscious (AVPU).

Prepare the casualty for transport. Splint any serious long-bone fractures with board or improvised splints, or by securing the affected limb to the body (Figure 8-4). If spine injury is possible, maintain manual stabilization, apply a cervical collar, and immobilize the casualty to a long spine board by securing the torso, then the head, then the legs, to the board. When packaging your casualty for movement, remember that evacuation may be prolonged and over less-than-ideal terrain, a rough and jostling experience. *Secure the casualty well to prevent any injury aggravation during transport.*

If the terrain is unsuitable for normal stretcher movement, such as a battlefield strewn with debris, dense forest, or rugged and rocky terrain, consider one-person or assisted-movement techniques. Two- and four-man stretcher carries may be too awkward and risk further casualty and rescuer injury. Direct the move to a staging point where you can then move to more normal stretcher carries or vehicle transport. Then move the casualty to a patient collection point (Figure 8-5). This location is prearranged by your operation plan, or you may designate it based on casualty numbers, their needs, and vehicle transport resources. Choose a patient collection point that you can associate

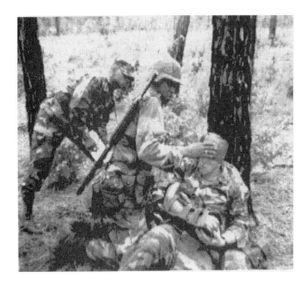

Figure 8-4 Preparing the casualty for evacuation.

with geographic landmarks, where ground or air vehicles can access it easily, and as close to the injured casualties as the terrain and hostile fire allows. Generally, you will locate patient collection points as close to the fire zone as vehicles can access without placing them in danger from enemy mortar or small-arms fire.

Depending on the circumstances, you may move the casualty from the fire zone to a patient collection point yourself, assign others to do it, or request help from the ambulance squads. Make such decisions, considering the potential need for your services during the continuing combat, the personnel resources available, and the time it might take for more rearward services to reach your location.

If the distance to the patient collection point or aid station is more than 30 minutes, plan for ongoing assessments, and if evacuation exceeds 2 hours, plan for interim care during the move. Again, these decisions and assessment and care offerings depend on the personnel, equipment, and supply resources available and the distances and terrain encountered.

Vehicular Evacuation

Vehicular evacuation is similar to rearward evacuation in that the casualty is immobilized to a movement device, and care during the move is minimized. However, care and assessment is further limited because access to the casualty is generally available from only one side, and there are often multiple casualties for each medic. *When you anticipate vehicle evacuation, assess and stabilize the casualty very well before the move and preplanning for ongoing care en route.* This is essential to simplify care en route and improve casualty mortality and morbidity (see chapter 9, Evacuation Care, for medical care activities provided during evacuation).

As you prepare and load the casualty into the vehicle, assure that there is documentation defining what field and vehicle-side assessment found as well as any care

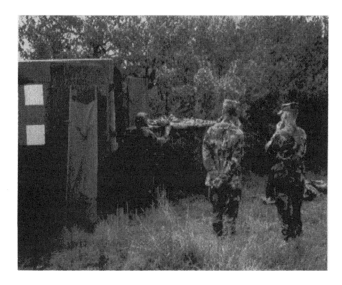

Figure 8-5 Casualties are loaded onto an ambulance at a casualty collection point.

given. Assure that documentation details the effects of any intervention as well as the trending of the patient's condition based on the results of ongoing assessments.

PRINCIPLES OF LIFTING AND CASUALTY MOVEMENT

Lifting and moving patients can subject you to potential disabling injury, especially during conflict. It is important to maintain yourself in good physical condition and use proper lifting techniques to reduce the risk of injury. Keep your feet about 8-12" apart both as you lift and walk with a patient. A narrow stance permits an easier loss of balance and greater possibility of a fall. *Lift with your major body muscles and not your back.* Use your legs, arms, and shoulders to do all the lifting. Keep your back straight and in the direction of the lift at all times. Do not twist your body before, during, or after the lift. This motion may subject some muscles to extreme strain. Grip any stretcher with the hands about 12-18" apart with the fingers gripping around the entire surface of the stretcher pole. If you or bearers are carrying a stretcher for a long distance and supporting just one side, change sides frequently. Try to match bearer height so that similar bearers are together or taller ones carry on the low side or end of the stretcher when on uneven ground (Figure 8-6).

Select lifting and carrying techniques to accommodate the ground to be covered. **Drags** generally keep the center of gravity of both you and the casualty close to the ground, making them very stable and unlikely to endanger your control or balance. Drags also require you to pull the casualty along the ground. This minimizes exposure to enemy fire. However, with uneven terrain, this may expose the casualty to further injury. When using drags, always move the casualty in the direction of the long axis of the body and head first. This approach aligns the limbs and minimizes any further injury body movement may cause during the drag.

Carries move the center of gravity of both you and the casualty higher than drags, and though they allow quick transport over an area, they predispose you to stumbling and falls. Carries also expose more of you and the casualty to enemy fire than drags. They may be a better choice for rearward evacuation over uneven terrain or very quick extractions. If personnel resources are adequate, stretchers or specialized equipment like the SKED may be the best selection for patient movement, especially for distances more than a few hundred meters. Using these multiple rescuer carries to accomplish patient movement makes the moves safer and more rapid (see Appendix E, Manual Carry and Lift Procedures).

When you employ a lift or carry that uses more than one rescuer, carefully explain to the rescuers what is about to happen and the cadence you will use to begin the move. The coordination of the move is essential to assure the patient is shifted as little as possible and that rescuers move together to limit the possibility of their injury or a fall. The rescuer at the casualty's head is a likely choice for coordinating the move since he or she can see the entire casualty and can watch the alignment of the nose, sternum, navel, and toes during the move. This careful observation assures a smooth and proper positioning, lift or carry.

Casualty Positioning

Frequently, you encounter a casualty that is not in position for assessment or application of movement techniques. Assess the exposed body area first, then gently move or roll the casualty to the full supine or prone position. In preparation for the roll, move the casualty's arm on the roll side, over his or her head. This provides the least displacement as the body turns on its side. Align the limbs with the arms to the body and the legs straight and together. Secure them as needed to expedite the move.

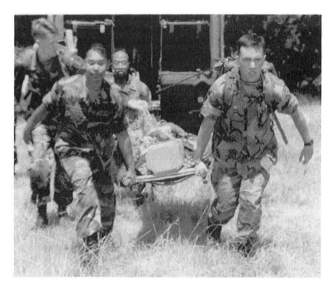

Figure 8-6 Four-man stretcher carry.

Lifts

Lifts are techniques that move casualties to a position where you can place them on a movement device or position them for a carry. Single-person lifts generally use body mechanics of both the casualty and rescuer to bring the casualty up to a position where the rescuer can get under and then carry the casualty. Multiperson lifts are generally designed to lift the casualty vertically enough to permit the insertion of a long spine board or litter or the casualty's movement to an awaiting stretcher. They are elective and offer very limited manipulation of the casualty (see Appendix E, Manual Lift and Carry Procedures). Casualty lifts generally accomplish one of two resulting positions: horizontal or vertical.

Lifts that bring the casualty to a vertical position generally use body mechanics and momentum to move the patient. When the casualty is prone, you approach from the head, squatting and placing your arms under the casualty's arms and around his or her back. You then move toward the casualty, shift to a full standing position, and lift the casualty to his or her knees. Then lift the casualty to his or her feet and draw him or her to the standing position, face to face. An alternative technique positions you straddling the casualty and reaching around his or her chest from the behind. You pull the casualty to his or her knees by lifting and moving backward. Then lock your arms around the casualty's chest, lift him or her toward the standing position and move backward a few feet, then move slightly forward. This locks the casualty's feet straight and in the standing position.

Consider lifts that position the casualty horizontally to place a stretcher, spine board, or other device under him or her. Horizontal lifts use two or three rescuers with their hands placed under the casualty. They then lift the casualty 4-6" as you place the stretcher or spine board beneath him or her. You can also use this lift to shift the casualty to an awaiting movement device. As with all multirescuer techniques, coordination is critical.

Drags

Drags involve moving a casualty along the ground without lifting him or her. However, this unprotected movement exposes the casualty to some risk of further injury aggravation. These moves do keep the casualty's weight close to the ground, limiting the chances of a trip or fall, and reduce exposure to enemy fire. Drags generally try to move the casualty along his or her long axis, by the head, neck, and shoulders, which helps keep the body in-line and reduces some of the risk of further injury.

Common drags include the cradle drop, sling, and neck drag. The cradle drop drag uses the fabric of the casualty's shirt as a harness to distribute the drag forces over the shoulder girdle and uses the rescuer's forearms to support and passively immobilize the head and neck. It keeps both the casualty and rescuer low but is difficult to accomplish with a heavy casualty, over rough terrain, or up an incline. You can effect this drag by either crouching low while dragging the casualty or moving backward while on your knees. The sling drag uses a short length of large diameter rope, twin pistol belts buckled together, or fabric, slung across the casualty's chest, under his or her arms, and then behind the head and neck to distribute the drag's force to the shoulder girdle. Using this technique, you can maintain a better grasp on the casualty and keep his or her body closer to the ground. You may also drag the casualty by passing the free loop through your head and shoulder, pulling him or her as you crawl toward safe cover. Use caution here because the casualty's head and neck are unsupported. Like the cloths drag, it may be difficult to execute this technique over rough ground or up an incline.

The neck drag ties the supine casualty's hands and slips your neck between the casualty's arms. You then crawl forward pulling the casualty by the arms. The casualty's head and neck are unsupported, and the associated motion may further aggravate any head, neck, or spine injury. This technique is very stable and gives you good control and mechanical advantage over the casualty during the drag (see Appendix E, Manual Carry and Lift Procedures).

Carries

Carries are designed for more rapid casualty movement than drags, and shift the casualty's weight higher above the ground. This permits you to move quickly over debris; however, it makes you more prone to stumbling and falls. Carries also expose you and the casualty to greater enemy fire. Hence limit their choice as a movement technique to quick moves under fire or when you are remote from the danger of enemy fire.

The carries you use most commonly for casualty movement are the saddleback, fireman's, and pack-strap carries. Each has advantages and disadvantages for your field use. The saddleback carry requires a semicooperative patient who is able to hold on to your shoulders and neck during the transport. You grasp the casualty's legs just above the knees as he or she straddles your back. This supports the casualty's weight on your lower back and hip. It is a quick and effective movement technique. The fireman's and pack-strap carries do not require a conscious casualty, and both permit quick movement with one of your hands relatively free to help with balance and casualty control. The fireman's carry places the casualty's torso across your shoulders while you hold his or her wrist with a hand coming behind and around his or her knee. The pack-strap carry supports the casualty by extending his or her arms over your shoulders while you pull the arms downward. This lifts the casualty's body as you bend at the waist. Although this lift keeps the casualty's weight lower than the fireman's carry, it is still somewhat unstable.

Two-rescuer moves, like the fore and aft, seat, and assisted carry, give greater stability than the one-rescuer carries. The fore and aft carry positions one rescuer at the head and another at the feet of the supine casualty. The rescuer at the head reaches around the casualty's chest from behind and under his or her arms, locks the hands, and lifts. The second rescuer stands between the casualty's feet, facing the same direction as the first rescuer, and grasps the legs just above the knees, and lifts. This provides very stable movement down a narrow trail or hallway. The seat carry places one rescuer on each side of the supine casualty. You bend the casualty's knees, and elevate his or her head and chest to a seated position. Then you and another lock one set of hands under the buttocks and one set behind the midback, and then lift the casualty until you and the other rescuer are standing. This technique is acceptable for short distances, but since you are walking sideways, you may stumble easily and fatigue quickly. The assisted carry is for a semiambulatory casualty who can walk with some assistance. It places the upright casualty's arms over your and another rescuer's shoulders. With your outside hand, you can hold the casualty's wrist and help assume some of the casualty's weight on your shoulders. You also place your inside hand on the casualty's back to help stabilize his or her walk.

Stretcher Carries

Stretcher carries require at least two bearers placed at the head and foot. More bearers are required when the casualty is large, when you will be traversing uneven or debris-strewn ground, or when traveling long distances. Then place bearers at the four corners or front, back, and each side of the stretcher. You can overcome obstacles by moving bearers ahead of the moving litter and lifting or lowering the casualty in anticipation of the obstruction. Here keep the casualty as level as possible during the move and the exchange of litter bearers. Stretcher transport is a good method for moving casualties long distances. However, frequent rest stops and calling for bearers to switch from side to side and end to end reduces fatigue (see Appendix E, Manual Lift and Carry Procedures and Figure 8-7).

Some specialized stretchers include the KED, long spine board, SKED, and stoke's basket. The KED is a semirigid short spine board designed to immobilize the cervical spine by affixing the head, shoulders, and pelvis to the device. It helps move the spine-injured casualty from a seated position to supine where you can then immobilize him or her to the long spine board. The long spine board is a full-length rigid board that provides definitive spinal immobilization when you use it with strapping and a cervical immobilization device (to assist with the immobilization of the head). The SKED is a flexible (usually plastic) semirigid stretcher that wraps the casualty for both immobilization and evacuation. The stokes basket is a wire or plastic basket shaped to accommodate and protect the casualty during evacuation. These devices can be very helpful in assisting you to evacuate casualties from areas where the terrain does not permit easy use of the stretcher or other carries.

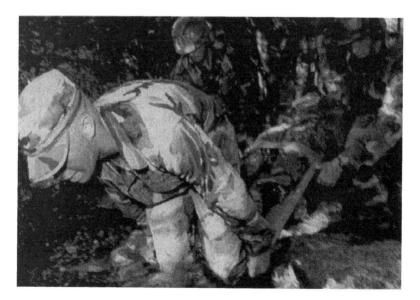

Figure 8-7 Two-man stretcher carry.

SPECIAL EVACUATION CONCERNS

Several special concerns are associated with the tactical environment. These include the casualty's equipment, prisoners of war, and the NBC environment.

Casualty's Equipment

Observe special considerations when handling a combat casualty's equipment. Return any weapons and munitions to the casualty's unit so that they can be re-utilized by the fighting force. This also limits the chance of injuries associated with accidental weapon discharge. Transport clothing, personal effects, and any specialized gear, such as NBC suit, dosimeter, Mark I kits, or other personal protective equipment, with the casualty. These materials pose no risk to care providers and will likely be lost if separated from the casualty.

Prisoners of War

If you are called upon to treat prisoners of war or other detained or arrested personnel, ensure that they are unarmed and do not pose a threat to you or injured personnel. Search them thoroughly and remove all weapons and potential weapons, and assure that there are enough armed personnel to prevent their escape. Keep all personal materials with prisoners, and be watchful for any potential intelligence or criminal evidence, such as maps, rank, unit designations, or contraband. Report such information to the unit commander.

NBC Environment

The nuclear, biologic, or chemical weapon environment creates some obstacles to, and special considerations for, evacuation. Personnel attempting to effect rescue or litter transport of a casualty out of the contaminated area are under increased stress while working in the NBC suit. Moderate their actions with frequent rest periods, and provide adequate hydration, especially in a warm environment.

The NBC environment also dramatically influences how you use medical transport vehicles. The danger of cross contamination restricts vehicles from crossing from the contaminated zone to the clean zone. This reduces the flexibility of movement resources and the transportation choices available to you. It is important to balance the resources between the two zones with a probable error on the side of keeping vehicles on the clean side. Keep any already contaminated vehicles on the contaminated side, and consider using nontraditional resources (tactical vehicles or commercial trucks) in the hot zone. Ground vehicles are best for contaminated zone use because they do not generate as much dust, debris, and contamination as a helicopter. Helicopters are also much more difficult to decontaminate. Do not use them near the transitional area from the contaminated zone to the clean zone since their rotor wash will spread contamination. Use ground vehicles to shuttle casualties to and from landing zones, placed remotely to the decontamination area. During the operation, perform frequent, though superficial, vehicle and personnel decontaminations to limit care provider and casualty cross contamination (Figure 8-8).

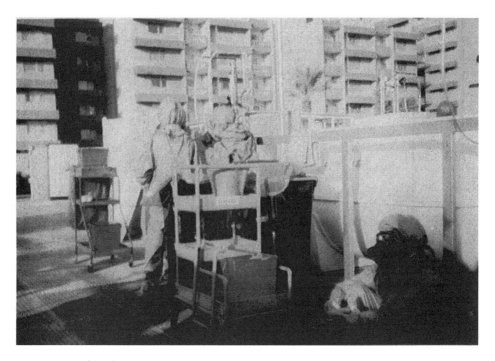

Figure 8-8 Perform frequent personnel and equipment decontaminations to prevent cross-contamination.

REQUESTS FOR EVACUATION

Evacuation from the tactical operation is an important and resource-consuming task. To assure you accomplish it efficiently and in a coordinated fashion, use the preestablished evacuation request process. The military standard request process uses nine items to describe your location and needs for evacuation services.

You will likely request evacuation via radio during both the wartime and peacetime operation. The major difference is that any radio request for wartime evacuation carries the hazard of giving the enemy intelligence and drawing hostile fire or forces. Hence *it is important to modify wartime evacuation requests to assure secrecy and security.* During wartime, your will encrypt your evacuation requests and use secure radio channels when possible (Figure 8-9).

The operations order for the engagement includes an evacuation plan and several important details relating to the evacuation process. It designates the radio channels to use when requesting evacuation, recommends evacuation routes, and may predesignate patient collection points. The plan may also identify available means of transport.

During the engagement, the unit commander makes requests for evacuation based on your advice. This advice must take into account the casualty's condition, his or her triage priority, and the tactical situation. Additionally, you must have the casualty ready for evacuation and identify any needs for replacement supplies. To assure that the request

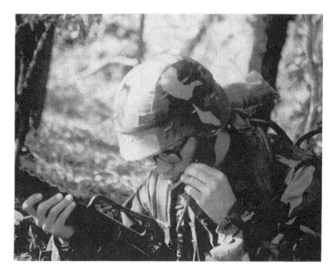

Figure 8-9 Using the radio to request evacuation.

contains all the necessary information, it is provided in a standard, nine-line format. This format varies only slightly between wartime and peacetime operations (see Table 8-1).

In the tactical engagement, assure the message is sent via secure means or is encrypted. Each item number remains in clear text. Allow no more than 20-25 seconds of message transmission time using clear, slow speech. Use the military phonetic alphabet to assure complete communication of the information. In cases where time is important, transmit the first five items initially, and then transmit the remaining information as soon as it is available. Assure the request is confirmed by the receiver.

VEHICLE EVACUATION

Evacuation may take place via ground, ship, or air. Each presents some advantages and obstacles to assessment and care and special considerations for evacuation.

Ground Evacuation

Ground evacuation is normally conducted using stretchers to move casualties from the fire zone to prearranged patient collecting points or aid stations. There the casualties, if not rendered fit to return to duty, are moved via ambulance to a medical treatment facility. From there, casualties are transported by ambulance, or other vehicle, out of the theater of operation, usually back to the continental United States.

The military ambulance is frequently staffed with two medics (one drives) and carries supplies and equipment to provide care and restock (backhaul) field medics as they expend their patient care supplies and equipment. When the vehicles are located close to the fire zone, pay special attention to using concealment and safe cover when possible, and cover the vehicle when it is stationary near or in the fire zone. However, covering the ambulance's red and white crosses will lose any protection they receive under the Geneva Conventions.

TABLE 8-1

9-LINE MEDEVAC REQUEST

Line 1   Location of Casualty Pickup

The location of the patient pickup site is given in grid coordinates from the operations map and is encrypted during a hostile engagement.

Line 2   Radio Frequency and Call Sign

The radio frequency and the call sign of the entity requesting the evacuation are identified and, in wartime, encrypted. A call sign suffix may be used to specify the individual requesting the evacuation.

Line 3   Evacuation Precedence

Item three identifies the number, then the evacuation precedence of the casualties. The letter A stands for urgent, B for urgent/surgical, C for priority, D for routine, and E for convenience. Each letter is preceded by the number of casualties in the category. If there are more than two precedence categories of casualties, they are separated by stating "break" between them. In combat, encryption is required.

Line 4   Special Equipment Requests

Item four requests special equipment for evacuation or patient care, either encrypted when security is needed or identified narratively during peacetime. A identifies none, B identifies hoist, C requests extraction equipment, and D requests a ventilator.

Line 5   Number of Litter and Ambulatory Casualties

This item defines the number of casualties in each of the litter and ambulatory categories for the purpose of transport, delineated as L 2 and A 4, or similar configuration. This information helps determine the number of vehicles needed for evacuation.

Line 6   Evacuation Site Security

Item six of the evacuation request identifies the level of hostile threat at the designated evacuation site. The absence of enemy is designated N; possible enemy, P; enemy in the area, E; and the need for armed escort , X. In peacetime, where there is no danger from unfriendly forces, use this item to narratively describe the nature of the casualty's wounds or illnesses.

Line 7   Designation of Evacuation Site

Item seven identifies the marking you use to designate the patient transfer point, usually a landing zone. Designate colored panels, A; pyrotechnic devices, B; smoke, C; no designation, D; or other designation, E. Do not transmit the color of panels or smoke until the evacuation vehicle is en route.

Line 8   Casualty Nationality and Combat Status

Item eight lists the casualties nationality and status: U.S. military (A), U.S. civilian (B), non-U.S. military (C), non-U.S. civilian (D), or enemy prisoner of war (E).

Line 9   NBC/Terrain Specifics

Use item nine, in wartime, to denote either nuclear (N), biologic (B), or chemical (C) threat. In peacetime, narratively denote any terrain specifics regarding the patient exchange point or landing zone, such as flat, sloped, or wooded. You may also use this item to identify the landing zone's relationship to local landmarks and prominent terrain features.

Three major types of ground ambulances are used in the tactical theater: the M-113, the HMMWV ("humvee"; Figure 8-10), and the more conventional ambulances. The **HMMWV** also can be configured as an ambulance and is the mainstay for tactical evacuation from patient collection points and aid stations to field hospitals. It has a wide wheel base, four-wheel drive, and high ground clearance to allow it very good off-road performance that you frequently need in the tactical environment. The low-profile version (M996) accommodates two stretcher patients, whereas the higher-profile vehicle (M997) can handle four stretcher patients. Transport from and between medical treatment facilities is accomplished by HMMWVs or older, more obsolete ambulances such as the M1010 (Figure 8-12). The **M-113** armored and tracked vehicle (when configured for casualty transport) carries 4 stretcher or 10 ambulatory patients, one medic, a driver, and the necessary medical supplies and equipment.

When using the M-113 and HMMWV, load the least serious casualties first so as to unload the most serious first. The loading order is upper right, lower right, upper left, and lower left with unloading following the reverse order. Place casualties with chest and abdominal wounds and IV fluids running in the lower berths. This will assist you in providing care during transit and permit enough elevation to accommodate IV fluid flow. The M-113 requires four personnel (Figure 8-11) for proper loading, and the HMMWV requires three.

Amphibious Evacuation

Amphibious evacuation will likely use landing craft specifically designed to drop off and pick up troops in shallow water. Their discharge gates drop into the water and provide ramps to facilitate loading and offloading (Figure 8-13). Surf, tides, currents, and variable water depths can make vehicle loading hazardous, especially under the threat of enemy

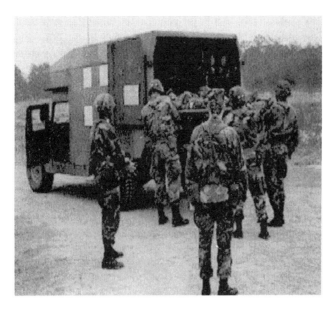

Figure 8-10 HMMWV or "humvee".

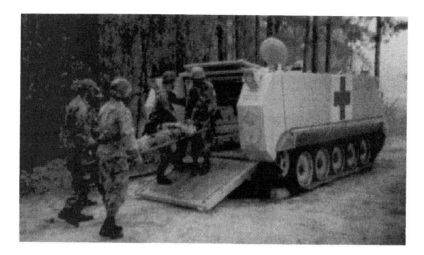

Figure 8-11 M113.

fire. In cold climates, the water temperature may rapidly draw heat from the litter bearers, limit their lower leg sensitivity and make casualty movement awkward. It may also expose you, the litter bearers, and your casualties to hypothermia.

Most large naval support and amphibious assault vessels have significant medical capacity. They can accept landing craft and airlift casualties, and are at least the equivalent of a field or surgical hospital. Naval hospital ships are the equivalent of general hospitals with a significant capacity for accepting and treating very large numbers of casualties.

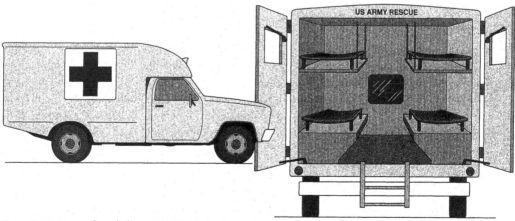

Figure 8-12 Box-style ambulance (M886, M1010).

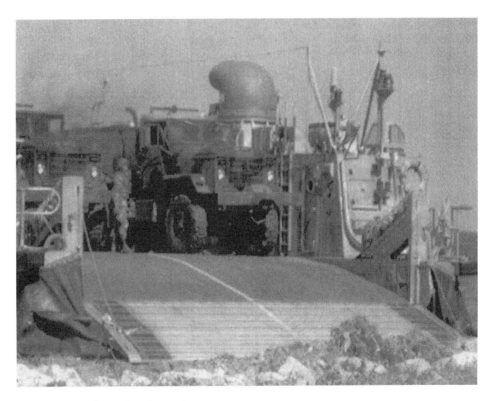

Figure 8-13 Landing craft with ramp down.

Helicopter Evacuation

The helicopter has revolutionized the care and transportation of field casualties since the Korean conflict. The ability of this specialized vehicle to land in otherwise inaccessible areas and to move a patient rapidly from the front line to a field hospital reduces the time from injury to definitive care to a minimum. The helicopter flies in a straight line, above normal obstacles and at speeds well above those of ground vehicles. In trauma, where rapid access to the surgical repair of penetrating injury is essential, the helicopter brings the patient and definitive care together very quickly.

The primary mission of the medical evacuation (medevac) helicopter is to move urgent casualties needing operative intervention to a surgical hospital and then other urgent casualties to the field or surgical hospital. They are also able to move medical personnel and equipment into, and in some circumstances, may move casualties from, otherwise remote and inaccessible points about the combat zone. Finally, they provide air crash rescue services and rescue downed air crews.

Medical evacuation uses two primary helicopters: the **U-60 Blackhawk** and **UH-1 Iroquois** (better known as the "Huey"). The Blackhawk transports from four to six litter patients or up to seven ambulatory casualties, and can be loaded from either side. When the hoist is in place, the Blackhawk's litter capacity shrinks to three or four casualties

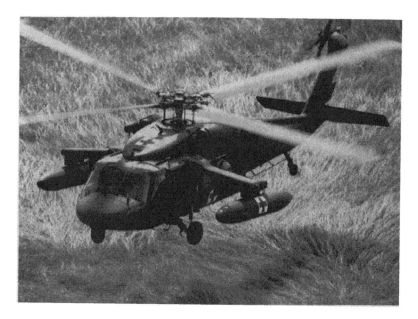

Figure 8-14 UH-60 Blackhawk.

(Figure 8-14). The Iroquois accommodates three to six litter patients or up to nine ambulatory casualties with half of the patients loaded from each side (Figure 8-15).

Evacuation by helicopter places three responsibilities upon you, as the medic: establish a landing zone, prepare the casualty for transport, and under the direction of the flight crew, assist with loading the helicopter.

Establishing a Landing Zone

When selecting a location for a landing zone, choose an area protected or remote from enemy fire and with a relatively flat, firm surface area clear of loose brush, debris, and overhead hazards (Figure 8-16). Nonlevel landing areas risk an unstable helicopter once on the ground, and the rotors may be dangerously close to the ground on the high side of the landing zone. Most military field evacuation helicopters require a landing zone of at least 100 feet (30 meters) in diameter.

Assure the pilot can easily identify the landing zone. If there is any question, mark the four corners with colored panels, staked firmly into the ground. At night, place flashlights or other nonflammable illumination at the four corners of the landing zone. Be careful not to shine any bright lights toward the pilot during landings or takeoffs since this reduces the pilot's night vision. Designate the wind direction by placing a small wind sock or light fabric on a tall stick. Smoke also designates wind direction well as long as it does not obscure the landing zone or any obstacles. Otherwise, stand with your back to the wind and arms extended forward to designate wind direction. Coordinate the aspects of the landing zone with the pilot by radio before he or she approaches.

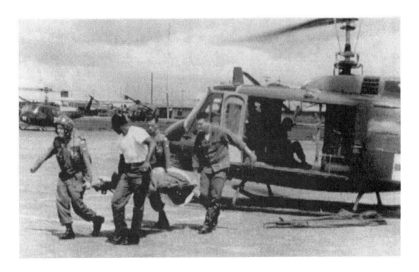

Figure 8-15 UH-1 Iriquois "Huey."

If the landing zone is not easily distinguishable, tell the pilot when you hear the rotors and from which compass direction the sound comes from. Also consider using colored smoke to more clearly identify the landing zone. In all operations where there is a chance of enemy fire, keep the landing zone as inconspicuous as possible while still making it visible from the helicopter.

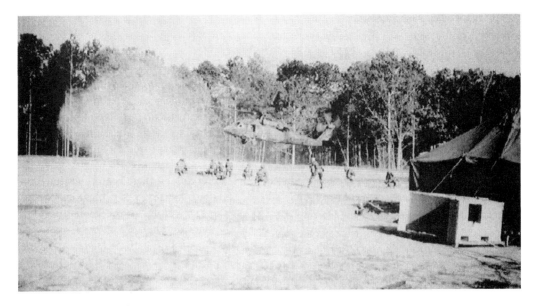

Figure 8-16 Typical landing zone.

Medevac helicopters generally land and take off into the wind. If you notice any fixed and unremovable obstacles to flight into and out of a landing zone, mark them clearly and alert the flight crew by radio before their approach. Position casualties perpendicular to the wind and at a good distance from the designated helicopter landing zone. This assures they are not adversely effected by the rotor wash and gives you rapid access to the landed helicopters for loading and unloading.

Casualty Preparation for Air Medevac

In preparing your patient for air medical transport, remember that *in-flight care is limited, and noise and vibration preclude some diagnostic evaluations.* Assure the patient's airway and consider endotracheal intubation if the patient is unable to control his or her own airway. Helicopter travel may induce nausea and vomiting in some patients because of the unusual aircraft movements. Be especially careful to establish a good airway and assure it can be cleared of emesis quickly should the casualty vomit. Make sure to tape all IV catheters securely in place and secure the administration set firmly to the catheter and solution bag. Recheck all bandaging and splinting, and take a final set of vital signs just before loading the patient into the helicopter. If the patient is in danger of moving deeper into shock, consider administering a bolus of 500 to 1000 ml of normal saline before the flight.

Air evacuation also moves the casualty to a higher elevation and reduces the atmospheric pressure. This reduces the pressure pushing oxygen into the hemoglobin and reduces the efficiency of respiration. This is of greatest concern for the patient that is seriously injured. Here this reduced efficiency may be all it takes to turn dyspnea into hypoxia, or compensated shock into decompensated shock. Hence, it is important to assure good casualty oxygenation and monitor serious casualties carefully with pulse oximetry during flight. Be prepared to administer high-flow oxygen and, possibly, ventilate the casualty by bag-valve-mask or ventilator.

Altitude also affects air-inflated devices (air splint, PASG, or blood pressure cuffs) or air-related injuries (pneumothorax or air embolism). As the helicopter or aircraft rises, the air pressure decreases, and vise versa as the craft descends. Air-filled devices like the air splint, PASG, and a BP cuff used as a tourniquet will increase pressure with increasing altitude. On descent, they will lose pressure. Some injuries also undergo pressure changes with the changing altitude. Alert the flight medical crew if any casualty has or is suspected of having one of these conditions.

Approaching the Helicopter

As the helicopter lands, crouch down and watch the flight crew for signals while protecting your eyes. The prop wash will lift debris and blow it forcibly outward from the rotor area. If the rotors remain turning during casualty loading or unloading (a hot on- or off-load), approach the aircraft with great caution. Secure loose clothing, supplies, and other materials. Stay low and assure all IV stands are lowered and nothing is in danger of contacting the rotors. Approach the helicopter at a 45-degree angle from the front, under the flight crew's direction and in their clear view. If the helicopter lands on an incline, approach from the low side only. Load and secure the casualties under the flight crew's direction, then leave by your approach route while again staying low.

SUMMARY

Evacuation in the tactical environment is a complicated and risky process. To assure both your safety and that of the casualties you attend, carefully survey the battlefield for enemy fire and places of cover or concealment, evaluate the casualty for his or her ability to self-extract or his or her injury severity and survivability, and inventory the resources at hand to distract enemy fire or help with the extraction. If risk-benefit considerations suggest extraction is merited, then use safe cover or concealment to egress to, and then rapid movement techniques to extract, the casualty.

Once you isolate a casualty from enemy fire, assess, stabilize, and prepare him or her for evacuation. Prioritize the casualty for transport, employ movement techniques, and direct him or her to a patient collection point or aid station. Then request transport to a medical treatment facility, either a field hospital or surgical hospital. Evacuation may take place via stretcher, ground vehicle, water craft, or helicopter, each with its benefits and disadvantages during combat. If evacuation is well thought out and takes place in a logical and coordinated order, it can work to reduce the risk of further injury both to you, as a rescuer, and to the casualty, your patient.

FOR FURTHER READING

Field Manual 8-10-6, Medical Evacuation in a Theater of Operations: Tactics, Techniques and Procedures. Department of the Army, Washington, DC, 1991.

Soldier Training Publication, Soldier's Manual and Trainers Guide (MOS 91B, Medical NCO, skills level 2/3/4/5). Department of the Army, Washington, DC, 1990.

Field Manual 8-230, Medical Specialist. Department of the Army, Washington, DC, 1984.

9

EVACUATION CARE

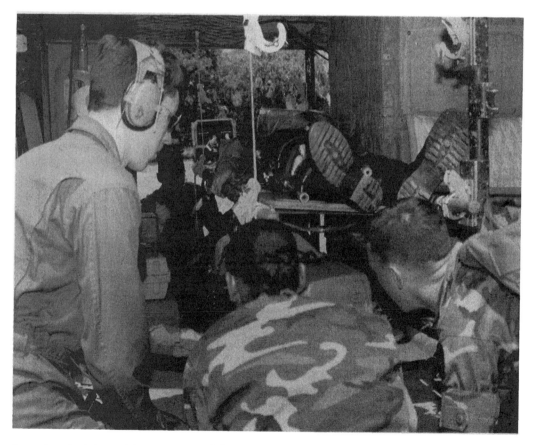

A casualty is loaded on a UH-1 "Huey" air ambulance.

OBJECTIVES

After reading this chapter, you will be able to:

1. Describe the role of the medic in prolonged evacuations and the focus of your care.
2. Describe the initial and focused assessments for a casualty undergoing evacuation.
3. Outline the priorities of the ongoing assessment in evacuation.
4. Describe the periodic assessments needed continually to monitor and assess the casualty.
5. List the electronic monitoring devices that can assist you in monitoring a casualty, and describe the function of each.
6. Describe the approach to ongoing care, and outline the priorities for this care.
7. Know the principles and procedures of providing oxygen therapy, positive pressure ventilation, suctioning, and bleeding control for evacuated casualties.
8. Know the procedures for providing fluid administration to treat casualties and provide maintenance hydration for evacuated casualties.
9. Describe how to provide for patient comfort and body-waste elimination during evacuation.

CASE

The company medics have just finished loading the last of four critical patients on your Humvee ambulance, and you are ready to depart. While your driver gets his bearings on the global positioning computer, you take a verbal report from the senior company medic. The first two patients have sustained gunshot wounds to the abdomen and have lost a lot of blood. Vital signs suggest early shock. The third patient has sustained a shrapnel wound to the chest and is having difficulty breathing. The third casualty has been ill with diarrhea for three days and is now dehydrated and very weak. You thank the company medic for his hard work and signal the driver to head out.

Recognizing the severity of the casualties and the need for immediate surgery for at least two of them (the abdominal wounds), you direct your driver to bypass the battalion aid station and plot a course for the medical company (clearing) where a forward surgical team has been established. You then begin a rapid but thorough assessment of all the casualties, focusing on the vital signs, mental status, patency of the airway, adequacy of breathing, control of all bleeding, and need for intravenous fluids. You also recheck all splints and bandages.

The chest wound casualty is having difficulty breathing, so you position his head to open the airway and apply oxygen. Breath sounds are diminished on the affected side, but tracheal deviation, neck vein distension, hyperresonance, and hypotension are all reassuringly absent. You cover the chest wound with gauze to avoid creating a seal that could lead to a lethal tension pneumothorax.

Both casualties with abdominal wounds exhibit anxiety, tachycardia, and mild hypotension (BP 86/50). Recognizing the signs of shock, you insert two large-bore IVs in each casualty and infuse a single bolus of 1000 ml of normal saline. This seems to improve the casualties' anxiety and reduces the tachycardia.

The last casualty (the one with diarrhea) is pale, diaphoretic, and anxious. He is also tachycardic and hypotensive. Recognizing shock from dehydration, you initiate two large-bore IV catheters and infuse several 1000-ml boluses of normal saline, reassessing the casualty between each bolus. This seems to improve the casualty's condition.

Once all the critical care is completed, you reassess each patient again, and then focus your attention on the comfort of the casualties for the long trip. Blankets, adjusting casualty positioning, small doses of intravenous morphine (for the three wounded casualties), and reassurance go a long way to relieve suffering.

At the clearing station, you help offload the casualties, giving a verbal report to the triage officer. You then complete the written record, update the field medical cards, and clean and restock your vehicle. With a few minutes to spare, you and your driver head to the chow hall for a cup of coffee, satisfied in your knowledge that you provided the best evacuation care possible for the four casualties.

INTRODUCTION

Tactical evacuation care is the ongoing assessment and care portion of casualty evacuation (see chapter 8, Tactical Evacuation). Casualties being moved from the point of injury or illness to definitive care (usually a hospital) will require periodic reassessment and adjustments to care. This section focuses on the need for providing care in prolonged evacuations.

Approach

The approach to evacuation care is very similar to tactical field care, except you and the patient are on the move (Figure 9-1). Furthermore, a prolonged evacuation requires you to address the ongoing needs of the patient during the time he or she is in your care. Your focus is on careful monitoring and reassessment of the casualty and instituting or

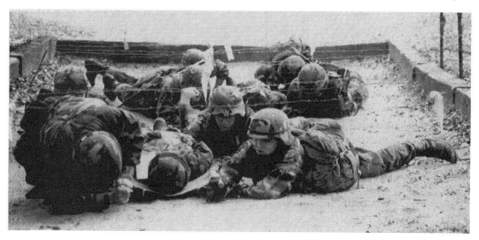

Figure 9-1 Providing care while on the move can be a tremendous challenge in the tactical environment.

changing treatment accordingly. In general, the goal of evacuation care is to maintain body systems until the destination is reached. Performing critical assessments or life-saving procedures in a cramped, moving, noisy vehicle, aircraft, or boat can be very challenging. Furthermore, the austere conditions of the tactical environment may require you to care for up to six critical patients. During this period, you will focus on the most important aspects of patient care.

Some casualties require rapid evacuation as a priority. The most common scenario in this case is the patient in shock from uncontrollable hemorrhage. The most important medical treatment for this casualty is rapid evacuation to a facility offering emergency surgery. *Prolonged attempts at field resuscitation (for example, initiating IV lines or continuing excessive and futile attempts to control bleeding) are not indicated when an ambulance is readily available. Instead, initiate IV lines and other supportive care while en route.*

ASSESSMENT

Repeat Initial and Focused Assessment

Provide a repeat of the initial and focused assessment just prior to moving. Secure the airway and position the casualty for gravitational drainage. If possible, place the patient in the recovery or left **lateral recumbent** position with the head facing at a downward angle. This permits oral secretions to drain and allows vomit to exit without filling the oral cavity. In the unconscious casualty, insert a nasal airway if he or she has an intact gag reflex, or an oral airway if he or she is without a gag reflex. Use of either the oral or nasal airway requires constant casualty monitoring. Consider endotracheal intubation for all unconscious casualty transports over any appreciable distance.

Administer oxygen to unconscious casualties or ones experiencing dyspnea, and guide its administration with pulse oximetry (if available) to a saturation of greater than 95%. Consider ventilatory support for any patient not moving an adequate volume of air or moving it at a very slow or very fast rate. However, remember that once you begin to ventilate a patient, you are obligated to continue until you arrive at a medical treatment facility. Oxygen-powered mechanical ventilators may be helpful but are usually in short supply and consume large amounts of oxygen (see Appendix D, Advanced Airway Procedures).

If the casualty may need fluid resuscitation during transport, as in penetrating body cavity trauma or uncontrolled external hemorrhage, *initiate intravenous therapy.* Use a large-bore catheter (14 to 18 gauge), and connect blood, trauma, or macro drip tubing between the catheter and a 1000-ml bag of normal saline. If there is a possible, yet future, need for fluid resuscitation, run fluids at a to-keep-open (TKO) rate, or establish a nonrestrictive flow saline lock (see Appendix C, Fluid and Medication Procedures). If the casualty displays the signs and symptoms of shock, then run the fluid wide open. Leave an additional bag of saline with the casualty, ready for administration. Current research suggests a maximum of 3000 ml of fluid is indicated during the first hour posttrauma if the casualty will receive definitive hemorrhage control (surgery) by the end of that hour. Otherwise, administer 250 to 1000 ml of solution to a casualty per hour in your care. Administer these fluids to maintain a suboptimal systolic blood pressure, not to return it to normal levels.

Consider using the Pneumatic Anti-Shock Garment (PASG), also known as a Medical Anti-Shock Trouser (MAST), for the shock patient. The device applies a circumferential pressure to the lower extremities and lower torso. This pressure effectively controls hemorrhage and, minimally, returns some blood to the critical circulation. Some authorities are questioning its use in penetrating injuries to the head and chest, so use it with caution, if at all, with these types of injuries. As with fluid resuscitation, inflate the device to maintain a subnormal blood pressure, not return it to preinjury levels.

Use the time since the injury and the current patient vital signs to determine how aggressive you will be in using IV fluids and PASG. If the injury occurred just minutes ago and the vital signs are already showing evidence of developing shock, be very aggressive in fluid administration and PASG inflation. If time has been great and the vitals are stable or just slightly subnormal, be conservative in both fluid administration and PASG inflation. However, carefully watch the casualty who suffers from a mechanism that could cause shock. The human body compensates very well for blood loss, to a point, then decompensates rapidly.

If the casualty is seen as a seizure or combative behavior risk, assure adequate restraint before loading him or her into a vehicle. If injuries permit, place the casualty face up on the stretcher and strap the arms, legs, and torso securely. Carefully monitor the airway, and be prepared to clear and suction it should vomiting occur. Wrapping the casualty in several layers of blankets may be helpful in dissipating the energy of the casualty's movements and may limit any harm restraint might cause him or her. Restraint is especially important for the combative or seizure patients who will fly in a helicopter. If the casualty breaks loose of the restraints, he or she may endanger the flight equipment and pilots.

As you prepare and load the casualty into the vehicle, assure that there is documentation describing the field assesment and care. Assure that documentation details the effects of any intervention as well as the trending of the patient's condition based on the results of ongoing assessments.

Ongoing Assessment

Reassess all critical (evacuation precedence urgent, or triage category immediate) casualties every 15 minutes or less. Quickly examine the ABCs and the casualty's mental status. Table 9-1 outlines the priorities of the ongoing assessments, and additional details follow.

Airway

Assure the continued adequacy of the airway. Listen for gurgling, snoring, or other sounds that may indicate upper airway obstruction. Supine patients maintain their airway best if the chin is tilted slightly up (as in the chin-tilt airway maneuver, Figure 9-2). However, unconscious supine patients are at greater risk of aspiration should emesis occur. Patients in the lateral recumbent (recovery) position can usually maintain the airway unassisted (Figure 9-3). This position is preferred because of the reduced risk of aspiration. *Place all unconscious casualties in the recovery position for transport unless contraindicated.* Possible contraindications include the need for spinal immobilization, airway control or mechanical ventilation, or other important medical need.

TABLE 9-1

PRIORITIES OF ONGOING ASSESSMENTS EVERY 15 MINUTES FOR CRITICAL PATIENTS

Airway
- Check for patency and obstruction
- Check artificial airway (e.g., ET tube) placement

Breathing
- Evaluate ventilation rate and depth (every 5 minutes)
- Reassess breath sounds or chest excursion bilaterally
- Reassess inspired oxygen concentration needs

Circulation
- Pulse and blood pressure (every 5 minutes)
- Capillary refill
- Evidence of bleeding

Mental Status
- AVPU (every 5 minutes)

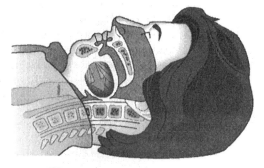

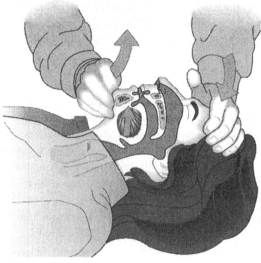

Figure 9-2 The head-tilt, chin-lift maneuver helps supine patients maintain a patent airway.

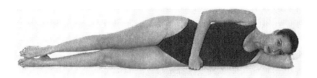

Figure 9-3 The recovery (lateral recumbent) position is optimal for patients unable to maintain a patent airway when supine.

If you have placed an oral or nasal airway (J-tube or trumpet), recheck its position and assess for obstruction (Figures 9-4 and 9-5). Gagging or choking indicates the oral or nasal airway is misplaced, too large (or possibly, too small), or the patient cannot tolerate it. Consider replacing an oral airway with a nasal one if gagging occurs.

Endotracheal tubes and other advanced airways should be carefully checked (Figure 9-6). Ensure that breath sounds and chest excursion are equal in both the left and right lung fields. Absent breath sounds and decreased chest excursion on the right frequently indicates inadvertent right mainstem bronchus intubation. Adjust the tube and reassess.

Breathing

Assure ventilation by measuring the respiratory or ventilatory rate and depth. The rate is simply the number of breaths per minute. Depth or adequacy can be estimated by auscultating good breath sounds or observing chest excursion (Figure 9-7). Listen for wheezing, crackles, or other abnormal breath sounds. In a noisy environment, auscultation can be difficult, and chest excursion may be preferred. Place the palms of both hands gently on the chest wall, and feel the chest wall expand and relax with each ventilation (Figure 9-8).

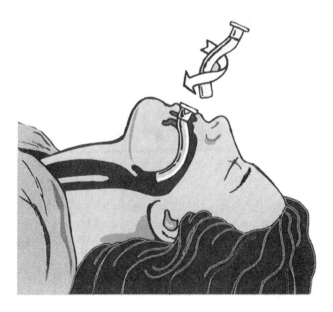

Figure 9-4 Proper positioning of an oropharyngeal airway.

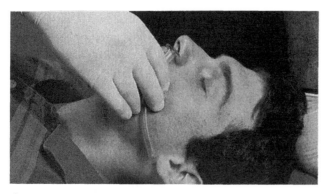

A.

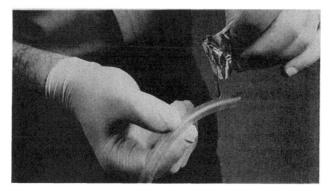

B.

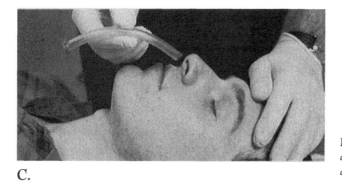

C.

Figure 9-5 Proper measurement and preparation of a nasopharyngeal airway.

Simultaneous visual inspection of the chest wall will help give a reliable estimate of ventilation volume. Unilateral absence of lung ventilation suggests simple pneumothorax, tension pneumothorax, or right mainstem bronchus intubation. Exclude or treat each as appropriate. Reassess the casualty's need for supplemental oxygen. *All critical casualties, especially those with dyspnea or respiratory failure, will benefit from high-flow oxygen.* Less serious

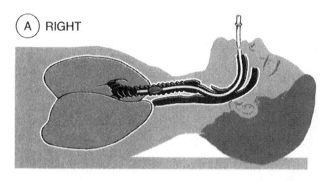

(A) RIGHT

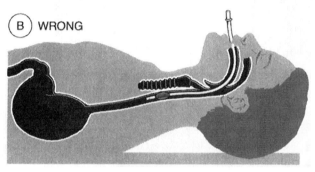

(B) WRONG

Figure 9-6 Proper positioning of the endotracheal tube is critical.

casualties may also benefit from oxygen therapy. Oxygen, however, is heavy and bulky, and can be a scarce commodity in the tactical environment. If supplies are limited, reserve oxygen for the most seriously injured or ill casualties. A useful tool to gauge the need for continued oxygen therapy is the pulse oximeter. Use supplemental oxygen to keep the peripheral oxygen saturation ≥ 95%. Adjust flow rates to maximize benefit and conserve oxygen. Remember, however, that peripheral blood oxygen saturation does not necessarily reflect tissue oxygen perfusion. Shock, toxins, and other factors may cause tissue hypoxia even in the face of good pulse oximetry readings (see Appendix D, Advanced Airway Procedures).

Circulation

Measure the pulse and blood pressure at least every 5 minutes for critical casualties or every 15 minutes for less serious casualties. Auscultation of blood pressure can be difficult in noisy environments, and palpation may be preferred. Although the information it provides is incomplete, palpation of blood pressure does provide the systolic BP, which is a useful indicator of perfusion pressure. Also useful and much easier to obtain is capillary refill. Gently depress the patients skin to cause blanching, release quickly, and observe the time until it refills to a pink color. Use central skin (neck, trunk, abdomen) to avoid false readings from cold extremities. Normal refill is < 3 seconds. Anything significantly prolonged suggests shock.

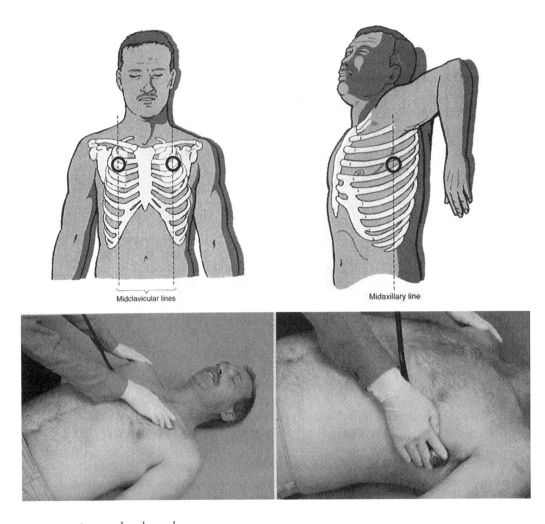

Midclavicular lines

Midaxillary line

Figure 9-7 Assessing breath sounds.

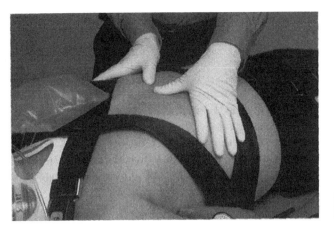

Figure 9-8 Assessing respirations by placing the hands on the thorax.

```
         Level of Consciousness
  ■ A  =  Alert
  ■ V  =  responds to Verbal stimuli
  ■ P  =  responds to Painful stimuli
  ■ U  =  Unresponsive
```

Figure 9-9 AVPU scale of level of consciousness.

Mental Status

Reassess the critical casualty's mental status every 5 minutes or less. Less serious casualties may be checked every 15 minutes. Assess orientation to person, place, and time and use the standard alert, verbal, pain, or unresponsive (AVPU) scale (Figure 9-9). More detailed scoring systems such as the Glasgow Coma Scale are useful but not required.

Trending the Patient

After each reassessment, compare the casualty's condition to previous assessments to determine a trend. Stable casualties may show some modest variability, but in general, will show no significant deterioration. Deteriorating casualties, on the other hand, may show decreasing mental status and progressive signs of respiratory distress or shock. *Increased respiratory rate together with decreased ventilatory volume is often an early sign of respiratory distress. Pulse rate may rise with impending shock, but may become bradycardic just before death. Capillary refill time usually increases to 3 seconds or more with progressive shock.* Casualties in shock or exhibiting deteriorating mental status or worsening respiratory distress need aggressive search for the causes of the problem and appropriate intervention.

Additional Ongoing Assessment

Casualties undergoing evacuation need more than just periodic assessment of the ABCs. Check all IV sites for patency, as well as other catheters (for example, needle thoracostomy). Check dressings for soakage of blood and any tourniquet for proper snugness. Recheck and adjust splints for snugness and immobilization, and assure that distal circulation and neurologic function is adequate. Include in this check cervical collars, head immobilization, and backboards and strapping. Be sure all are snug but not so tight as to restrict the airway or breathing. Recheck the pulse and capillary refill in all extremities with injuries (Figure 9-10). Don't forget the patient's safety and comfort. Be sure all straps are properly adjusted and the patient's body temperature is maintained. Table 9-2 outlines the additional considerations in the ongoing assessment.

Monitoring

Ideally, you will monitor all evacuated casualties. Monitoring devices are small, lightweight, rugged, and relatively inexpensive. Furthermore, machine monitoring frees you from many burdensome reassessments and allows greater attention to other critical

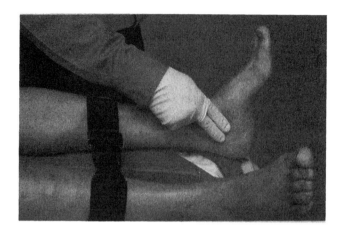

Figure 9-10 Assess pulse, capillary refill, motor and sensory function in all injured extremities.

TABLE 9-2

ADDITIONAL CONSIDERATION IN ONGOING ASSESSMENTS

- IV sites and catheter patency
- Dressing, bandage, and tourniquet effectiveness
- Splint adequacy (including c-collar and spineboard)
- Casualty temperature maintenance
- Waste elimination
- Casualty comfort

---

patient needs. Monitoring also serves as an early warning system, providing important patient information before it otherwise becomes apparent to you. These factors make monitoring an important element of any casualty evacuation system, and all tactical medics should be familiar with its use.

Several types of electronic monitoring systems are available for prehospital use (Table 9-3). This section briefly examines several of them with an eye toward their use in the tactical environment. If you require further information on electronic monitoring, please seek out one of the many fine emergency-care textbooks available.

TABLE 9-3

MONITORING OPTIONS IN EVACUATION CARE

- Automated sphygmomanometer (pulse and BP)
- Pulse oximeter (oxygen saturation)
- Electrocardiograph (ECG) monitor (heart rhythm)
- Capnometer (end-tidal CO_2)

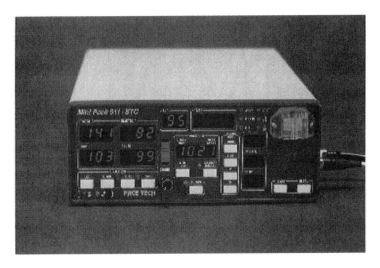

Figure 9-11 Automated sphygmomanometer can relieve the medic from having to retake frequent vital signs.

Automated Sphygmomanometer

These devices automatically obtain a noninvasive (cuff on the arm) BP and pulse (Figure 9-11). They can be set to measure the BP and pulse at any desired interval. Modern machines are reliable and relatively immune to noise and motion artifact, and they require little special training. The great advantage of these devices is to free you from the burden of frequent pulse and blood pressure checks. Additionally, some machines maintain a memory of previous readings for up to several hours.

Pulse Oximeter

After the automated sphygmomanometer, the most next useful monitor for tactical evacuation is the pulse oximeter (Figure 9-12). This device provides you with information otherwise not directly available through physical examination, namely, peripheral blood oxygen saturation. This device can report the delivery of oxygen to one of the most distal body organs, the skin. An important use in casualty evacuation is the conservation of oxygen supplies. Adjust oxygen flow rates to keep the oxygen saturation ≥ 95% (see Appendix D, Advanced Airway Procedures).

ECG Monitor

Electrocardiographic (ECG) monitoring is the traditional method of prehospital electronic monitoring (Figure 9-13). It provides a continuous measure of heart rate and rhythm. It is most valuable in patients at risk for cardiac dysrhythmias such as suspected myocardial infarction (heart attack). It is less valuable in the tactical setting since few casualties will have cardiac dysrhythmias as their primary problem. An exception might be burn patients and chemical agent casualties, who may be prone to cardiac ischemia and dysrhythmias.

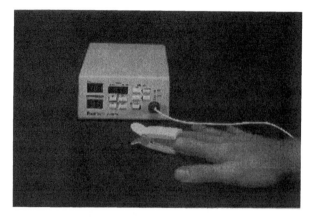

Figure 9-12 The pulse oximeter is a useful assessment tool in tactical evacuation.

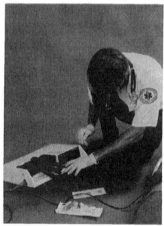

Figure 9-13 ECG monitor has limited value in tactical assessment, but may be useful in chemical agent casualties and burns.

Capnometer

Capnometry is the measurement of expired CO_2 ($ETCO_2$). In the prehospital arena, you will use the **capnometer** almost exclusively on intubated patients (Figure 9-14). For this purpose, capnometry is very useful in assuring the patency of the airway and ventilation.

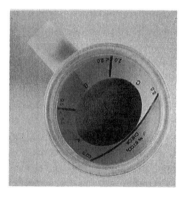

Figure 9-14 Colorimetric capnometer (end-tidal CO_2 detector) for use in intubated patients.

Perform capnometric monitoring on intubated casualties during evacuation. This is especially important if you cannot give constant attention to the casualty, as may occur when you are treating multiple casualties. Capnometry can also help you overcome some of the difficulties in assessing the respiratory system in a moving, noisy evacuation vehicle.

ONGOING CARE

The other major component of casualty evacuation is ongoing care. This component requires you to synthesize the information obtained from the ongoing assessments and apply it to change or maintain patient treatment. This approach is not different from the ongoing care in traditional, short-transport prehospital care, except that tactical evacuation can stretch for hours or even days.

Approach

The approach to ongoing care is to provide the care necessary to maintain critical body systems and general patient comfort throughout the evacuation process. The evacuation environment is frequently noisy and bumpy, and constantly in motion. This, combined with the austere conditions in the tactical environment, limits the care that you can provide. Thus, you must focus on those elements of care that are most important. In general, these important elements of care parallel the treatment in the tactical field care stage of tactical care (see chapter 1, Tactical Environment of Care). Concentrate on the ABCs, fluid management, medications, and patient comfort. Tables 9-4 and 9-5 describe the approach to ongoing care and the general management of patients in evacuation care.

Airway and Breathing

The same approach to care is employed during evacuation as in tactical field care (see chapter 1, Tactical Environment of Care). Perform interventions such as endotracheal intubation and assisted (overdrive) ventilation for the same indications. During long evacuations, intubated patients may require periodic suctioning of the endotracheal tube. The indications for this procedure include copious endotracheal secretions, increasing ventilatory pressures (increasing difficulty bagging), and suspected endotracheal tube plugging. Casualties most at risk for this problem are victims of pulmonary and nerve agents.

TABLE 9-4

APPROACH TO ONGOING CARE IN TACTICAL EVACUATION

- Provide care necessary to maintain critical body systems and ensure patient comfort
- Focus on the most important elements of care
- Recognize the limitations of the tactical evacuation environment when providing care

---

TABLE 9-5

GENERAL OUTLINE OF CARE FOR CASUALTY EVACUATION

Airway
- Proper patient positioning
- Manual airway methods and suction
- Naso or oropharyngeal airways
- Endotracheal intubation
- Cricothyrotomy or cricothyrostomy

Breathing
- Bag-valve-mask ventilation
- Mechanical (automatic) ventilator
- Needle thoracostomy (pleural decompression)
- Oxygen therapy in hypoxemic or critical patients

Circulation
- Control bleeding with pressure dressings or tourniquet
- Maintain large bore IV access
- Intermittent fluid boluses (maintenance IV)

Disability and Drugs
- Maintain splints and dressing
- Repeat dosing of selected medications
- Antibiotics in selected cases

Adapted, in part from Butler KF, Hagmann J, Butler EG: Tactical Combat Casuality Care in Special Operations. Milit Med 1996; 161 (s): 3-16.

Endotracheal Suctioning

To perform this procedure, first assemble all necessary equipment: sterile whistle-tip flexible suction catheter (Figure 9-15) sized to fit the endotracheal tube, suction device and tubing, and sterile gloves.

1. Don sterile gloves and use sterile technique.
2. Hyperventilate the patient for 15-20 seconds.
3. Measure the catheter to the length of the ET tube (approximately from tube adapter to sternal notch).
4. Insert catheter into ET tube (without suction operating) as far as the carina (Figure 9-16).
5. Apply suction for 10 seconds while you twist the catheter back and forth.
6. Continue suction and rotation as catheter is withdrawn.
7. Hyperventilate the patient again for 15-20 seconds.

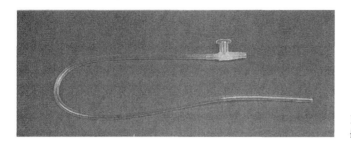

Figure 9-15 Whistle-tip flexible suction catheter.

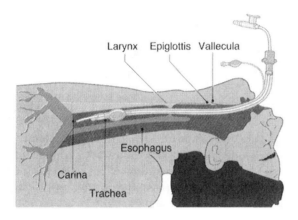

Larynx Epiglottis Vallecula

Esophagus

Carina

Trachea

Figure 9-16 Endotracheal suctioning.

There are some risks to endotracheal tube suctioning. Stimulation of the lower airway can cause serious bradycardia and stimulate cough. Treat bradycardia by aborting the procedure and, if it continues, by administering intravenous atropine. Cough is not a serious problem except in closed head injury, where the rise in intracranial pressure can be life threatening. Avoid suctioning the ET tube of closed head trauma casualties unless clearly indicated. The most common risk of suctioning (this includes routine oral and nasopharyngeal suctioning in patients without ET tubes) is hypoxia from prolonged or too frequent suctioning. Hypoxia can be minimized by (1) hyperventilating before and after suctioning, (2) minimizing suction time to 10 seconds, (3) providing 100% oxygen, if available, and (4) monitoring by pulse oximetry.

Ventilation

Patients with inadequate respirations or respiratory failure require assisted or overdrive ventilation or complete ventilatory support. Provide this by bag-valve-mask or an automatic mechanical ventilator. The prolonged evacuations in the tactical setting virtually compels the use of automatic devices (Figure 9-17). Each ventilator manufacturer will specify the unique operating requirements, and you must be familiar with the available equipment (see Appendix D, Advanced Airway Procedures).

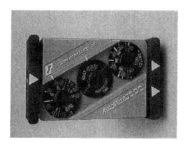

Figure 9-17 Portable mechanical ventilator for prehospital use.

Ventilate adult casualties at a rate of 12 per minute (once every 5 seconds) during evacuation. Head-injured casualties and children require faster rates. Tidal volume is approximately 800 ml for the adult or 10-12 ml/kg for children (see Table 9-6).

Oxygenation

It is standard prehospital care to provide high-flow oxygen to all serious and potentially serious patients. This practice is based on the need to maximize tissue oxygenation in critical patients and the virtual lack of risk of administering high concentrations of oxygen. Unfortunately, this practice of universal oxygen administration consumes large volumes of oxygen and is not suitable to the tactical environment. Therefore, only selected casualties will receive oxygen. In general, severe respiratory distress, respiratory failure, and uncompensated shock are indications for oxygen therapy. Use a nonrebreather mask (Figure 9-18). The pulse oximeter is a useful tool to estimate oxygenation. Oxygen saturation levels ≥ 95% do not require supplemental oxygen in the tactical setting. Conversely, saturation levels < 95%, particularly if associated with serious signs and symptoms, are an indication for oxygen therapy. Table 9-7 outlines the indications for supplemental oxygen.

When administering supplemental oxygen, use a nonrebreather mask at 10-15 lpm (sufficient to keep the reservoir filled) for spontaneously breathing adults. In casualties receiving positive pressure ventilation, use 100% oxygen (use a reservoir). If a pulse oximeter is available, adjust the oxygen flow rate just to keep the saturation at or above 95% (Table 9-7).

TABLE 9-6

VENTILATION RATES AND VOLUMES IN EVACUATION CARE

CATEGORY	RATE/MINUTE	TIDAL VOLUME
Most adults	12 (every 5 s)	800 ml
Head-injured adults	15 (every 4 s)	800 ml
Pediatric	20 (every 3 s)	10-12 ml/kg

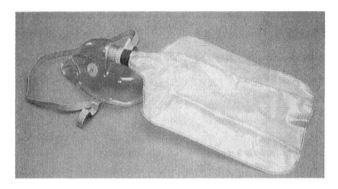

Figure 9-18 Nonrebreather mask should be applied on all critical casualties.

TABLE 9-7

USE OF SUPPLEMENTAL OXYGEN IN TACTICAL EVACUATION

- Severe respiratory distress
- Respiratory failure or casualties receiving artificial ventilation
- Uncompensated shock
- Suspected cyanide poisoning and severe symptoms
- Pulmonary agent poisoning and severe symptoms
- If pulse oximetry is available, titrate oxygen flow rates to keep $SaO_2 \geq 95\%$

Circulation

Ongoing care for circulation includes continued measures to control bleeding. Maintain direct pressure, pressure bandages, and tourniquets already applied. If previously applied, maintain antishock (PASG, MAST) garment inflation at a constant pressure.

Maintain intravenous access through the use of saline lock devices. Constant drip infusion (keep vein open [KVO]) rates are less desirable in the tactical setting because they require frequent monitoring and consume scarce fluids.

Additional Fluids

Casualties undergoing relatively short (2-3 hours) evacuations do not usually require any additional intravenous fluids beyond that needed to treat shock or significant hemorrhage (see chapter 1, Tactical Environment of Care). Of course, if the casualty's condition changes (for example, compensated shock deteriorates into uncompensated shock), then additional fluid for treatment may be needed (Table 9-8).

Maintenance Fluids

In rare circumstances, evacuation may stretch into days. In this situation, casualties require maintenance fluid administration. Maintenance fluids are those fluids necessary to maintain basic body hydration requirements. This fluid is in addition to fluid needed

TABLE 9-8

ADDITIONAL FLUID ADMINISTRATION
IN CASUALTY EVACUATION ONGOING CARE
(INCLUDES FLUID ADMINISTERED IN THE TACTICAL FIELD CARE STAGE—ADULT DOSAGES)

CONDITION	FLUID ADMINISTRATION
Controlled or absent hemorrhage without shock	Saline lock
Controlled hemorrhage with shock	NS 1000 ml; may repeat up to 3000 ml total
Uncontrolled intraabdominal or intrathoracic hemorrhage with shock	NS 1000 ml total
Isolated head wound with shock	NS 1000 ml total
Shock from dehydration, diarrhea, vomiting, or sepsis (biologic agent)	NS 1000 ml; may repeat up to 5000 ml total

to treat hemorrhage, shock, and other medical problems. The average adult needs approximately 2500 ml of fluid per day to maintain optimal hydration.

To provide the fluid maintenance for prolonged evacuation, first determine if the casualty can drink orally. Most ambulatory casualties are able to drink and should be allowed to do so. (An intact thirst mechanism is an accurate barometer of hydration and should be used to determine the hydration needs of ambulatory casualties.) Unconscious casualties, intubated patients, and most critical casualties will be unable to drink. Any casualty who may need urgent surgery should not be allowed to drink. Casualties who cannot drink will require intravenous fluid maintenance (Figure 9-19).

Calculate the daily requirement based on the casualty's weight (Table 9-9). The typical adult casualty will require 2500 ml per day. It is easiest to administer this daily dose in four equally divided doses every 6 hours. It is also acceptable to provide this 24-hour fluid requirement as a constant drip rate. This latter method, however, is less desirable because constant infusions require frequent checks and accurate time-volume

TABLE 9-9

MAINTENANCE INTRAVENOUS FLUID REQUIREMENTS FOR CASUALTIES IN
PROLONGED (> 24 HOURS) EVACUATIONS IN THE AUSTERE TACTICAL ENVIRONMENT

PATIENT	24-HOUR REQUIREMENT
Adult	36 ml/kg (2500 ml)
PEDIATRIC	
0-10 kg	100 ml/kg
11-20 kg	1000 ml plus 50 ml/kg for weight above 10 kg
> 20 kg	1500 ml plus 20 ml/kg for weight above 20 kg

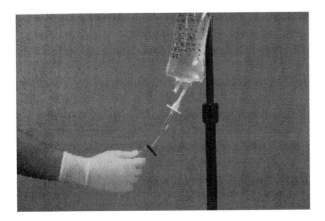

Figure 9-19 Many casualties will require intravenous fluids during prolonged evacuation.

calculations. In all cases, remember the goal of maintenance fluid infusions is to provide baseline levels of fluid to sustain body systems. Patients needing fluids for acute problems (continued hemorrhage, uncompensated shock, and so on) may require additional fluids beyond maintenance requirements (see Table 9-8).

For children, it is necessary to calculate carefully the maintenance rate based on weight. Depending on the size of the child, the rate varies (Table 9-9).

For example, a 5-kg child would receive:
5 kg x 100 ml/kg/day = 500 ml/day

A 30-kg child would receive:
1500 ml + 10 kg (the weight above 20 kg) x 20 ml/kg/day = 1700 ml/day

If available, use half- or quarter-normal saline for maintenance fluid administration. Five percent dextrose (D_5) added to the solutions is also acceptable. Infants should always have some dextrose added to their maintenance fluids to prevent hypoglycemia. If this is unavailable, normal saline (or Ringers Lactate) is an acceptable alternative for all patients anticipated in the tactical environment.

Disability and Drugs

Disability refers to the casualty's neurologic status and the immobilization of fractures and other injuries. The focus is on the adequate immobilization of the cervical spine, use of spineboard, and long-bone splints. Not all casualties require spinal immobilization (see chapter 1, Tactical Environment of Care), but if indicated, employ and maintain it throughout evacuation. Likewise, splints, bandages, and tourniquets should be applied and maintained.

Medications

In this section, drugs refer to medication redosing during evacuation. Some medications you initially administer in the tactical field care stage may require redosing if evacuation

TABLE 9-10

**MEDICATIONS COMMONLY USED IN THE TACTICAL
SETTING THAT MAY REQUIRE REPEAT DOSING**

- Atropine
- Pralidoxime
- Diazepam
- Morphine
- Albuterol

time exceeds a few hours. Medication redosing is based on two factors: (1) a continued need or indication for the medication, and (2) the appropriate time interval for redosing. Certain medications may require redosing. Table 9-10 lists common drugs used in the tactical setting that may need redosing. A thorough review of Appendix A, Medications for the Tactical Environment, is essential to identify the proper indications and dosing intervals for specific medications.

Waste Elimination

Casualties transported for any length of time may need to eliminate body waste through either urination or defecation. You must be prepared to handle this common clinical procedure for the comfort and safety of your patients. You should be familiar with urinals, bedpans, and foley catheters.

Urinal and Bedpan

The urinal is a tall and narrow container used to collect urine from male casualties (Figure 9-20). To use it effectively, the casualty must be cooperative and able to use at least one hand. The bedpan is used for collecting urine from female casualties and feces from both male and female casualties (Figure 9-21). It generally requires a cooperative patient who can also lift his or her buttocks high enough to get on the pan. Obviously, critically ill and spinal immobilized casualties cannot use a bedpan. Instead, lots of towels and barrier pads will be needed to contain the casualty's feces and urine. In all cases of waste elimination, record the volume eliminated.

Bladder Catheter

If a foley or bladder catheter (a soft rubber catheter inserted through the urethra into the bladder) is in place, be sure the tube is not stretched or pulling on the urethral opening (Figure 9-22). Check all connections for leaks. The bag can hold 1000 ml or more of urine and can be emptied when full. Be sure to record the urine volume and time when emptying the bag. If the foley catheter falls out during evacuation, it should not be replaced

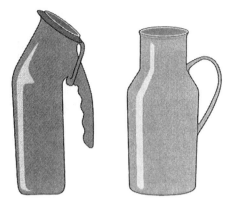

Figure 9-20 Male urinal.

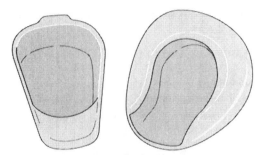

Figure 9-21 Bedpan.

unless you are trained in this procedure. Instead, you will need to use a bedpan, urinal, or lots of towels to catch the urine.

Patient Comfort

Attending to the casualty's basic comfort is an important component of evacuation care. *One of your prime functions as a tactical medic is to relieve pain and prevent suffering. Accomplish this through patient positioning, maintenance of body temperature, judicious use of analgesia, and psychological reassurance* (Table 9-11). Unless otherwise medically indicated (for example, the need to maintain cervical immobilization), allow the patient to assume a comfortable position. Keep the casualty warm, but avoid overheating him or her. Let the awake patient guide the need for additional blankets, and so forth. A good rule of thumb for unconscious casualties is to use slightly more blankets or coverings than necessary to keep you (the medic) comfortable. Redosing of morphine is important

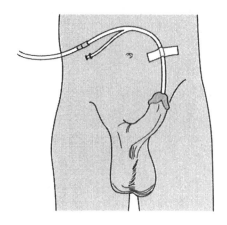

Figure 9-22 Foley catheter inserted into the male urethra.

TABLE 9-11

ELEMENTS OF PATIENT COMFORT IN CASUALTY EVACUATION CARE

- Patient positioning
- Maintenance of body temperature
- Judicious use of analgesia
- Psychological reassurance

to alleviate suffering. Reassess the casualty's level of consciousness, vital signs, and estimated degree of pain before each dose (see Appendix A, Medications for the Tactical Environment).

Lastly, do not forget the value of human compassion and reassurance. A few positive, caring words or a reassuring touch can immeasurably boost a casualty's morale. A caring, concerned attitude is a proud tradition among medical providers in the field, and its continued practice is encouraged.

SUMMARY

The tactical environment presents unique challenges to care during evacuation. You, the tactical medic, can overcome these challenges by applying the principles of assessment and treatment to achieve the best possible care for your patients. Repeat the initial and focused assessment before or soon after departure. In addition to checking the patient, also recheck the effectiveness of all bandages, dressings, tubes, and lines. During transport, reassess a critical casualty's vital signs every 5 minutes and a non-critical casualty's every 15 minutes. Initiate or adjust care as indicated by the trend of the casualty's condition. Provide for the casualty's fluid maintenance on long transport and assure casualty comfort through proper positioning, application of blankets, administration of analgesia, and above all, verbal reassurance.

FOR FURTHER READING

BUTLER FK, Hagmann J, Butler EJ: Tactical Combat Casualty Care in Special Operations. Military Medicine, 1996; 161, Suppl: 3-15.

DE LORENZO RA: Improving Combat Casualty Care and Field Medicine: Focus on the Military Medic. Military Medicine, 1997.

DE LORENZO RA: Military and Civilian Emergency Aeromedical Services: Achieving Common Goals with Different Approaches. Aviation, Space and Environmental Medicine, 1997; 68(1): 56-60.

BOWEN TE, Bellamy RF: Emergency War Surgery, 2nd ed. U.S. Government Printing Office, Washington, DC, 1988.

WEINER SL et al.: Trauma Management of Civilian and Military Physicians. WB Saunders, Philadelphia, 1986.

BELLAMY RF: Combat Trauma Overview, in Zajtchuk R, Bellamy RF (eds): Anesthesia and Perioperative Care of the Combat Casualty. Department of the Army, Washington, DC, 1995.

ZAJTCHUK R (ed): Conventional Warfare: Ballistic, Blast and Burn Injuries. Department of the Army, Washington, DC, 1991.

BLEDSOE BE et al.: Paramedic Emergency Care. Brady, Englewood Cliffs, NJ, 1997.

Field Manual 8-10-6, Medical Evacuation in a Theater of Operations. Department of the Army, Washington, DC, 1991.

O'KEEFE MF et al.: Emergency Care, 8th ed. Brady, Englewood Cliffs, NJ, 1998.

10

TACTICAL TRIAGE

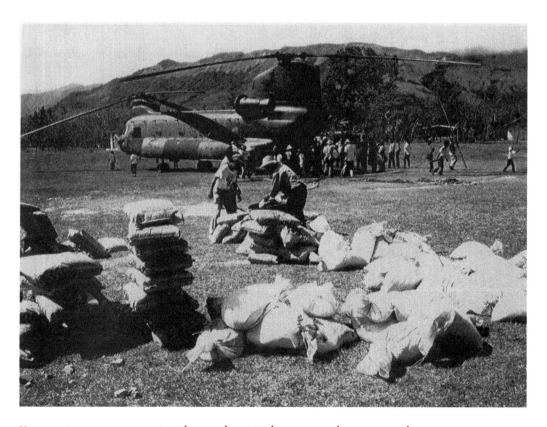

Humanitarian missions may require military medics to conduct mass casualty triage on civilians.

OBJECTIVES

After reading this chapter, you will be able to:
1. Describe the principles of triage, and apply them to the tactical setting.
2. Outline the NATO standard of triage, and describe the four standard triage categories.
3. Outline the principles of initial triage, and describe the START procedure as it applies to the tactical setting.
4. Describe the principles of ongoing and subsequent triage, and explain how this differs from START.
5. List some of the important medical conditions falling into the immediate, delayed, minimal, and expectant categories.
6. Describe the concepts of mass casualty incidents, including triage and treatment teams, incident command system, and triage tags.
7. List some important tips and pitfalls in triage.

CASE

You are the medic assigned to Alpha team. While on patrol in hostile territory, your unit is attacked and sustains heavy casualties. As the only medical person assigned to the team, you quickly realize there are more patients than you can possibly treat, and so you summon help. You then begin the process of triage, or sorting through the casualties to identify those most in need of immediate attention.

First, you call out to the wounded, instructing those who can walk or limp to move to a safe collection point. With these less-injured casualties moving toward safety, you turn to the remaining casualties lying on the ground. Approaching the first casualty, you rapidly assess ventilation, perfusion, and mental status. Using just this information, the casualty is assigned a triage category or priority, and it is noted on a field medical card or triage tag. You then move on to the next casualty and perform the same task. In this rapid fashion, a large number of casualties can be triaged in a relatively brief period. To save time, you take only the time necessary to make an initial categorization, and resist the urge to provide extensive care.

Only when all the casualties have been reached and triaged do you begin to provide medical care. First to be treated are casualties with acute airway obstruction, respiratory failure, uncontrolled bleeding, and severe shock. Less ill casualties will have to wait (this is the essence of triage).

Eventually, all the casualties will get treatment, and help will begin to arrive. At that point, you can begin to focus on making evacuation plans and extracting your patients from the zone of operations.

OVERVIEW

The term *triage* comes from French and means "to sort." The modern term *triage* can refer to a number of clinical situations, ranging from emergency department (ED) triage by nurses to the sorting of victims of disasters. This chapter focuses on triage as it applies to the tactical situation. In particular, the focus falls on the sorting of casualties as a result of hostile action. However, since many of the principles of tactical triage apply to other situations (terrorist attacks, urban mass casualty incidents, and natural disasters, for example), all EMS providers can appreciate the discussion.

History

The father of modern triage is Baron Dominique Jean Larre, a surgeon in Napolean's Army. His system of attending first to the soldiers most in need of care, regardless of rank, is still a basic tenent today. In the American Civil War, John Wilson observed that care to others could be expanded if care to those with likely lethal wounds was deferred. By World War I, military triage began to resemble modern methods in that motorized ambulances were sent to appropriate hospitals from distribution points. World War II brought dramatic improvements in survival, at least in part from better triage. Korea and Vietnam saw further refinements in triage and dramatic decreases in wound mortality. Rapid evacuation off the battlefield to field hospitals was felt to be a major factor in improving outcomes.

The history of civilian triage and natural disaster medical care is much less detailed. Until recently, little was written about these important situations. Nonetheless, we know the principles of triage remain the same, regardless if performed on the battlefield, barricade, or disaster zone.

Principles

The primary principle of triage is to accomplish "the greatest good for the greatest number of casualties." With this overriding principle in mind, it is easy to see the wisdom of categorizing or sorting patients by priority. This allows scarce medical care to go to those who will benefit the most.

The second principle of triage is to "employ the most efficient use of available resources." By definition, triage implies more patients than providers, equipment, and ambulances than are available to care for them. Efficiency stretches the available resources and helps to support the primary principle of caring for as many casualties as appropriate.

Although the first two principles apply to all triage environments, another principle applies primarily to the tactical situation. Because the ultimate focus of the tactical unit is to accomplish the mission, it follows that tactical triage should support this goal. *Therefore, the third principle of triage is to "return key personnel to duty as quickly as possible."* This gives the unit commander the maximum number of personnel possible to accomplish the mission. Table 10-1 lists the principles of tactical triage.

TABLE 10-1

PRINCIPLES OF TRIAGE

- Greatest good for the greatest number of casualties
- Employ the most efficient use of available resources
- Return key personnel to duty as quickly as possible

TABLE 10-2

FACTORS FOR SUCCESSFUL TRIAGE

- Focus on easily treated conditions
- Perform rapid, accurate but focused assessments
- Continually reassess and retriage

TRIAGE SYSTEMS

There are several accepted systems of triage, each with its own particulars. However, all share the same factors for success (Table 10-2). First is to focus on easily corrected medical problems while conducting triage. Since resources are scarce, only problems that consume limited amounts of time or supplies, or limited numbers of personnel, are addressed. More complicated problems will, by necessity, have to wait. Second, by performing rapid but accurate assessments, over and under triage will be avoided. The last factor highlights the dynamic, or ever-changing, conditions of the patient and situation. Continual reassessment is crucial to successful triage.

NATO Standard

The most widely accepted tactical triage technique is the NATO standard method. It is used by the military forces of the United States, Canada, and most of Western Europe. It has also been adopted or modified for use by many non-NATO nations and by many civilian agencies within the United States. Therefore, most of the emphasis of this chapter is on the NATO standard triage technique.

NATO Categories

NATO triage uses four levels of priority (Table 10-3). The highest priority category is termed **immediate** and refers to the urgent nature of the casualty. This category implies the need for rapid (within minutes to an hour) intervention to save life, limb, or eyesight. Not

TABLE 10-3

TRIAGE CATEGORIES IN THE NATO SYSTEM

- Immediate
- Delayed
- Minimal
- Expectant

all critically ill or injured patients are immediate. *Only those with an imminent threat and who also have a good chance of survival, given the available resources, are categorized as immediate.*

The second priority is termed **delayed** and refers to the need for treatment (usually surgery) that is required but can wait for a few hours. **Minimal** patients are those with minor problems requiring medical attention, but whose condition is unlikely to deteriorate over the next several hours to a day. The last category, **expectant** are patients who are so gravely ill or injured that survival is unlikely. These patients are expected to die.

Other Systems

Other methods of triage prioritization exist using three, four, or five categories. None has ever been shown superior to the NATO categories. Nevertheless, all EMS providers should be familiar with the system in place locally. Readers desiring details of other systems are referred to the reading list at the end of the chapter.

Initial Triage

The actual performance of triage requires more than an understanding of principles. It also requires a structured approach or procedure. Perhaps the best procedure is the START (Simple Triage And Rapid Treatment) method. Though originally developed for civilian responses to mass casualties, it is highly adaptable to all tactical situations, including combat.

START is simple, fast, reliable, and a good choice for initial triage. Its focused nature is particularly helpful in far-forward environments where resources are scarce. All levels of prehospital provider (basic EMT, paramedic) as well as nurses and physicians can employ it. It is the recommended technique for initial tactical emergency care.

Figure 10-1 depicts the basic START algorithm. START uses four key decision points (Table 10-4) to make a rapid, initial triage decision. Using these key decision points, the experienced medic can employ the entire algorithm and triage a patient in 10 to 12 seconds. This rapid speed is highly desirable in "care under fire" circumstances (see chapter 1, Tactical Environment of Care) or other situations of imminent danger. The speed of START triage also makes it ideal when large numbers of casualties must be triaged by a small number of medics.

TABLE 10-4

KEY DECISION POINTS FOR START TRIAGE

- Able to walk (ambulate)?
- Ventilation present?
- Capillary refill < 3 s?
- Follows simple commands?

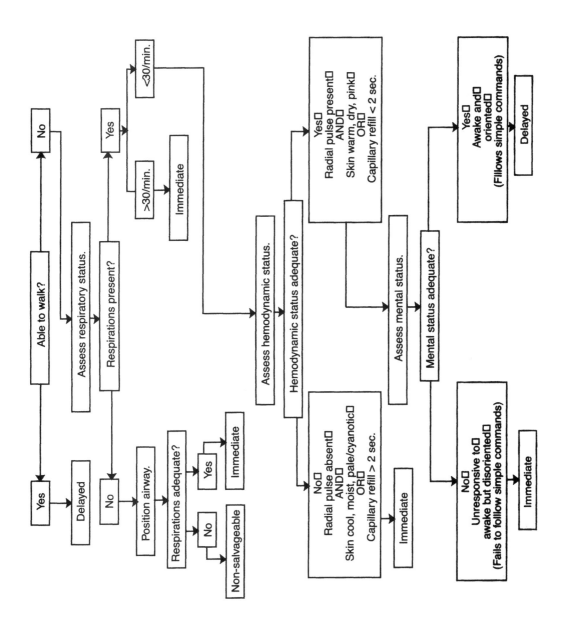

Figure 10-1 START method of triage.

Using START

The first step in START (after ensuring scene safety) is to remove all ambulatory (walking) patients to an area of relative safety. If the tactical situation allows, simply shout the instruction "If you can get up and walk, move immediately to the _____ area." If necessary, for tactical reasons, approach each casualty individually to whisper the instruction. If the threat of hostile fire or other danger is high, be sure all casualties who can walk, limp, or crawl are included in the command to move. The primary concern is to remove them from danger.

The net result of the "able to walk?" decision point is twofold. First, it clears the immediate area of all patients able to move to safety under their own power. Second, all ambulatory patients are now categorized as delayed or minimal. (This differs slightly from the original START method whereby ambulatory patients are all categorized as delayed.) If necessary, these walking casualties can be reassessed later when time permits.

Attention is now focused on the remaining, nonambulatory casualties. Using the START algorithm, each casualty is assessed for ventilation, perfusion, and mental status in sequence. Casualties with no ventilation are expectant. Casualties with tachypnea (>30 respirations per minute for adults) are immediate. A similar process is used for assessment of perfusion and mental status. In this fashion, all casualties are rapidly triaged and assigned an initial category.

Ongoing Triage

START is an excellent technique for initial triage. Its primary purpose is to clear the battlefield, disaster site, or mass casualty site. However, since triage is a continual, dynamic process, it does not end with START. Additional triage is needed to retriage and possibly reclassify patients. This can take place at the aid post, casualty collecting point, aid station, hospital, or any stage in between. The closer the casualty arrives to the hospital, the more detailed the triage assessment and the more complex the decision making. The next section briefly outlines the stages or echelons of care, and subsequent sections provide more detail on triage decisions after START.

Echelons of Care

Echelon refers to stage, as in different levels or points of care, from scene of injury to hospital. In the military, five echelons of care are identified (Table 10-5). For this discussion, we focus on the first two levels because these echelons are found far-forward on the battlefield. Traditional civilian EMS providers operate in similar echelons although the parallel is not exact. Prehospital care and EMS (to include first responders) comprise echelon I (Table 10-6). Echelon II does not usually have a civilian correlation. In disasters and in mass-gathering medical care, however, an echelon II facility might be a field treatment site staffed with physicians, nurses, and limited diagnostic support. Echelon III and IV represent local hospitals and regional trauma centers, respectively.

Civilian EMS providers on large tactical missions are probably familiar with the military version of echelons of care. Tactical medics provide echelon I care, whereas the command post probably has a co-located echelon II medical station, perhaps staffed with

TABLE 10-5

MILITARY ECHELONS OF CARE

ECHELON	LEVEL OF CARE
I	Emergency medical treatment
II	Resuscitative treatment
III	Resuscitative surgery
IV	Reconstructive surgery
V	Rehabilitation

TABLE 10-6

ECHELONS OF CARE AND CORRESPONDING CIVILIAN ELEMENTS

ECHELON	MILITARY	CIVILIAN*
I	Self and buddy aid, medic	First responder, EMT, paramedic
II	Medical company	Treatment area in mass casualty incident
III	Combat support hospital	Community hospital
IV	General hospital	Regional hospital
V	Military or VA hospital	Regional trauma center

*Comparison is for illustration only.

a physician. In sea or air operations, echelonment may take a different form. Echelon I still represents the most forward elements of care, usually a Navy corpsman or an Air Force medical technician. Echelon II might be at a beachhead or airstrip, or onboard a ship (such as an LST or helicopter carrier). Echelon III facilities exist on larger ships, typically aircraft carriers. A hospital ship is a full-service medical facility and can provide the equivalent of echelon IV care.

TRIAGE DECISION MAKING

Triage is a dynamic process with constant reevaluations, assessments, and decisions made on patient classification. At each stage of care, the medic should make every effort to retriage, and if necessary, recategorize the patients in his or her care. Once all patients are triaged, begin treating the highest priority patients (if tactical circumstances allow). This process is repeated at each stage or echelon of care, all the way to definitive care at the hospital. Because patient conditions can change with time and treatment, retriage patients after long transports or other lengthy intervals.

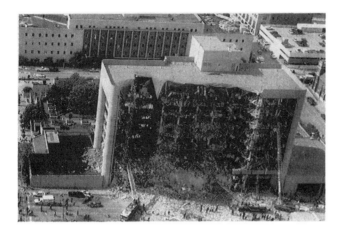

Figure 10-2 A mass casualty incident can involve both military and civilian medical providers. Oklahoma City bombing, April 19, 1995.

Initial Triage

The best guideline for initial tactical triage is the START method. START is most useful in initially clearing the battle zone or disaster sites (Figure 10-2). It focuses on airway, breathing, perfusion, and mental status. Of great importance, it also helps clear the site of ambulatory (walking-wounded) patients, dramatically reducing evacuation resources.

Subsequent Triage

START is an excellent method for initial triage. However, once the patient begins to move toward higher echelon care (evacuation), a more detailed approach to triage is needed. This is particularly true if the treatment capabilities improve as the patient is evacuated. With more advanced and complex treatments, more detailed and accurate triage is needed to identify casualties most likely to benefit.

Table 10-7 outlines a more detailed approach to triage. Similar to START, this outline follows the ABCs of prehospital care, but requires a more thorough assessment of the patient's condition. With practice, an experienced medic can accomplish most of the assessment in under 1 minute.

Immediate

When conducting triage, it is helpful to focus on the few medical conditions warranting the immediate, or highest priority, category. Table 10-8 lists several conditions fitting this category. Knowledge of these problems can help focus the brief and rapid history and physical examinations required for effective field triage.

Delayed

Table 10-9 list conditions fitting the delayed category. Many of these conditions are serious and potentially life threatening. They may require extensive and intensive treatment. However, they are not expected to significantly deteriorate over several hours and, therefore, can safely wait until the immediate category of patients can be stabilized. Of course,

TABLE 10-7

SUBSEQUENT TRIAGE REQUIRES A FOCUSED ASSESSMENT

- Airway
- Verbal response (talking/crying phonation)
- Evidence of obstruction
- Breathing
- Rate, depth (chest expansion)
- Breath sounds bilaterally
- Circulation
- Pulse rate
- Capillary refill
- Gross bleeding
- Disability (neurological)
- Level of responsiveness (AVPU)
- Ability to move all four extremities
- Expose
- Undress patient
- Examine for major problems

TABLE 10-8

SOME MEDICAL CONDITIONS WARRANTING "IMMEDIATE" CATEGORIZATION (HIGHEST PRIORITY)

- Upper airway obstruction, stridor
- Life-threatening bleeding
- Tension pneumothorax
- Extensive second- or third-degree facial burns
- Untreated poisoning (chemical agent) and severe symptoms
- Heat stroke
- Severe respiratory distress
- Decompensated shock
- Complicated obstetrical delivery (e.g., breech, associated seizures, prolapsed cord)
- Rapidly deteriorating level of responsiveness
- Any life-threatening condition that is rapidly progressing

TABLE 10-9

SOME MEDICAL CONDITIONS WARRANTING
"DELAYED" CATEGORIZATION (NEXT HIGHEST PRIORITY)

- Compensated shock
- Fracture, dislocation, or injury causing circulatory compromise
- Severe bleeding controlled by tourniquet or other means
- Suspected compartment syndrome
- Open fractures and dislocations
- Penetrating head, neck, chest, back, or abdominal injuries without airway or breathing compromise or decompensated shock
- Severe headache with altered mental status
- Severe abdominal pain with abdominal wall rigidity and no shock
- Uncomplicated, immobilized cervical spine injuries
- Fever (rectal) > 40°C or 104°F in child < 3 years old or > 38°C or 100°F in child < 3 months old
- Large, dirty, or crushed soft tissue wounds
- Moderate dyspnea (not rapidly worsening)
- Severe combat stress symptoms or psychosis
- Other conditions that are unlikely to worsen over the next several hours

a delayed patient can unexpectedly deteriorate (or, perhaps, improve) and may need to be recategorized as appropriate. This again underscores the need for constant retriage.

Minimal

Patients falling into the minimal category are those who still need treatment but have conditions unlikely to deteriorate over a day or so. Table 10-10 outlines just a few of the conditions meeting this requirement. Most of these patients will be ambulatory and, in fact, may be capable of assisting with the relief operation.

In military operations, it is important for triage personnel to identify minimal casualties who can be returned to duty with little or no treatment. In a dire military circumstance where the mission is in jeopardy, it may be necessary to take these patients out of order and treat them first. This returns to the commander the maximum fighting strength available to accomplish a critical mission. This may be the only exception to treating a minimal casualty before an immediate one.

Expectant

Expectant patients are, by definition, expected to die, unless maximal resources are expended. Since triage implies multiple patients and few resources, the maximal resources are unavailable. Table 10-11 outlines medical conditions fitting the expectant

TABLE 10-10

SOME MEDICAL CONDITIONS WARRANTING
"MINIMAL" CATEGORIZATION (THIRD HIGHEST PRIORITY)

- Closed fractures and dislocations, uncomplicated
- Uncomplicated or minor lacerations (including those involving tendons, muscle, and nerves)
- Burns involving < 20% BSA in an adult
- Frostbite
- Dental pain
- Strains, sprains, bruises
- Minor head injury (LOC < 5 min, now with normal mental status)
- Mild respiratory distress
- Chest pain in person < 40 years old
- Penetrating injuries to extremities (bleeding controlled)
- Other conditions not likely to deteriorate

category. *Notably, expectant does not mean "no treatment." Rather, it means intensive time-consuming treatment will be withheld until higher priority patients are cared for first. Basic comfort care, such as blankets and parenteral analgesia (IV or IM morphine, for example) should be provided.* If all other higher priority patients are stabilized, attention can then be given to the expectant patient. If tactical conditions are favorable, it may be worthwhile attempting a resuscitation on an expectant patient if no higher priority patient demands care.

Flexibility in Triage

It cannot be overemphasized that triage is a dynamic process. The standard four categories are merely a convenient tool for the medic to use in rapidly and effectively conducting triage. Depending on circumstances and the tactical scenario, casualties may

TABLE 10-11

SOME MEDICAL CONDITIONS WARRANTING
"EXPECTANT" CATEGORIZATION (LAST PRIORITY)

- Cardiac arrest from any cause *
- Respiratory arrest (except when caused by drugs, poisons, or airway obstruction)
- Massive brain injury
- Second- or third-degree burns > 70% BSA (> 50% for elderly or chronically ill individuals)
- GSW to head with GCS = 3
- Cardiogenic shock (decompensated)

*See Table 1-8 for possible exceptions.

need to be upgraded or downgraded. Tables 10-8 to 10-11 are merely guides and are not meant to replace good tactical medical judgment.

MASS CASUALTY INCIDENTS

Mass casualty incidents (MCI in civilian parlance or MASCAL in the military) are characterized by an overwhelming number of patients (usually all at once) compared to available medical personnel and resources. In the military, this can be a result of an intense fire fight, artillery attack, shipboard fire, or aircraft crash, for example. Civilian disasters range from natural events such as hurricanes, tornadoes, earthquakes, and volcano eruptions to floods, avalanches, and epidemics. Man-made events include radioactive and chemical releases, airplane crashes, and multiple-car collisions. Large structure fires and industrial accidents can also result in multiple casualties. Terrorist attacks (Figure 10-2), regional wars, and famine represent emerging concerns with great potential to generate multiple simultaneous casualties. Despite this wide array of causes, common principles still apply to all MASCAL events. This section provides an overview of MASCAL operations with an emphasis on the tactical perspective.

Concept of Operation

The first step when faced with a MASCAL is to ensure scene safety. This may entail engaging the enemy with return fire, putting on NBC protecting garments and mask, or other measures to ensure team safety. The second step is to estimate roughly the size and scope of the MASCAL, and communicate this information to the mission commander. Be sure to include requests for additional support (such as more litter bearers) or for special resources (a hazardous materials team or NBC decontamination unit, for example). Since this is a preliminary report, speed of communication takes precedence over exact accuracy. Subsequent reports can always be transmitted that update or refine the information.

Once scene safety and initial communications are achieved, the medical personnel should assemble into triage and treatment teams, and plans should be made for evacuation. Triage, treatment, and evacuation then commence. Since additional resources will usually begin to arrive, these assets are added, and the process develops. Afterward, retrograde or cleanup operations begin and the MASCAL ends.

Triage Teams

In general, the most highly trained and experienced field personnel should lead triage. In the tactical setting, this will often be the senior medic. In large operations, a field-experienced physician may be triage team leader. The leader's role is to make the actual triage decisions and direct the other team members. (In many tactical situations, there will be only one medic, and thus the "team" will be an individual.) For initial field triage, use the START method. Move quickly, spending no more than 10-12 seconds per patient. Remember, by definition, triage is a rapid decision made on incomplete information. Subsequent iterations of triage at higher echelons will adjust patients' categories as appropriate.

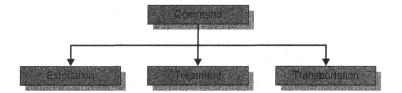

Figure 10-3 Incident command system.

Treatment Teams

Treatment teams, evacuation, and staging areas and other support elements will be employed only in large MASCAL. In the tactical environment, such elaborate setups are rarely encountered at the first echelon of care. Instead, the focus is to clear the MAS-CAL site and evacuate casualties by whatever means possible. Readers wanting more information on treatment teams, staging areas, and other elements of large MASCAL are invited to consult the reading list at the end of the chapter.

Incident Command System

The incident command system (ICS; Figure 10-3) is a civilian method of organizing the personnel and equipment employed at a MASCAL or other large incident. It defines command, control, and communication relationships, and establishes areas of responsibility. For example, the medical branch is responsible for triage and treatment of patients. ICS allows different agencies in different parts of the country to operate together in support of large incidents.

ICS is a civilian method of command and control. Tactical medics need to be familiar with it, however, because they may be deployed in support of a civilian disaster. Also, tactical medics supporting law enforcement will be operating under ICS from time to time. Fortunately, tactical medics can easily adapt to ICS because the principles borrow from military command and control procedures. First, the ICS commander has overall responsibility for the incident, just as the tactical mission commander is the ultimate authority for the mission. Medical needs may not necessarily take priority if mission or incident needs take precedence. Second, ICS follows the chain of command, a concept to which all tactical medics are accustomed. Last, ICS is built on flexibility to allow for a wide variety of incidents. Tactical training, too, encourages flexibility and improvisation. Thus the basic principles of ICS should come easy to the tactical medic.

Triage Tags

Triage tags are designed to communicate the triage category, treatment rendered, and other medical information. By necessity, the information on tags is brief. Triage tags are usually placed on the casualty by the triage officer although other members of the team may place or add information to the tags.

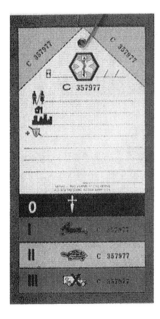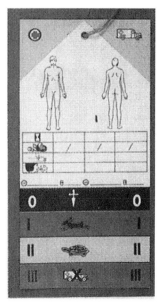

Figure 10-4 Civilian
METTAG triage tag.

The tactical medic must be familiar with two different types of triage tags. The first is the civilian tag, of which the METTAG is the most popular (Figure 10-4). The tag has color-coded perforated tabs that make it easy to identify a casualty's category quickly. Since these color codes correspond with the NATO classification system (Table 10-12), tactical medics should easily adapt to using METTAGs.

The other tag in widespread use is the military field medical card (FMC; Figure 10-5). Although the FMC serves a similar purpose as METTAG triage tags, the design is less intuitive and more difficult for the novice to use. (The design is limited, in part, by international agreements.) Nonetheless, with practice, the FMC can be as effective as fancier designs.

Not all portions of the FMC need to be completed at the time of triage. In fact, in a MASCAL, only the triage category would be recorded. If possible, however, the medic

TABLE 10-12

METTAG AND NATO CATEGORIES

METTAG COLOR	METTAG DESCRIPTION	NATO
Red	Urgent	Immediate
Yellow	Nonurgent	Delayed
Green	No hospital treatment	Minimal
Black	Dead or unsalvageable	Expectant

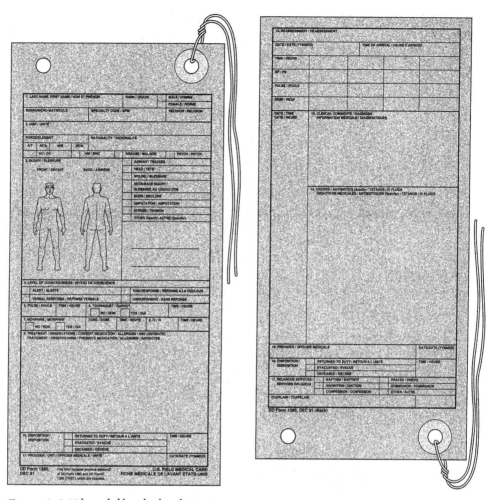

Figure 10-5 Military field medical card (FMC).

should attempt to complete all the information outlined in Table 10-13. The other portions on the FMC can be safely ignored until later. They will be completed once the casualty reaches a higher echelon facility such as a hospital.

When writing on an FMC or triage tag, use indelible ink. Attach the tag to the casualty's wrist or ankle. Attaching the tag to the casualty's shirt buttons is risky if his or her clothing is removed during tactical field care or evacuation. Both the FMC and METTAG allow the medic to maintain patient accountability. The FMC has carbonless copies, whereas the METTAG has detachable, numbered tabs. After each casualty is triaged and tagged, keep one copy or tab. Later, these can be used to reconcile patient counts, and so on.

TABLE 10-13

DESIRABLE INFORMATION TO INCLUDE ON THE MILITARY
FMC AT TIME OF INITIAL FIELD TREATMENT

Name
Service number (Social Security Number)
Age
Grade and unit
Date and time of encounter
Assessment
Field treatment

TIPS AND PITFALLS IN TRIAGE

Move Quickly

The most common error in MASCAL situations is moving too slowly. Do not dwell on any one patient. Make the initial triage decision based on a rapid assessment of airway, breathing, perfusion, and responsiveness (Table 10-4). Avoid any temptation to assess for other injuries, or worse, to treat injuries. Once all patients are triaged, a second round of triage can be performed with more focus.

Do Not Second-Guess

Trust your medical instincts. Do not go back to retriage until all casualties have been triaged. Remember, the goal is the greatest good for the greatest number of casualties.

Let the Most Experienced Lead

The medical team member with the greatest training and experience (relevant to tactical emergency care) should be triage leader, regardless of rank or position. Do not allow petty power concerns to get in the way of good patient care.

Plan Ahead

Have a plan or SOP for dealing with triage and mass casualty situations. Identify areas of responsibility, evacuation and treatment procedures, communications links, and other essential procedures.

SUMMARY

Triage is a method of sorting patients by order of priority. The overriding **principle** of triage is the "greatest good for the greatest number of casualties." Triage, like **all medical** procedures, requires training and experience to perform well. Mass casualty **situations** overwhelm the available medical resources and require the use of triage to set patient priorities.

FOR FURTHER READING

KENNEDY K et al.: Triage: Techniques and Applications in Decision **Making. Annals** Emergency Medicine, 1996; 28: 136-144.

RYAN JM et al.: Assessing Injury Severity During General War: Will the **Military Triage** System Meet Future Needs? Journal Royal Army Medical Corps, 1990; 146: 27-35.

AUF DER HEIDE E: Disaster Response. CV Mosby Co., St. Louis. 1989.

LLEWELLYN CM: Triage: In Austere Environments and Echeloned **Medical Systems.** World Journal Surgery, 1992; 16: 904-909.

EASTMAN AB et al.: Field Triage, in Feliciano DV et al. (eds): **Trauma, 3rd ed.** Appleton & Lange, Stanford, CT, 1996.

11

TACTICAL ENVIRONMENTAL AND PREVENTIVE MEDICINE

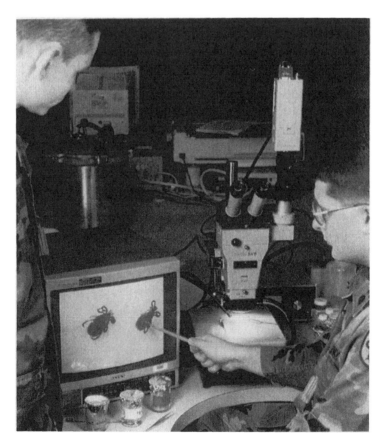

Medics use computer technology to identify potential disease vectors.

OBJECTIVES

After reading this chapter, you will be able to:
1. Describe the medical threat assessment, and list the major medical threats in the tactical setting.
2. Outline the risks of heat injury, and describe the strategies of minimizing this risk.
3. Demonstrate knowledge of the wet bulb globe temperature (WBGT) index, and apply it to work-rest cycles in the tactical setting.
4. Outline the risks of cold injury, and describe the strategies of minimizing this risk.
5. Demonstrate knowledge of the wind-chill chart, and apply it to cold injury countermeasures in the tactical setting.
6. Describe the methods of the water purification recommended for use in the tactical environment.
7. Outline the principles of safe food handling, serving, and storage.
8. Describe the importance of good personal hygiene and handwashing in the prevention of disease.
9. Outline the major types of tactical field latrines and the situations for which they are suited.
10. Describe the normal and abnormal responses to psychological stress, and outline the key clinical findings and treatment of abnormal reactions.
11. Outline the principles of vector control in the tactical setting.

CASE

You are a medic assigned to a joint task force providing humanitarian assistance to disaster areas. In addition to your regular medical duties, you are responsible for preventive medicine operations in your unit. Your job is to assure the food is safe to eat, the water is clean and uncontaminated, latrine facilities are sanitary, and the spread of contagious diseases is minimized. In effect, you are the public health representative for your commander and unit. Their safety and well-being depend largely on your skills in preventive medicine.

Effectively accomplishing your preventive-medicine tasks requires constant vigilance. Water sources and containers must be inspected and checked for chlorine residual, food serving and storage temperature must be measured, and latrine facilities planned and constructed in a sanitary fashion. Disease-spreading insects and rodents must be controlled, and strict hand washing enforced among food handlers. To extend your positive influence as far as possible, you must be both a medical expert and diplomat. Communication with cooks, food handlers, latrine diggers, and field sanitation teams is essential. You must regularly consult the unit physician for specific preventive medicine advice, and keep your leaders informed. The success of the mission depends on a healthy force, and effective preventive medicine can help accomplish this.

INTRODUCTION

Medical personnel operating in a field or tactical environment face challenges not encountered in ordinary prehospital operations. Extremes of the environment, including weather, insects, and disease, pose concerns not only for patient care but also for the effectiveness of the medical team and operational unit members. Keeping clean and hygienic in the field is not merely a matter of comfort, but of health, too. Lastly, the extreme emotional stress possible on tactical missions requires the medic to be prepared to deal with the effects of combat stress.

This chapter explores this diverse array of problems with a focus on prevention. Thus, this chapter is an introduction to preventive medicine in the field. Although treatment is certainly important for the medic, prevention is better. Prevention preserves the strength of the unit to accomplish its mission while conserving medical resources. For this reason, preventive medicine is essential for all medics or prehospital personnel operating for any period in field or tactical conditions. Readers desiring a more detailed discussion of treatment are referred to general texts on emergency care.

History

Historically, disease and nonbattle injuries (for example, heat or cold injuries) have claimed far more casualties than actual combat during war. In the past 200 years, the United States has sustained 80% of its casualties this way. Only 20% occurred from bullets, munitions, and the like. Major battles of this century have been won and lost by these effects. The German invasion of Russia in World War II was halted mostly by the harsh Siberian winter (cold injuries). Trenchfoot was a significant problem for both the British and Germans in World War I. Insects posed a major challenge to forces operating in the Pacific during World War II and in Vietnam. On the civilian front, lengthy standoffs between barricaded suspects and law enforcement (for example, Waco, Texas) have forced tactical medics to spend many hours facing the harsh elements.

MEDICAL THREAT ASSESSMENT

The medical threat comprises both potential enemy or hostile actions and environmental conditions that reduce the effectiveness of the tactical unit. Essentially, it is those medical conditions that tactical medics must be familiar with to be effective in their mission. Significant medical threats are weapons or environmental conditions that keep unit members from returning to duty.

Elements

The elements of the medical threat include a range of hostile actions such as battle injuries and NBC threats and environmental extremes such as heat and cold (Figure 11-1). Table 11-1 lists the elements of the medical threat. This chapter focuses on the environmental and preventive medicine aspects of the medial threat.

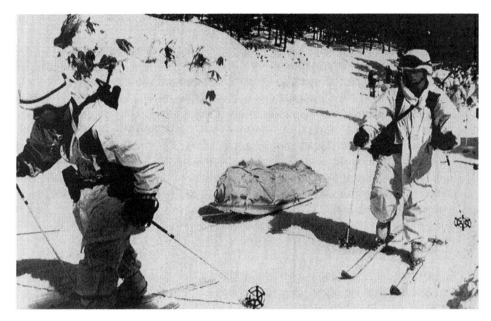

Figure 11-1 Extremes of weather are common in the tactical environment.

Medical Threat Assessment

The medical threat assessment is a tool used by unit leaders and medical personnel to prepare for the most likely threats. With advanced knowledge of the likely threats, the unit leader can take steps to minimize or avoid the threat. *Ideally, the medical threat assessment takes place well before the start of the operation.* This affords the greatest opportunity to plan,

---

TABLE 11-1

ELEMENTS OF THE MEDICAL THREAT

- Naturally occurring disease
- Environmental extremes and hazards
- Battle injuries
- Direct energy weapons
- Blast effect munitions
- Flame and incendiary weapons
- Missiles
- Nuclear weapons
- Biological weapons
- Chemical weapons
- Combat and psychological stress

---

train, and equip to meet the threat. However, even a short notice can be helpful to the unit leader or commander.

The most senior-level medical person in a unit is usually responsible for preparing the medical threat assessment. For small units, this may be the individual tactical medic. Ordinarily, the threat assessment need not be complex or lengthy. In military operations, much of the information needed to formulate a medical threat assessment can be a gleaned from the operations order (Op Order). The Op Order contains information about enemy forces, terrain, weather, and other details that provide the specifics about likely threats. For example, if the Op Order states the unit will be breaching a minefield, and the weather will be cold and wet, then likely threats include blast and shrapnel injuries and hypothermia. In turn, this information can be used to supplement stocks of bandages and initiate refresher training on the warning signs of hypothermia.

Medical Intelligence

Medical intelligence includes not only the medical threat assessment but also information on medical facilities, evacuation assets, and other factors that may affect the availability of tactical care. Again, the senior medic is responsible for investigating what is already in place for a given operation. For example, a nearby civilian hospital with a reputation for good care may be available to use during the operation. Alternatively, a complete lack of indigenous medical infrastructure may compel the unit to bring complete medical teams and evacuation capabilities.

In summary, the medical threat assessment and medical intelligence gathering is the process of gathering essential medical information before an operation begins. Good medical information will allow unit leaders and medics to tailor the operational plan in the most effective and efficient manner.

HEAT INJURIES

Heat injuries usually occur in hot climates such as deserts and jungles but can also occur in temperate and even cool climates. The extra exertion common on tactical operations coupled with heavy, dark uniforms, body armor, helmets, and lots of extra gear compounds the risk. For this reason, all medics should be alert to the possibility of heat injury in all but the coolest of conditions.

Heat Injury Risk

The risk of heat injury rises with increasing temperature and humidity. Hot, humid conditions can combine to present great risk. The wet bulb globe temperature (WBGT) index is a measure of the heat burden that takes into account temperature, humidity, and sunlight. WBGT is frequently available from the weather service or installation operations center.

TABLE 11-2

WATER INTAKE AND WORK-REST CYCLE
RECOMMENDATIONS FOR HOT CONDITIONS AND HEAVY WORK

WBGT (°F)	WBGT (°C)	WATER INTAKE (QT/HR) (L/HR)*	HOURLY WORK-REST CYCLES (MIN)
Below 82	Below 27.5	0.75	40/20
82-84	27.5-29	1.0	30/30
85-87	28-30.5	1.0	30/30
88-89	31-31.5	1.0	20/40
90 above	32 above	1.0	10/50

*Do not exceed 1.5 qt/hr (l/hr) or 12 qt/day (l/day).
WBGT= wet bulb globe temperature index. Adapted from FM 21-1, Dept. of the Army, Washington, D.C., and other sources.

Strategies

The more strenuous the activity, the greater the body's heat production. Thus a key way to reduce the risk of heat injury is to reduce exertion. *Without a doubt, the most effective strategy to reduce the risk of heat injury is to drink plenty of water and rest often.* Table 11-2 provides water intake and work-rest cycle recommendations for hot conditions and heavy work. Do not exceed 1.5 qt/hr (l/hr) or a total of 12 quarts (liters) in 24 hours. Table 11-3 lists other strategies to avoid heat injury. Be particularly cautious when fully suited in an NBC protective ensemble. The ensemble adds 5°-9°C (10-15°F) to the WBGT index when calculating the heat injury risk.

Acclimatization

Given several weeks' time, the human body can become acclimatized or adapted to hot environments. The kidneys will conserve water while the heat-loss mechanisms (primarily sweating) become more efficient. If at all possible, allow the team to work moderately

TABLE 11-3

STRATEGIES TO PROTECT AGAINST HEAT INJURY

- Drink plenty of water
- Enforce work-rest cycles
- Stay in shade
- Choose evening or morning for strenuous work
- Avoid tight, nonbreathable clothing
- Maintain physical fitness
- Avoid medications that increase heat injury risk

in the hot environment (with frequent rest and plenty of water) for 2 to 3 weeks before embarking on strenuous activity. *Acclimatization, though helpful in reducing heat-related injuries, does not entirely reduce the risk of heat injury.* Careful attention to the medical threat of heat injury must always be considered in hot conditions.

COLD INJURIES

Cold injuries have plagued tactical forces for centuries. Many operations, by necessity take place outside, exposed to the elements. Long periods of inactivity, such as guard duty, surveillance, and intelligence-gathering operations, coupled with physical exhaustion provide many opportunities for cold injuries to occur. Waterborne operations, including amphibious landings, river fording, or swamp crossings are at particular risk, owing to the dangerous capacity of water to hasten cold injuries. Even simple exposure to rain or a sweat-soaked uniform can turn an otherwise benign climate into a dangerously cold one. Therefore, all medics must be thoroughly versed in the prevention, recognition, and treatment of cold injuries. This section outlines the preventive strategies needed by medics to avoid cold injuries for themselves and their teams.

Cold Injury Types

There are 3 major types of cold-related injuries to be concerned about: (1) hypothermia, (2) frostbite, and (3) immersion foot. Although the three types of injuries have different presentations and symptoms, they all share similar risk factors and similar prevention strategies. Thus, by preparing and avoiding one cold injury type, all will generally be avoided.

Cold Injury Risk

Cold injury risk increases as the air temperature declines. However, air temperature is not the only factor to consider. Two other factors, moisture and wind speed, can dramatically increase the cold injury risk. Remember, it does not have to be below freezing for you to suffer severe cold injury. Temperatures as high as 10°-15°C (50°-60°F) can cause cold injury under the right conditions!

Temperature and Wind

Wind increases cooling of exposed body surfaces through convection and evaporation. As wind speed increases, so does cooling. This effect is known as windchill. For example, a 20 mph (30 km/h) wind on a 32°F (0°C) day can make it feel as cold as 7°F (-14°C). Figure 11-2 shows the windchill for various temperatures and wind speeds. Any exposed flesh, including skin surfaces inadequately covered by effective, wind-breaking material, will be affected. Commonly exposed areas include all parts of the face, neck, and hands.

Moisture and Water

Moisture is a significant threat in any operation occurring in cool or cold conditions. *Water conducts heat many times faster than air, and the evaporative effects of water can cause*

WIND CHILL CHART											
	LOCAL TEMPERATURE (°F)										
	32	23	14	5	-4	-13	-22	-31	-40	-49	-58
Wind Speed (MPH)	**EQUIVALENT TEMPERATURE (°F)**										
CALM	32	23	14	5	-4	-13	-22	-31	-40	-49	-58
5	29	20	10	1	-9	-18	-28	-37	-47	-56	-65
10	18	7	-4	-15	-26	-37	-48	-59	-70	-81	-91
15	13	-1	-13	-25	-7	-49	-61	-73	-85	-97	-109
20	7	-6	-10	-32	-44	-57	-70	-83	-96	-109	-121
25	3	-10	-24	-37	-50	-64	-77	-90	-104	-117	-117
30	1	-13	-27	-41	-54	-68	-82	-97	-109	-123	-137
35	-1	-15	-29	-43	-57	-71	-85	-99	-113	-127	-142
40	-3	-17	-31	-45	-59	-74	-87	-102	-116	-131	-145
45	-3	-18	-32	-46	-61	-75	-89	-104	-118	-132	-147
50	-4	-18	-33	-47	-62	-76	-91	-105	-120	-134	-148
	LITTLE DANGER FOR PROPERLY CLOTHED PERSONS*			**CONSIDERABLE DANGER***			**VERY GREAT DANGER***				
*DANGER FROM FREEZING OF EXPOSED FLESH											

Figure 11-2 Wind-chill chart.

rapid body cooling. Measures to prevent the soaking of clothes from the outside (from rain, sleet, snow) and the inside (perspiration) will be critical to avoiding cold injury. Operations occurring in water (scuba, river fording, swamp crossings) are at high risk for hypothermia, even at temperatures well above freezing.

Strategies

Measures to decrease cold injury risk primarily involve controlling or avoiding cold, wind, and moisture. Proper clothing and equipment is critical in this regard. The tried-and-true strategy of wearing multiple thin layers of clothing instead of one bulky layer remains true today. As temperatures and comfort levels change, layers can be added or taken away. New, lightweight "breathable" shells offer the best of both worlds: repelling water while allowing perspiration to escape. This reduces the danger of moisture buildup next to the skin.

Acclimatization

The human body has little or no capacity to adapt or acclimatize to a cold environment. In other words, the physiological response of the body does not improve over time. The risk of cold injury is just as great after the team has spent days or weeks in the cold environment as when the operation began. What does improve is the team member's strategies and coping skills to avoid cold injury. Protection from the cold is a learned skill. Training and experience are important.

Human Differences

Research has shown that different people have different risks for cold injury. The very young and old, as well as the ill or injured (for example, the medic's patients) are more susceptible than young, healthy adults. Different races and ethnic backgrounds also influence cold risk. The important message for leaders and medics alike is to maintain a high degree of vigilance when assessing team members for cold injury. It is entirely possible for just one team member to sustain cold injury even when all team members share similar exposure to the cold.

The Feet

Special attention should be paid to the feet. Because of their contact with the cold ground, tight fitting boots, and constant perspiration, the feet are at great risk for frostbite and immersion foot. Even a minor cold injury to the foot can incapacitate a person; therefore, prevention is crucial. Despite high-technology boots, moisture-wicking socks, and other innovations, there remains no substitute for frequent sock changes in the field. Under normal conditions, this should be a matter of routine once or twice daily. Under very cold or wet conditions, three to four times daily is not unreasonable. Table 11-4 lists some strategies to prevent cold injuries.

TABLE 11-4

STRATEGIES TO AVOID COLD INJURY

- Avoid cold, wind, and moisture
- Wear multiple layers of loose-fitting clothing
- Wear a water repellent but "breathable" shell
- Change socks frequently
- Drink plenty of fluids
- Get plenty of rest, and eat all meals
- Avoid alcohol and tobacco

TABLE 11-5

COLD INJURIES COUNTERMEASURES

WIND-CHILL	TEMPERATURE COUNTERMEASURE
30°F (-1°C) and below	• Remind personnel of cold injury risk
25°F (-4°C) and below	• Team leaders and medics inspect personnel for proper wear of protective clothing
	• Provide warm-up shelters and warm beverages
0°F (-18°C) and below	• Team leader and medics inspect personnel for early signs of cold injury
	• Rotate exposed and stationary personnel frequently
-10°F (-23°C) and below	• Ensure all personnel are paired and establish "buddy checks" for early signs of cold injury
-20°F (-29°C) and below	• If possible, modify or curtail mission to avoid cold exposure

Adapted from FM 21-10, Field Hygiene and Sanitation, Dept. of the Army, Washington, DC, 1983

Additional Strategies

In addition to proper clothing, modification of the mission and increased vigilance can reduce the risk of cold injury in severe conditions (Table 11-5). Furthermore, be sure to drink plenty of water, eat all meals, and get plenty of rest. Resistance to hypothermia and comfort levels all increase in well-rested and fed personnel. Just as important is avoidance of alcohol and tobacco. Alcohol not only impairs judgment but also causes vasodilatation, which increases the hypothermia risk. Tobacco (in any form, including smoking and chewing) can vasoconstrict the small vessels, greatly increasing the risk of frostbite in the hands and feet. Table 11-4 outlines some additional strategies to reducing the risk of cold injury.

DIARRHEA AND FOODBORNE ILLNESS

Tactical units operating in the field for anything beyond a day or two are at risk for diarrhea and foodborne illnesses. The risk rises dramatically the more food and water is procured locally rather than brought with the team or supplied directly from the base of operations. If possible, pack-in all the necessary food and water for the operation. However, this is not practical on an operation exceeding a few days. In this situation, the medic must be skilled in preventing diarrhea and foodborne illnesses in his or her unit. Diarrhea and foodborne illnesses usually strike a group of personnel or even the whole unit. Unit effectiveness can be greatly compromised. This section introduces the concepts of water purification, safe food preparation, and personal hygiene measures to reduce the risk of disease.

Water Purification

In the United States and most developed countries, the water supply is safe for drinking and cooking. In these countries, it is usually safe to trust the water supply. However, if in doubt, the water can be field tested and treated as outlined later. *If the safety of the water source cannot be assured, then it must be sanitized by either boiling or chemical means.* Boiling water for at least 5 minutes is very effective at removing diarrhea-causing organisms, but is not practical for large quantities of water. (In an emergency, boiling for only a few seconds is still very helpful.) The chemicals chlorine and iodine are the other preferred field methods of sanitizing the water. Chlorine, in particular, is very effective for purifying large quantities of water. Incidentally, chlorine purification is used by virtually every municipal water supplier in the United States, and billions of gallons of chlorine-treated water are consumed every day by most of the U.S. population. It is both safe and effective when used properly. Table 11-6 outlines several methods to sanitizing water for drinking and cooking.

Chlorine Levels

To ensure the continued safety of the water supply, periodically check the chlorine residual in the water using a water-testing kit. These kits are easy to use and readily available through military supply channels or from commercial suppliers (Figure 11-3). All field medics should be proficient in using these kits. Table 11-7 shows the recommended chlorine residuals for various water sources for field use. If the chlorine residual is too low, add more chlorine, mix the water thoroughly, and retest after 10 minutes. If the level is too high, no action is required. The water is safe for consumption as long as the chlorine residual is less than 15 ppm. Chlorine dissipates over time, so periodic rechecking is needed every few days.

TABLE 11-6

SEVERAL METHODS TO SANITIZING WATER FOR DRINKING AND COOKING

METHOD	AMOUNT	NOTES
Boiling	5-10 minutes	
Iodine tablets	1 tablet per quart/liter, wait 35 minutes	2 tablets for cloudy or very cold water
Chlorine ampule	1 ampule in canteen cup (8 oz or 0.25 l) to make solution.	Pour 1 tablespoon or 15 ml (1 canteen capful) of solution per quart/liter, wait 30 minutes
1 ampule	5 gallons (20 l)	Mix and check residual in 10 minutes (Table 11-7)
3 ampules	36 gallons (lister bag)	
Calcium hypochlorite	1 heaping tablespoon or 25 ml (1 messkit spoonful) per 400 gallons (water "buffalo" trailer)	Same as above

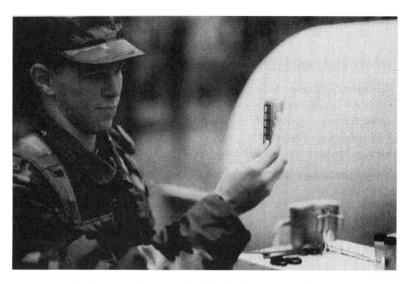

Figure 11-3 Checking the chlorine residual of a drinking water supply.

TABLE 11-7

CHLORINE RESIDUAL LEVELS OF DRINKING
AND COOKING WATER FOR FIELD OPERATIONS

SOURCE	CHLORINE RESIDUAL (PPM)
Municipal water at source (spigot, faucet)	0.5-1
Municipal water in storage containers	1-2
Other water, routine field conditions	5
High-risk situations (consult medical authority)	10

FOOD PREPARATION AND HANDLING

Just as a properly treated water supply is essential for field operations, so is a safe food supply. Food preparation in the field is inherently risky. The challenges of providing power, light, fuel, water, heat, and pest control make safe and efficient food preparation difficult. However, careful attention to just a few simple principles can dramatically reduce the risks of diarrhea and other foodborne illnesses in field kitchens. Table 11-8 outlines these principles.

TABLE 11-8

REDUCING DIARRHEA AND FOODBORNE ILLNESS RISKS IN FIELD FOOD OPERATIONS

- Use prepackaged meals designed for field use (MRE, precooked canned foods)
- Observe strict handwashing
- Avoid unapproved sources of food
- Keep hot foods hot—at or above 140ºF (60°C)
- Keep cold foods cold—at or below 40ºF (4.5°C)

Field Foods

The safest approach to providing food in the field is to use prepackaged meals designed for field use. The military Meal, ready to eat (MRE) is widely available, compact, nutritious, and available in a number of entrees. It can be eaten hot or cold, and has an exceptionally long shelf life (3-6 years). These characteristics make MREs ideal for short field operations. Alternatives or supplements to MREs include a wide variety of precooked and canned or shelf-stable products available at any supermarket.

Local Food Sources

Most prolonged operations will require the preparation of meals in the field from basic ingredients. Here, the source of the foodstuffs is important. Any locally procured foods must be from a reliable source. In the United States, most jurisdictions have adequate food safety laws and regulations in place to assure food safety. Outside the United States, it may be necessary to consult professional food inspectors or medical authorities to get information on local food safety.

Food Temperature

Careful attention to food temperature is a crucial element in any field food operation. Temperature greatly affects the growth rate of dangerous bacteria in food, the leading cause of foodborne illnesses. By regulating the temperature at which food is cooked, maintained, and stored, bacteria growth can be minimized. *Hot foods should be at least 140ºF (60°C). Cold foods should be kept at or below 40oF (4.5°C).* By adhering to these temperature requirements, the risk of promoting dangerous levels of bacteria is reduced. To measure food temperature, use any ordinary food thermometer. Place it in several portions of the food, and wait 1 to 2 minutes for the reading to stabilize.

Handwashing

To avoid the spread of diarrheal disease, all food handlers must observe strict handwashing. The hands must be washed for at least 2 minutes with warm water and soap after every bathroom use or contact with raw or undercooked meats, poultry, or fish. The use of disposable

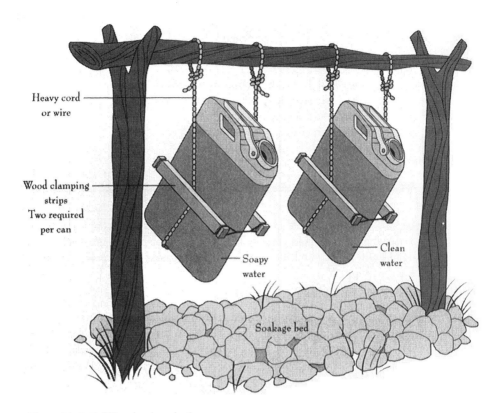

Figure 11-4 Field handwashing facility.

gloves can help reduce contamination of food but is not a substitute for thorough hand-washing by food handlers. Just as food handlers must wash their hands, so too must the personnel eating the food. Handwashing points should be established at the beginning of the food line and near all bathroom facilities (Figure 11-4).

FIELD SANITATION

Field sanitation is practically a discipline unto itself, requiring a diverse knowledge of biology, medicine, construction, and engineering. The medic plays an important role in assuring his or her unit complies with the basics of field sanitation. Good sanitation practices will not only improve the comfort of personnel in the field, but will reduce the risk of debilitating disease. Field sanitation involves topics already discussed, including food and water supply safety, as well as the content of this section: personal hygiene, latrine and bathroom facilities, and waste disposal. Insect control is discussed separately.

Personal Hygiene

Proper personal hygiene can go a long way toward improving comfort out in the field and even prevent debilitating and uncomfortable disease. Field conditions, by their very nature,

TABLE 11-9

PERSONAL HYGIENE IN THE FIELD

- Wash hands after bathroom use and before all meals
- Change socks at least once or twice daily
- Change underclothes daily
- Brush teeth daily
- Sponge bath daily
- Bath and change uniform twice weekly

make personal hygiene difficult. However, the medic can set the example for the unit by diligently following the basic guidelines in Table 11-9. Only a few minutes each day are needed to accomplish these tasks, and all can be completed without compromising the mission.

Latrines and Bathrooms

Properly prepared and marked latrines or bathrooms are essential to avoiding contaminating personnel, equipment, or worse, the food and water supply. *The practice of eliminating body wastes in the open (such as "behind a tree") is unsightly, smelly, and hazardous to all, and must be discouraged.* Instead, the following paragraphs describe some simple techniques for use as field latrines.

The most convenient choice for a field latrine is the portable toilet. This device is readily available from commercial vendors and has the advantage of being easy to clean, comfortable (compared to more expedient toilets), and self-contained. The primary disadvantage is lack of availability in remote locations. When available, however, the commercial portable toilet is the first choice for field latrine service.

In the absence of a portable toilet, a field expedient latrine must be constructed. Depending on the size of the unit, the length of the operation, and the degree of mobility expected, simple or elaborate toilets can be devised.

Site Selection

All latrines should be located as far away as practical from any food service, preparation, or storage areas. The minimum distance is 100 meters. Choose level ground, and avoid sites that are uphill from the primary campsite or water supply. Avoid sites that are close to streams, lakes, or ponds (including dry lakebeds or streambeds). As much as possible, locate latrines downwind from sleeping and food preparation areas.

Latrine Types

Field expedient latrines range from simple cat holes to multiple-hole deep pit latrines. This section focuses on the simpler types that are more practical for tactical teams on the move. Readers wishing additional details are referred to the sources listed at the end of the chapter.

TABLE 11-10

FIELD LATRINE TYPES AND USE

TYPE	TYPICAL USE
Cat hole	One-time use when on the move
Straddle trench	Several uses for short stay
Deep pit	Many uses for extended stay
Portable toilet	First choice, if available
Burn-out latrine	Same as deep pit

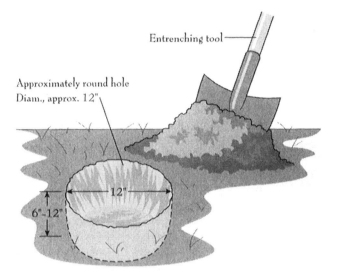

Figure 11-5 Cat hole latrine.

Table 11-10 lists field latrine types and their typical use. The cat hole (Figure 11-5) is the quickest of all latrines. It is simply a 12" diameter, 6-12" deep hole that is filled back after use. It may be used by two or three people and then closed. The straddle trench (Figure 11-6) is really just an elongated cat hole and allows use by several people simultaneously. It is dug as a 4' trench that is 2 1/2' deep and 1' wide. A good rule of thumb is to dig approximately 4 trenches per 100 males (1 trench for up to 25 men) and 6 trenches per 100 females.

The deep pit latrine (Figure 11-7) is more elaborate than trench latrines and is designed for longer-term use. If unable to dig the required 6' deep hole (water-logged ground or shallow bedrock), use the burn-out latrine. The large pails substitute for the deep pit and are periodically removed, and the waste is either burned or hauled to a sanitary facility.

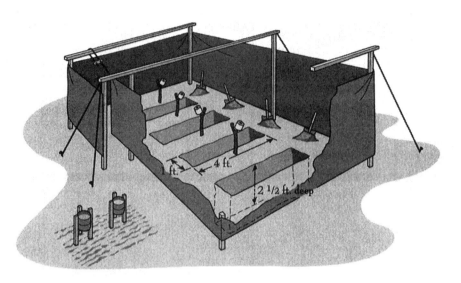

Figure 11-6 Straddle trench latrine.

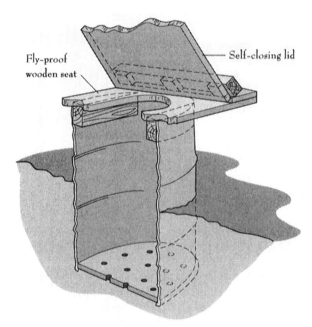

Figure 11-7 Deep pit latrine.

Latrine Sanitation

It is the responsibility of the medic periodically to inspect latrine facilities. Adequate toilet tissue is an obvious need, as are nearby handwashing facilities (Figure 11-4). Periodic spraying with insecticides will reduce housefly infestations. Full latrines need to be

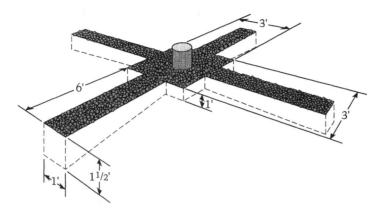

Figure 11-8 Soakage pit.

closed by filling with dirt and then marking the latrine (unless the mission prohibits this marking). Adequate latrine sanitation can reduce the spread of disease and improve the comfort of field operations.

Waste Disposal

Nonhuman waste includes food scraps, cooking grease, waste water, and ordinary trash. This waste requires proper disposal to avoid attracting flies, generating foul odors, and transmitting disease.

Ideally, waste should be hauled out of the field and sent to appropriate disposal facilities. If this is not possible, a field expedient method of disposal must be used. A garbage pit can be dug (4' x 4' x 4' deep hole) for the disposal of solid waste. Liquid waste requires a soakage pit (Figure 11-8). All waste pits should be periodically sprayed with insecticide and closed by burying. Solid waste may be burned if operational requirements permit. Never locate waste pits closer than 30 meters from food service, but do locate the pit sufficiently close to be convenient.

VECTOR CONTROL

Overview

In the tactical environment, **vector** refers to an animal, usually an insect, that transmits disease. Disease-carrying insects are a significant environmental threat to tactical units. Controlling these vectors can help prevent disease and have the added benefit of controlling annoying, but nondisease-carrying, biting insects and other pests.

Vectors and Disease

Table 11-11 outlines some typical insect vectors and the diseases they transmit. Though not all diseases are endemic to all parts of the world, the examples given illustrate the wide distribution of vector-borne diseases.

TABLE 11-11

VECTOR-BORNE DISEASES: TYPICAL EXAMPLES

VECTOR	DISEASE	DISTRIBUTION
Mosquito	Malaria	Tropics
Mosquito	Encephalitis	N. America, Asia, Europe
Tick	Rocky Mountain Spotted Fever	N. America
Tick	Lyme	N. America, Europe
Housefly	Diarrhea illness	Worldwide
Tse tse fly	Sleeping sickness	Africa

Control

The mainstays of vector control are proper sanitation, protective clothing, and chemical repellents (Table 11-12). Proper sanitation includes the use of properly constructed field latrines, good handwashing practices, and proper disposal of garbage. The previous sections of this chapter provide details on field sanitation.

Protective clothing is a critical element in preventing biting insects from getting to the skin. Long-sleeved shirts and long pants are a must in the field, as are adequate head and foot gear. Collars and cuffs should be snug (but not too tight). For sleep, blankets, mosquito netting, or indoor accommodations are needed.

Properly applied, chemical repellents can be a highly effective and safe means of preventing insect bites. Many commercial and government issue products are available, but the best products contain the repellent N,N diethyl-meta-toluamide, or DEET. Apply as directed, paying special attention to collar and cuff areas and any exposed skin. Avoid contact with the eyes, mouth, or other mucous membranes. Concentrations up to 25% may be used on adults, however, avoid concentrations exceeding 10% on children. Permethrin or other pyrethroid-containing products are also effective, but are applied to clothing only. They have the advantage of lasting through several washings. In all cases of applying chemical repellents, follow the manufacturer's directions carefully to avoid inadequate or toxic application.

TABLE 11-12

MAINSTAYS OF VECTOR CONTROL

- Proper sanitation
- Protective clothing
- Chemical repellents

PSYCHOLOGICAL STRESS

Stress, as used in this section, refers to the mind and body's natural reaction to environmental conditions. Stress is a normal and natural process, and occurs on a routine, daily basis. Operations in the field can frequently amplify stress because of austere, uncomfortable conditions, physical exhaustion, lack of sleep, and boredom. Later, when the "shooting starts," the psychological stress can be overwhelming and occasionally disabling. This section explores the stress of tactical operations, describing normal and abnormal responses. Emergency care is outlined and prevention strategies are discussed.

History

Psychological stress in tactical operations has been studied for years, mostly as it relates to military action and wars. In World War I, soldiers with abnormal psychological response to combat stress were termed *shell-shocked* for the unrelenting artillery shelling suffered by the troops. In World War II, the terms *combat fatigue* and *thousand-yard stare* emerged to describe the abnormal reactions to the horrors of war. More recently, the military has used the term *combat stress* to describe these effects. The civilian EMS profession has adopted a similar term: *critical incident stress*.

Normal Response

Anyone facing a serious life-threatening situation such as a gun battle, firefight, or NBC attack will normally feel the effects of fear, fright, and horror. This normal stress reaction is largely mediated by adrenaline, the "fight or flight" hormone. Table 11-13 lists the common symptoms of the normal reaction to acute stress.

The fight or flight reaction is a natural, protective reflex shared by all mammals. It is nature's way of mobilizing the organism to deal effectively with the threat. Its positive effects include enhanced alertness, vision, strength, and speed. These can certainly be an advantage when performing a tactical mission. Under most conditions, the majority of individuals will be able to channel this stress reaction appropriately to deal better with the threatening situation.

TABLE 11-13

NORMAL SYMPTOMS OF ACUTE PSYCHOLOGICAL STRESS

- Feelings of fear and anxiety
- Rapid, pounding heartbeat
- Sweaty palms and forehead
- Nausea and vomiting
- Rapid, shallow breathing
- Trembling, shaking
- Dilated pupils

TABLE 11-14

ABNORMAL FINDINGS OF ACUTE PSYCHOLOGICAL STRESS

MILD FINDINGS	SEVERE FINDINGS
Aches and pains	Significant personality change
Jumpiness and anxiety	Rapid, pressured talking
Cold sweat, dry mouth	Memory loss
Short of breath	Seeing or hearing things that aren't there (hallucinations)
Diarrhea or constipation	Complete withdrawal or constantly silent
Fatigued and tired	Complete lack of interest in food or sleep
Difficulty concentrating	Panic running or hysteria under fire

Abnormal Response

On occasion, a person facing a highly stressful situation will react with unhelpful, and sometimes debilitating, signs and symptoms. In severe cases, these symptoms can be life threatening. Table 11-14 outlines the spectrum of findings that may occur. Early recognition of these signs and symptoms is critical because most are treatable. Early intervention may improve the outcome and allow an earlier return of the casualty to duty.

Treatment

The principles of treating an acute stress reaction in the field are outlined in Table 11-15. The key point is to treat mild casualties as far forward as possible and with the expectation of recovery. By itself, this positive expectation can boost the casualty's morale and improve outcome. Severely affected casualties, on the other hand, need acute intervention and prompt evacuation. Severely affected casualties are treated just like ordinary psychological or psychiatric emergencies-with reassurance, compassion, and in extreme cases, restraint. Severely affected casualties are evacuated as expeditiously as possible.

TABLE 11-15

PRINCIPLES OF TREATING ABNORMAL REACTIONS TO ACUTE STRESS

- Expectation of recovery
- Short period of rest ("good night's sleep")
- Assign routine, productive duties to keep casualty busy (personal hygiene, helping with sick call, etc.)
- Treat forward; avoid evacuation unless symptoms interfere with mission
- Rapidly evacuate casualties when symptoms jeopardize the mission or pose a risk to self or others

TABLE 11-16

PREVENTION OF ACUTE STRESS REACTION IN THE TACTICAL ENVIRONMENT

- Enforce sleep discipline
- Reduce uncertainty by keeping unit informed
- Promote cohesion among unit members
- Promote health, safety, and welfare

Prevention

Simple steps can frequently reduce the risk of acute stress reactions in tactical situations. Perhaps most important is ensuring adequate sleep. Sleep deprivation markedly increases the risk of developing problems. At least 5 hours of uninterrupted sleep each day will allow for continuous operations. However, for short periods, even an hour or two of sleep can be helpful. Attention to unit and individual morale and welfare will also alleviate stress. Adequate food, water, and shelter can help resist the stress of hostile operations. Assimilate new members into the unit rapidly to avoid feelings of isolation. Table 11-16 outlines strategies to prevent acute stress reactions.

SUMMARY

Despite the harsh conditions of the tactical environment, the medic can learn to cope with the conditions. The primary environmental threats are heat and cold injuries, diarrhea and foodborne illness, and insect vectors. Preventive medicine for the tactical medic includes understanding the principles of field sanitation and safe food and water preparation. Attention to these principles will help ensure a safe and effective tactical operation and mission success.

FOR FURTHER READING

Field Manual 21-10 (Air Force Manual 161-10). Field Hygiene and Sanitation Department of the Army and Air Force, Washington, DC, 1983.

Field Manual 8-33, Control of Communicable Disease in Man, 13th ed. Department of the Army, Washington, DC.

Technical Bulletin TB MED 81. Cold Injury. Department of the Army, Washington, DC.

Technical Bulletin TB MED 507. Occupational and Environmental Health Protection, Treatment and Control of Heat Injury. Department of the Army, Washington, DC.

Technical Bulletin TB MED 576. Sanitary Control and Surveillance of Water Supplies at Fixed and Field Installations. Department of the Army, Washington, DC.

ZAJTCHUK R, Bellamy RF (eds): War Psychiatry. Department of the Army, Office of the Surgeon General, Washington, DC, 1995.

12

BASICS OF TACTICAL AMBULATORY CARE

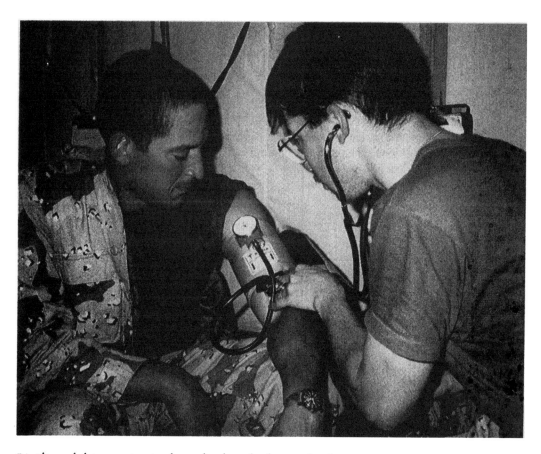

Providing ambulatory care is a time-honored tradition for the tactical medic.

After reading this chapter, you will be able to:
1.   Discuss the principles of tactical ambulatory care to include scope of practice, importance of physician supervision, and the approach to ambulatory care.
2.   Understand the parameters for the medic practice of ambulatory care.
3.   List the scope of practice elements for medic performance of ambulatory care for minor problems.
4.   List the minor complaints the tactical medic is likely to encounter.
5.   Discuss the specific fundamentals of identifying each of the uncomplicated minor problems listed in the chapter.
6.   Discuss the danger signals of each of the minor problems listed in the chapter.
7.   Discuss the specific fundamentals of treating each of the uncomplicated minor problems listed in the chapter.
8.   List the over-the-counter drugs on the medic formulary, and discuss their use.

CASE

You are a hospitalman 2nd class (HM2) aboard a Navy frigate cruising the Indian Ocean. While making your morning rounds inspecting the galley, you are approached by a sailor. He is requesting "aspirin" for a headache.

Because of your training and experience, you are authorized to provide advice and care for these types of minor complaints. Since the scene is safe, you immediately conduct an initial assessment, which shows a 22-year-old male sailor complaining of headache. He appears comfortable and his airway, breathing, and circulation are all intact. Vital signs are normal.

Focused assessment reveals the headache is neither severe nor sudden, and today's headache is similar to all previous headaches. The sailor denies loss of consciousness, recent trauma, fever, stiff neck, or vomiting. Physical examination is unremarkable, with normal neurologic examination.

The patient appears to have a mild, uncomplicated headache, for which he is requesting aspirin. Your protocol authorizes the dispensing of acetaminophen (aspirin-substitute) 650 mg by mouth, and the patient accepts the tablets. Before the sailor departs, you caution him to return if symptoms persist or worsen. You make a note in your logbook to check back with the sailor later in the day to see how he's doing. You also thoroughly document the patient's encounter and plan to discuss the care with the fleet medical officer later that afternoon.

INTRODUCTION

It is a time-honored tradition for the military medic to tend to the troops' minor medical needs (as well as providing emergency care). This minor, routine care goes by several names, including sick call, ambulatory care, and acute minor care. The common theme among these terms is the medical care of minor aches, pains, and ailments that the troops suffer during the course of normal duty.

This chapter introduces the basic principles of ambulatory care, with an emphasis on common problems encountered in the tactical environment. It is intended to give the medic a basic foundation for providing "first aid" for these problems. It is not intended as a substitute for a comprehensive text in ambulatory medicine or a formal course in the care of minor complaints. In all cases, medics providing ambulatory care must ensure they are operating within their scope of practice and under the supervision of a physician or PA.

SCOPE OF PRACTICE

Providing ambulatory care is outside the traditional bounds of prehospital care. Prehospital care is usually concerned with emergencies, and the goal is transportation or evacuation of the patient to the hospital. Ambulatory care differs in that the patient has a nonemergency minor complaint, and evacuation is usually not necessary. In the military, medics have a longstanding role in providing and assisting in ambulatory care. In the civilian sector, this concept is new, so civilian readers are urged to move carefully when considering this mode of practice.

Whether or not the medic practices in the military, the practice parameters of the ambulatory care are constant (Table 12-1). *The central parameter is that ambulatory care, like emergency care, is performed as an extension of the physician's services. The medic is a physician extender, and as such, acts as the eyes, ears, and hands of the physician.* Therefore the physician (or the PA) must be integrally involved in all aspects of the medic's care. Depending on the circumstance, this may include "over-the-shoulder" supervision or indirect supervision and guidance through the use of protocols. Physician involvement in training, evaluation, and quality assurance is also required. In fact, all the principles of medical control and prehospital practice apply to ambulatory care.

Practicing within your scope of practice (Table 12-2) implies written protocols and guidance on what can be treated by the medic and what must be referred to the physician or PA. It is mandatory to review all cases with the supervising physician or PA. Depending on circumstances, this can occur while the patient is still present or at the end of the day. In all cases, this should occur within 24 hours of treatment. To ensure accurate review, all patient encounters require documentation to include name, time of encounter, chief complaint, focused assessment, and treatment rendered. Of course, all questionable or suspicious cases should be referred to the physician or PA immediately.

TABLE 12-1

PARAMETERS FOR THE MEDIC PRACTICING AMBULATORY CARE

- All care is an extension of the physician's care.
- Always practice within your scope and ability.
- Review *all* cases with the supervising physician or PA.
- Document all care.
- Refer all questionable or suspicious cases to the physician or PA.

TABLE 12-2

- Only treat simple (uncomplicated) minor problems.
- Only treat otherwise healthy adults.
- Only treat minor problems the patient would ordinarily self-treat, but for the tactical situation. (The lack of an available drug store compels the patient to request medic assistance.)
- Immediately refer all cases of complicated, worsening, or persistent symptoms.
- When in doubt, refer immediately to a physician.
- All serious or potentially serious symptoms (e.g., chest pain, shortness of breath) are treated as emergencies.

THE APPROACH TO AMBULATORY CARE

The approach to an ambulatory patient is much the same as the approach to an emergency patient, but without the pressure of urgency. Since the patient comes to the medic (rather than vice versa) and is relatively comfortable and ambulatory, the scene survey and initial assessment are abbreviated or omitted. Instead, move to the focused assessment to get information on the patient's chief complaint. Check for danger signals and render treatment. Always advise the patient to return if symptoms persist or worsen.

COMMON COMPLAINTS

This section introduces several common minor complaints and provides brief guidance on how to treat them. This guide is not intended as a substitute for a comprehensive text on ambulatory care. Furthermore, all care must be reviewed with the supervising physician or PA. Lastly, this guide is intended only for use on healthy adults who have been periodically screened for serious underlying disease (through routine physical examination). Use of this guide in patients not meeting this criteria may result in adverse outcomes. (Even under optimal conditions, some patients will fail to improve, or worsen, and the medic must be alert to this possibility. Physician referral is mandatory in all suspicious cases.)

FORMULARY

The formulary or list of drugs authorized for medic use in ambulatory care is restricted to over-the-counter medications (see Appendix A, Medications for the Tactical Environment). Prescription drugs are not authorized for use by the medic in ambulatory care. Of course, in emergencies and in accordance to protocol, medics will frequently administer prescription drugs, usually by the intravenous route (for example, atropine and epinephrine). Use of prescription drugs requires the direct authorization (for example, written protocol) of an individual with a license to practice medicine (a physician or PA).

Appendix A, Medications for the Tactical Environment, lists the drugs on the formulary and provides details on their use. All over-the-counter (OTC) drugs come labeled with instructions for use. The medic must always check the label and ensure the intended use is consistent with the labeling. Use of an OTC drug in a manner not consistent with the labeling is dangerous and should never be attempted except under direct physician supervision.

USING THIS GUIDE

This guide is further intended solely to address minor complaints. Anything more than mild, common symptoms must trigger a referral to a physician. Perhaps the best guide is to judge whether the patient, if he or she had access, would have treated himself or herself with common remedies. In other words, if not for the tactical situation and lack of a nearby drug store, the patient would've taken care of himself or herself. This test helps ensure the medic practices well within his or her scope of practice and reduces risk of missing a serious problem.

The medic should treat only "simple" or uncomplicated symptoms in otherwise healthy patients. Be alert for warning signs or "danger signals" (Table 12-3) that suggest serious disease. Multiple symptoms, or symptoms lasting beyond a few hours or so, are also suspect. Obviously, any worsening symptoms should immediately signal a physician referral.

Table 12-4 outlines the common complaints addressed in this chapter. Following are additional comments and tips to treating these minor problems.

Headache

Headaches are quite common and can be caused by a variety of factors. Tension headache is the most common form and is caused by physical or emotional stress. Tension headaches tend to develop gradually. Sudden onset headache suggests a serious cause. Uncomplicated tension headaches are similar to the patient's previous headaches and are not the worst ever. Treatment is acetaminophen 650-1000 mg po q 4 hours.

A word about a similar drug, aspirin, is needed. Because aspirin can significantly interfere with blood clotting, its use in the tactical environment should be avoided. Acetaminophen is just as effective and does not have the undesirable side effects of aspirin.

Any headache that is new, different, or worse, or has any associated symptoms (especially loss of consciousness, nausea, vomiting, fever, or stiff neck) mandates immediate physician referral. Another serious cause of headache is carbon monoxide poisoning. These headaches are severe and frequently associated with nausea or vomiting. Be suspicious of carbon monoxide poisoning if more than one person is affected or if symptoms develop in an enclosed area (particularly if an engine, furnace, or generator is operating nearby) such as a tent or vehicle.

Cough

Cough represents irritation of the respiratory tract from a number of causes. Viral infections, seasonal allergies, irritating dust, and smoke are common causes of mild cough. More serious causes include pneumonia, asthma, bronchoconstriction, and pulmonary edema. Mild

TABLE 12-3

SELECTED MINOR PROBLEMS AND DANGER SIGNALS

SYMPTOM	UNCOMPLICATED FEATURES	DANGER SIGNALS
Headache	Mild, similar to previous	New, different, worst. Fever, reduced LOC
Cough	Mild, absence of other symptoms	Fever, sputum, pain, SOB
Runny nose	Absence of other symptoms. Clear/pale yellow discharge	Fever, pain, headache, greenish/bloody discharge
Sore throat	All cases to physician	Fever, stiff neck, drooling, dyspnea
Stomach upset	Caution in patients > 35 years, may be a sign of cardiac disease.	Pain, vomiting, fever, failure to improve in 1-2 hours
Nausea and vomiting	Mild, patient can easily consume water, absence of other symptoms	Pain, fever, lightheadedness
Diarrhea	No more than 1-2 BMs per hour for 2-3 hours	Cramps lasting longer than a few moments. Pain, tenderness, bloody stool, fever
Fever	Mild, absence of other symptoms	Chills (rigors), headache, pain
Rash	Small patches, mild itching	SOB, fever, diffuse/widespread patches, joint pain, rash on palms/soles
Bug bites	Few, localized bites or stings	SOB, fever, pain away from site, significant swelling, redness
Blisters	Small, few, clear fluid	Large (> 2 cm) or multiple, redness, yellowish/greenish fluid
Bumps and bruises	Small, mild discomfort no function loss	Large, painful, or multiple
Cuts and scratches	Shallow, not through dermis, gap < 2 mm, not over face, neck, hand, feet, or genital area	Large, deep, multiple, functional loss, gap > 2 mm, located over functional area of body (Table 12-6), signs of infection (Table 12-8)
Dental pain, toothache	Single tooth. Absence of swelling, fever; able to drink easily	Swelling, fever, suspicion of airway obstruction
Chipped tooth	Single tooth, small fragment. Absence of tooth, red spot, or bleeding (exposed pulp)	Multiple teeth, loose or avulsed teeth, exposed pulp, choking/coughing associated with dental trauma
Mouth sores	Single, small (< 1 cm). Absence of other symptoms	Multiple, large (> 1 cm). Fever, swelling, difficulty swallowing, dyspnea

cough in healthy adults without associated symptoms may be treated with dextromethorphan cough syrup and, if the patients smokes, cessation of smoking. Occasionally, an uncomplicated cough will be accompanied by a mild scratchy throat or runny nose. *Danger signals include fever, sputum (phlegm) production, pain, and shortness of breath.* Uncomplicated cough is treated with dextromethorphan syrup, 10 ml (2 teaspoons) every 6-8 hours.

TABLE 12-4

COMMON COMPLAINTS ENCOUNTERED FREQUENTLY IN THE FIELD

- Headache
- Cough
- Stomach upset
- Nausea and vomiting
- Diarrhea
- Fever
- Bumps and bruises
- Minor scratches and cuts
- Rash
- Runny or stuffy nose
- Sore throat
- Bug or insect bites
- Blisters
- Dental pain

Runny Nose

Runny nose and nasal congestion is usually caused by the common cold or seasonal allergies. Uncomplicated cases are painless although mild discomfort or scratchy throat are common. More significant symptoms should be absent. Nasal discharge is clear or pale yellow. *Danger signals include fever, headache, pain, or greenish or bloody nasal discharge.* Tactical treatment is pseudoephedrine 60 mg po every 4-6 hours.

Sore Throat

Sore throat has a variety of causes, several of them serious. For this reason, tactical treatment by the medic is for temporary relief only. All cases need physician referral within 24 hours. *Danger signals necessitating more immediate referral include fever, stiff neck, drooling of secretions, and dyspnea.* Temporary tactical treatment is Tylenol 650-1000 mg po q 4 hours and throat lozenges as needed. However, temporary treatment is not a substitute for prompt referral.

Upset Stomach

"Stomach upset" is a lay term for dyspepsia, or acid indigestion. The usual cause is overeating or consumption of disagreeable foods. Uncomplicated cases are very mild and are promptly relieved by antacids. *Danger signals include abdominal pain, chest pain, vomiting, fever, and failure to improve within 1-2 hours.* In persons more than 35 years old, the symptoms could be confused with myocardial infarction, so extra caution is warranted. Antacids (one or two tablets, chewed) containing calcium, aluminum, and/or magnesium are effective for uncomplicated dyspepsia.

Nausea and Vomiting

Nausea and vomiting are very nonspecific findings with causes ranging from uncomplicated viral infection, food poisoning, and pregnancy to pancreatitis. Only the mildest symptoms should be treated by the medic. *Symptoms preventing the patient from easily drinking water warrants immediate referral. Other danger signals include abdominal pain, fever, or light-headedness.* Field treatment involves switching to clear liquids (for example, apple juice, Gatorade) and saltine crackers for 12-24 hours. Medications are not indicated for tactical treatment by the medic.

Diarrhea

Diarrhea is the passage of multiple, liquid stools. A single liquid or soft bowel movement without any other symptoms is likely normal and requires no treatment. True diarrhea, however, can be a big nuisance in the field at best, and life threatening at worst. The usual cause is viral or bacterial, and a case of diarrhea may herald other cases of food-borne or waterborne diseases. If two or more patients have diarrhea symptoms, immediate physician consultation is warranted.

Uncomplicated diarrhea is fewer than one or two bowel movements per hour for not more than 2-3 hours. Symptoms exceeding this value should prompt a referral to the physician. Mild cramping may accompany the bowel movements, but this discomfort should pass within a few moments. *Danger signals include prolonged cramps, pain, abdominal tenderness, bloody stool, or fever.* Treatment is attapulgite, 30 ml (2 tablespoons) after each bowel movement. Food handlers with diarrhea must be restricted from work until cleared by a physician.

Fever

Fever is defined as a rectal temperature greater than 38.3ºC (101ºF). An oral or tympanic temperature greater than these values may also be considered a fever for purposes of tactical care. Axillary temperatures are unreliable. Thermometers are standard equipment (Figure 12-1) and should be carried by all medics in their aid bags.

In young, healthy adults, fever is usually caused by an infection. Uncomplicated fever might be accompanied by fatigue (malaise). *Complicated fevers are those with any other significant symptoms, including chills (rigors), headache, or pain. Because of the difficulty*

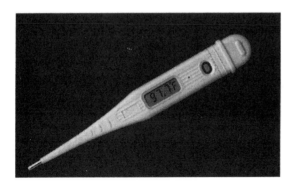

Figure 12-1 An electronic thermometer for field use.

in pinpointing the cause of a fever, all patients with fever should see a physician within 24 hours. Uncomplicated fevers may be treated temporarily with acetaminophen 650-1000 mg po q 4-6 hours while awaiting arrival of the physician. All cases of complicated fevers should be referred immediately to the physician.

Rash

Rashes have a whole host of causes, most of which are benign, but a few are serious. The rashes with relevance to tactical medical care are localized and usually caused by irritating chemicals (chemical dermatitis). More diffuse rashes can represent infections, allergies, or other serious diseases and are referred to the physician. *Rash danger signals include widespread or diffuse patches, shortness of breath, fever, joint pain, or rash on palms or soles.* All uncomplicated rashes not improved within 48-72 hours should be seen by a physician.

Among the most common rashes in the field are those caused by poison ivy, poison oak, and poison sumac (Figures 12-2, 12-3, and 12-4). Small patches of reddish, itchy bumps (papules) are usually located on the hands, arms, and legs. A similar pattern can be mimicked by multiple insect bites. Poison ivy is treated with calamine lotion liberally applied (and allowed to dry) to the affected areas. Avoid the eyes, mouth, and mucous

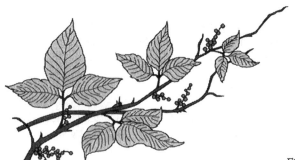

Figure 12-2 Poison ivy.

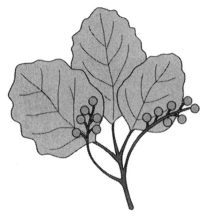

Figure 12-3 Poison oak.

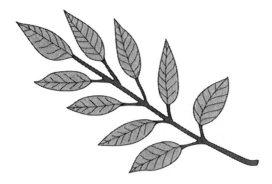

Figure 12-4 Poison sumac.

membranes. Reapply as needed. Itching can be controlled with diphenhydramine 25-50 mg po q 6 hours. This medication can induce drowsiness, so driving, shooting, and any other activity requiring alertness must be curtailed.

Bug Bites

"Bug bites" is the generic term for minor bites and stings of insects, spiders, and other small pests. The best method of controlling bug bites is prevention. Knowledge of proper clothing, use of repellents, and insect behavior is important for the tactical medic (see chapter 11, Tactical Environmental and Preventive Medicine).

A few bites or stings on an otherwise healthy adult usually causes mild pain and irritation at the site, plus a small bump (papule) or red spot (macule) may form. Systemic or generalized symptoms are absent in uncomplicated cases. If a stinger remains at the site, gently scrape it off with a piece of cardboard, credit card, or similar stiff object.

Danger signals include fever, significant swelling or redness, pain away from the bite or sting site, and more important, shortness of breath. Any dyspnea may herald serious anaphylaxis, and this situation must be treated as an emergency. Treatment for anaphylaxis may include subcutaneous epinephrine, IV or IM diphenhydramine, IV fluids, and immediate evacuation.

Uncomplicated bug bites are treated like minor rashes, with topical calamine lotion and oral diphenhydramine. Cool packs may ease the discomfort associated with bee stings.

Blisters

Blisters are the bane of ground troops and can affect anyone forced to walk or run more than they are used to. *The best method of blister control is prevention* (see chapter 11, Tactical Environmental and Preventive Medicine). Despite the best efforts of individuals, however, the medic will inevitably be faced with caring for blisters in the field. Successful treatment of blisters can restore an individual's effectiveness and improve morale. Therefore, all tactical medics should be skilled and equipped to deal with blisters.

Blisters are caused by repetitive friction on a small area of skin, usually the foot. Tight or ill-fitting boots or shoes, infrequent sock changing, or excessive wetness all can contribute to blister formation. Once formed, blisters are painful and can impede mobility, agility, and speed. In extreme cases, the affected individual may require evacuation. Proper treatment in the early stages can prevent most bad outcomes, however.

If the affected area is tender and red, but not yet formed into a blister, treatment is directed at drying and padding the area. Cut a generous (at least two or three times the diameter of the affected area) piece of "moleskin" or similar padding (in a pinch, gauze or an adhesive bandage will suffice), and place it over the area. A sock change is mandatory to reduce wetness. Changing footwear will also help. In most cases, this is all that will be needed.

Once a blister has formed, there are two approaches to treatment. If the mission is nearly completed and some degree of rest or reduced walking is anticipated, then the optimal treatment is the same as the preceding paragraph. Padding and drying of the feet are all that is needed, and the treatment is effective until rest occurs.

If the affected individual cannot reduce activity enough to alleviate significantly the blister pain, it may be advisable to drain the blister. Draining has the advantage of reducing pressure and pain and improving the effectiveness of padding. The chief disadvantage is the remote risk of infection and potential worsening of the blister since the patient is likely to continue the activity that caused the blister in the first place.

Draining a Blister

Blister drainage is an easy procedure. Technically, though, it is a minor surgery that mandates strict attention to procedural details. Universal precautions are required throughout the procedure. Equipment needed is (one) alcohol or Betadine prep, (one) 2 x 2 sterile gauze pad, and (one) 20-25 gauge sterile needle (such as an angiocatheter or injection needle; Table 12-5). First, reassure the patient and explain the procedure. Prep the blister with the Betadine or alcohol pad. Insert the needle near the margin of the blister dome keeping the needle parallel to the skin (Figure 12-5). The dome of the blister has no nerve endings, so introducing the needle should be painless. Pain suggests the entry point was on the skin rather than the dome, or the needle trajectory is not parallel to the skin. Insert the needle 4-5 mm into the dome, and then withdraw. Then apply gentle pressure to the blister dome, expressing the clear blister fluid. Wipe up any excess with the gauze. Properly dispose of the equipment, exercising caution with the sharp needle. Then pad the blister as described in the previous sections.

TABLE 12-5

EQUIPMENT NEEDED TO DRAIN A BLISTER

- Alcohol or Betadine prep
- 2 x 2 sterile gauze
- 20-25-gauge sterile needle

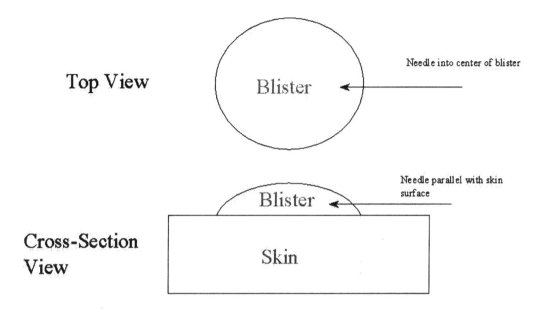

Top View

Blister

Needle into center of blister

Cross-Section View

Blister

Skin

Needle parallel with skin surface

Figure 12-5 To drain a blister, insert the sterile needle at the base of the blister dome, keeping the needle parallel to the skin surface.

Blister danger signals include large (greater than 2 cm in diameter) and multiple blisters. Blisters with more than a thin (2-3 mm) rim of redness surrounding the blister dome, or yellowish/greenish fluid, suggest infection. All complicated blisters require the patient to be seen by a physician.

Bumps and Bruises

Bumps and bruises are lay terms for minor contusions and are used to convey the mild nature of injury that may be safely treated by the medic. Bumps and bruises differ from more serious injury (requiring standard emergency care) by the severity of injury. For purposes of primary treatment by the medic in tactical field care, bumps and bruises must cause only mild pain to the patient, but no restriction of mobility or function. That is, the patient must retain full use of the affected body part and suffer only mild discomfort from the bump or bruise. This distinction is important because any functional loss from an injury implies more serious underlying damage that must be evaluated by the physician. If, after assessment, the medic finds only mild discomfort and no functional loss (for example, the patient can walk, run, and jump on a bruised leg), then field treatment is indicated. As with all ambulatory care performed by the medic, the case must be documented and discussed with the supervising physician.

Danger signals include large, painful, or multiple bumps and bruises, and any loss of function, no matter how slight. Treatment is with cool packs and elevation, if possible. Always wrap ice or cold packs in cloth, and never place ice directly to the skin. Ibuprofen 200-400 mg po q 6 hours may also provide temporary relief. Ibuprofen is contraindicated in patients with previous peptic ulcers and in pregnancy (see Appendix A, Medications for the Tactical Environment, for additional details).

Cuts and Scratches

The term *cuts and scratches* is used in place of the technical terms *lacerations and abrasions* to emphasize the minor nature of conditions suited for primary medic treatment. Cuts and scratches includes the whole host of minor wounds, including laceration, incisions, and abrasions. Uncomplicated cuts and scratches that are indicated for primary medic treatment must be shallow and not go completely through the skin (dermis). Bleeding must be easily controlled with direct pressure and must stop after a few minutes of pressure. There can be no foreign bodies or gross contamination with dirt or other matter. Wound gape is the spread of the wound margins. Anything greater than 2 mm requires a physician referral, except on the face, where gape is never tolerated, and any such wound should be referred. Critically, there must be no bodily function loss (for example, inability to bend a finger). Because function is such a critical factor, any lacerations located on the face, neck, hands, wrists, feet, ankles, or genital area (critical function areas of the

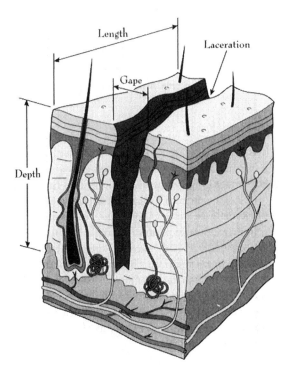

Figure 12-6 Laceration depth is measured from skin surface to bottom of wound. Gape is the spread of the wound edges.

body) require consultation with the physician to ensure a thorough wound examination. (This list of body parts requiring consultation with the physician is easy to remember. It is the same list as high-risk burn areas discussed in emergency-care textbooks.)

Treatment of cuts and scratches outside the scope of primary medic practice includes deep (through the dermis) or gaping (> 2 mm) lacerations (Figure 12-6). A clue to laceration depth is the presence of subcutaneous fat, tendons, or other structure in the wound depths. Because visualization of many wounds is difficult without adequate light and homeostasis (control of oozing or bleeding), any wound in doubt must be referred immediately to the physician for examination and possible suture repair. Wounds on a body part listed in Table 12-6 always require the input of a physician. Remember, primary medic treatment of cuts and scratches is aimed at identifying minor wounds that can be treated safely without sutures or other surgical repair.

Danger Signals

Danger signals for cuts and scratches include any loss of bodily function, uncontrolled bleeding, or any signs of infection. Signs of infection include redness, pus, swelling, fever, or red streaks (lymphangitis) from wound proximally.

Irrigation

Treatment of cuts and scratches is simple and involves two steps: (1) cleaning or irrigation, and (2) dressing. Irrigation is performed using sterile saline (normal or 0.9% saline) under gentle pressure (Table 12-7). Using sterile technique and taking universal precautions (splash hazard), fill up a 20-ml syringe (or any handy 10-50-ml sterile syringe with luer-lock). Attach the flexible catheter from an 18-gauge anigiocatheter, discarding the steel needle in a safe manner. Avoid using catheters larger or smaller than 18 gauge since this will result in improper water pressure. Squirt the saline stream into the wound. Keep the catheter tip just a few millimeters from the wound. It is acceptable and desirable to insert the catheter into the wound depths. Use just enough force on the syringe to ensure a steady stream, but avoid significant splashing. Collect waste fluid in the basin, and dab the wound gently with sterile gauze when done to absorb excess saline.

TABLE 12-6

AREAS OF THE BODY WHERE MINOR LACERATIONS
REQUIRE A PHYSICIAN EXAMINATION

- Face
- Neck
- Hands and wrist
- Feet and ankles
- Genital area

TABLE 12-7

EQUIPMENT NEEDED TO IRRIGATE A MINOR WOUND

- Sterile saline
- 20-ml syringe (any size 10-50 ml)
- Flexible catheter from 18-gauge angiocatheter
- Basin to collect waste fluid
- Sterile gauze or sponges

A rule of thumb is to use 100 ml of saline per each centimeter (cm) of laceration length (250 ml per inch). Since primary treatment by medics is limited to minor cuts and scratches, most irrigation should be in the range of 50-100 ml. However, when the medic is directly assisting the physician in wound care, larger lacerations may require more extensive saline irrigation.

Dressing

Following irrigation, reinspect the wound. If there is any doubt that it is more than a minor, uncomplicated cut, immediately refer it to the physician. Otherwise, place a small dab of bacitracin ointment on the cut, and dress it with an adhesive bandage (or sterile gauze and tape). If bacitracin ointment is unavailable, plain sterile white petrolatum is an acceptable substitute, as is polymyxin B/neomycin ointment.

Pitfalls

The primary pitfall in managing minor cuts and scratches is attempting to treat wounds that are beyond the scope of medic practice. Careful attention to the limitations and danger signals outlined previously will minimize risk. Any suspicious, unusual, or doubtful cases must be brought to the attention of the physician.

Other pitfalls in minor wound care center on the techniques used in irrigation and dressing. Always perform irrigation in the manner described. Do not soak or immerse wounds in any liquid. Similarly, never scrub a wound with a bristle brush. These time-honored traditions are now known to be ineffective and damaging to tissues. Avoid any irrigating solution except sterile saline. Plain or sterile water, Betadine, soaps, detergents (for example, Hibiclens), and alcohol are all toxic to tissues and delay healing. Perhaps one exception is the poloxamer surfactants (Sur Clens), which are safe for most minor wounds. Lastly, be sure to instruct the patient to keep the wound clean and dry (frequent dressing changes are a must in the field), and report any signs of infection immediately (Table 12-8).

TABLE 12-8

SIGNS OF WOUND INFECTION

- Redness (erythema)
- Pus
- Swelling
- Fever
- Red streaks (lymphangitis)

Dental Pain

Dental pain includes toothache, chipped teeth, and minor gum or lip sores. It is a common complaint in the field or aboard ship. The best method to control minor dental problems is prevention. All persons, military or civilian, should see their dentist regularly. Military experience has shown that virtually all emergency dental problems can be avoided through regular checkups.

The tactical approach to dental pain is to provide temporary relief until the patient can see a dentist. Since a physician can also treat or temporarily repair many dental problems, refer all patients complaining of dental pain to the physician (or dentist, if available) within 24-48 hours.

Toothache

Toothache is pain in a single tooth. Usually, gentle tapping on the affected tooth (with a wooden tongue blade) will illicit severe pain. Uncomplicated cases have no swelling or fever, and the patient can drink easily. *Danger signals include fever, swelling inside the mouth or visible in the face or neck, or any suspicion of airway obstruction.* Temporary relief can be obtained by applying eucalyptus oil to the affected tooth and surrounding gums, and ibuprofen 200-400 mg po q 6 hours. Referral to a dentist within 48 hours is desirable; the supervising physician should examine the patient sooner, if possible, to confirm the problem. Lastly, be concerned with any toothache or jaw pain associated with chest pain or shortness of breath. In this case, toothache may be a sign of cardiac problems (for example, myocardial infarction), especially in patients >35 years old.

Chipped Teeth

Small chips in teeth occur from minor trauma or from chewing hard food. Tactical treatment focuses on providing temporary relief and identifying those cases in need of immediate dentist or physician attention.

Minor uncomplicated chipped teeth have small fragments and cause only mild discomfort. Loose fillings also fall into this category. Examine the patient's teeth carefully to identify where the chip came from. Using universal precautions gently wipe the tooth (the portion still in the patient's mouth) with gauze. If a red spot or bleeding is visible on the tooth, this suggests exposure of the pulp in the root canal (Figure 12-7). Immediate referral is necessary in these cases. If possible, use a flashlight to obtain clearer visualization. If there is no red spot or blood, temporary relief may be provided with eucalyptus oil and ibuprofen (as described previously). Physician or dentist referral is required within 24-48 hours.

Danger signals for chipped teeth include a red spot or blood on the surface of the chipped tooth. This suggests exposure of the tooth pulp. Failure to promptly treat this injury may result in infection and tooth loss. Check for loose or missing teeth. All require referral to the dentist or physician. Any avulsed (missing) teeth should be located and immediately placed in a tooth-preserving solution (for example, Sav-a-Tooth). Do not scrub or excessively handle avulsed teeth. Alternative tooth-preserving methods, in order of preference, are (1) held in between the patient's gum and cheek (requires a cooperative patient not at risk for swallowing or aspirating the tooth), (2) milk, and (3) sterile saline. If evacuation time to a dentist or physician is greater than 1 hour, it is reasonable to attempt tooth reimplantation. Consult a standard emergency care textbook for details on this procedure. Lastly, question any patient with a chipped tooth about choking or gagging associated with the dental trauma. This suggests aspiration of a tooth fragment and warrants referral to the physician.

Mouth Sores

Mouth sores can occur on the lips, gums, or tongue. They have multiple causes, ranging from viral infections to trauma from teeth (accidental tongue biting). Because of the rich nerve supply to the oral cavity, even small sores can be quite annoying. Mouth sores that may be primarily treated by the medic are single and small (<1 cm) and have no associated intraoral or facial swelling. Fever, difficulty swallowing, or dyspenea are likewise absent.

Danger signals are large (> 1 cm) or multiple sores, or any intraoral or facial swelling. Fever, difficulty swallowing (dysphagia), or difficulty breathing (dyspnea) are danger signals

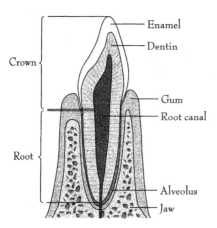

Figure 12-7 Structure of the tooth. Exposure of the pulp in the root canal demands referral to a dentist or physician.

suggesting serious disease. Uncomplicated oral sores are treated the same as for toothache. Apply topical oil of eucalyptus every hour or so for pain relief. Ibuprofen 200-400 mg po q 6 hours is also effective. If the patient smokes, advise him or her to quit or cut down.

SUMMARY

This chapter introduced the concept of ambulatory field care for minor problems. Key to the success of this care is awareness of the medic's scope of practice and strict adherence to the principles outlined in this chapter. Careful attention to detail and identification of danger signals improves outcome and minimizes risk. Critical to the process is the active involvement of the physician, both to establish treatment protocols and to review each case treated by the medic within 24 hours.

FOR FURTHER READING

DE LORENZO RA: Military Medic: The Original Expanded Scope EMS Provider. J Emerg. Med Serv (JEMS), 1996.

Health Services Command, Ambulatory Patient Care: Algorithm—Directed Troop Medical Care HSC Pam 40-7-21, US Army AMEDDC&S, FT. Sam Houston, TX, 1992.

HAMILTON GC (ed): Presenting Signs and Symptoms in the Emergency Department. Williams & Wilkins, Baltimore, 1993.

BARKER LR, et al. (eds): Principles of Ambulatory Care, 4th ed. Williams & Wilkins, Baltimore, 1995.

BACKER HD, et al. (eds): Wilderness First Aid. Jones and Bartlett Publishers, Sudbury, MA, 1998.

AURBACH PS, et al. (eds): Management of Wilderness and Environmental Emergencies, 2nd ed. Mosby, St. Louis, 1989.

Field Manual 8-230, Medical Specialist. Department of the Army, Washington, DC, 1984. (historical purposes only)

13

TACTICAL LAW ENFORCEMENT MEDICAL SUPPORT

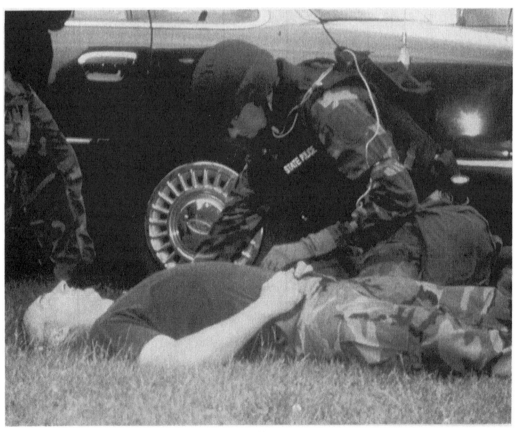

Tactical law enforcement medic providing care to a fallen officer.

OBJECTIVES

After reading this chapter, you will be able to:

1. Describe the concept of Tactical Emergency Medical Support (TEMS) for law enforcement operations, and explain how it fits in with the overall concept of tactical emergency care.

2. Describe the "zones of care" and their importance to tactical EMS decision making.

3. List the components of transit risk, and accurately determine transit risk for a given tactical operation.

4. Determine the disadvantages and benefits of providing various types of care in the warm zone, and make correct decisions about which interventions should be initiated in the warm zone.

5. List the key concepts of the Rapid and Remote Assessment Methodology (RAM).

6. Describe the 13 steps in the process of conducting Medicine Across the Barricade (MAB).

7. Describe the patterns of injury one is likely to see while supporting a tactical law enforcement operation.

CASE

The SWAT team you support has been called to the scene of a hostage situation. The hostage taker is a 28-year-old male who is involved in an acrimonious custody dispute with his former spouse. Their three-year-old daughter and one-year-old son live with her, and all three are being held hostage. Negotiators have been talking to the subject for almost 3 hours, but have made little progress. He states that he will kill any police officers who try to approach the house. Negotiators tell you that they fear for the safety of the wife and children. Countersniper/observer teams have confirmed that the subject has two semiautomatic handguns in the waistband of his pants.

The SWAT commander is formulating emergency assault plans in case negotiations break down. He wants to know if using the incapacitating agents CS or OC will be dangerous for the children in the house since one of them has a history of asthma. He also wants your suggestions on how the child's medical history might be used to the negotiator's advantage.

Suddenly, a shot rings out, and the negotiator hears the phone drop on the other end. The SWAT team commander decides to approach the kitchen window with a periscope instead of inserting tear gas because of the presence of children. With the periscope mirror in place, what appears to be a large amount of blood is visible on the floor, along with one of the handguns. The subject cannot be seen. The team commander inquires whether the loss of that amount of blood would be incapacitating. You respectfully point out that it is sometimes difficult to determine how much blood has been lost by just looking at a puddle on the floor. Besides, no body is visible, so you must assume that the subject is still able to move.

Fearing for the safety of the wife and two children, an emergency assault is ordered. Upon entry, the hostages are found unharmed in the bedroom. The subject is located on the basement floor with a close-range gunshot wound to the shoulder. "Medic up!" is shouted, and you quickly move to the patient who has been cleared for weapons and possible booby traps by SWAT officers. He has no pulse and no spontaneous respirations. There is a large amount of additional blood loss on the floor, and it has been about 50 minutes since the gunshot was first heard. With help from your partner, you simultaneously intubate and attempt a large bore IV at the antecubital fossa. However, your venipuncture attempt produces only a nonbleeding puncture wound. An external jugular stick yields the same results. A glance under the patient shows early signs of lividity. In compliance with your protocols, you elect not to attempt any further resuscitation and advise the team commander.

The wife and children are very concerned about the subject despite being held hostage. They resent the presence of the police, who they feel are responsible for the subject's death. Recognizing a deteriorating situation, the incident commander instructs the detectives to delay their interviews and asks you and one of the negotiators to talk with the family. As soon as the family realizes that you are a medic and have been assigned to help them, their attitude changes, and they become more cooperative. Eventually, the investigation confirms that the subject died of a self-inflicted gunshot wound from his own handgun.

INTRODUCTION

Medical support for law enforcement special operations is a science that has achieved a status of legitimacy and recognition in recent years. Widely known as Tactical Emergency Medical Support (TEMS), the appellation specifically denotes emergency medical support and not emergency medical services, in recognition of the wide range of activities that the tactical medic provides beyond management of acute trauma. Much like military tactical emergency care, TEMS focuses on injury control, preventive medicine, performance decrement, and health maintenance initiatives. Documented experience has shown that, though the tactical medic must be fully prepared to deal with acute trauma, serious injury is uncommon in this setting. On the other hand, minor injury and illness occur frequently and can seriously degrade the tactical team's capability of achieving mission success. So, although less alluring and dramatic than trauma care, this focus is likely to improve the team's probability of meeting its law enforcement and public safety objectives.

These are principles that have been developed and validated through centuries of military experience, and modern TEMS borrows heavily from the science of military medicine. However, conventional war and law enforcement special operations differ in important ways, and the transfer of military tactical care must be done with careful modification. For example, in law enforcement operations, there is no such thing as "acceptable casualties." The public and political expectation is that law and order will be restored and maintained without "collateral damage." Ironically, modern military operations have recently taken on the appearance of police actions or humanitarian missions. Although military and law enforcement operations seem to be on a convergent course, the two will never be identical, and models drawn from one environment must be cautiously applied to the other.

The essence of the difference between TEMS and everyday EMS is not the specific treatment procedures employed, but rather the context in which medical decision making is done. For example hemorrhage control is achieved by applying direct pressure in both environments, but in TEMS, there is an inclination to move quickly to a tourniquet in the tactical setting if initial attempts at direct pressure fail. (See discussion in chapter 1, Tactical Environment of Care, for more detail on this topic.)

ZONES OF CARE

Two Zone Concept

The area of operation in the law enforcement tactical setting is normally defined by the terms *inner perimeter* and *outer perimeter*. Although different meanings are ascribed to these terms in various regions of the country, the inner perimeter is generally a geographically defined area in which subjects are contained, with entrance and egress controlled by the Special Weapons and Tactics (SWAT) team. The outer perimeter is a larger area, encompassing the inner perimeter, which is controlled by the law enforcement agency and from which the public is excluded. These areas are frequently thought of as concentric circles with the tactical target lying in the center.

Three Zone Concept

The two zone approach of inner and outer perimeters is critical to the containment of an incident and has utility in planning and implementing tactical options. However, it is limited in direct application to TEMS decision making. Instead, a three zone concept is used for clarity (Figure 13-1).

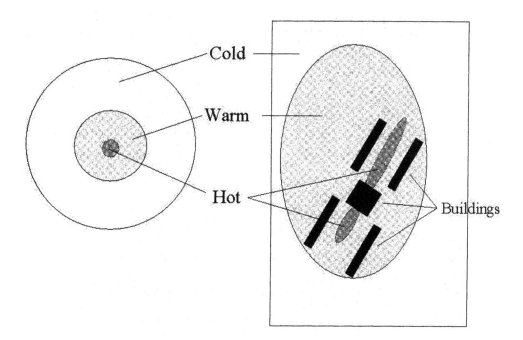

Figure 13-1 The three zones of medical support for law enforcement. The concentric circles are useful for discussion; however, in real life, they are likely to be irregular as shown.

Hot Zone

The hot zone is that area in which the tactical medic and the patient are subject to a direct and immediate threat. What constitutes a direct and immediate threat is subjectively determined and depends on the specific mission circumstances. A subject with a gun and a clear line of fire would certainly qualify as a direct and immediate threat. Exposure to an area where the subject *might* be located, but has not yet been seen, would be insufficient by itself to constitute a direct and immediate threat.

Assessment and treatment in the hot zone incurs enormous risk. This is the same concept as "care under fire" discussed in chapter 1, Tactical Environment of Care. *Usually, extraction, whether by self or others, is the only appropriate intervention in the hot zone* (Figure 13-2). Extraction includes rudimentary procedures manually to maintain an open airway and spinal alignment. In some cases, extraction may need to be deferred because of extraordinarily high risk to the provider or low probability of a successful extraction.

Cold Zone

The cold zone is that area where no significant danger or threat can be reasonably anticipated for the provider or patient. This may be due to the interposition of distance, time, terrain features, or firepower between the provider and the threat. TEMS decision making in this circumstance is almost identical to everyday EMS decision making, with the

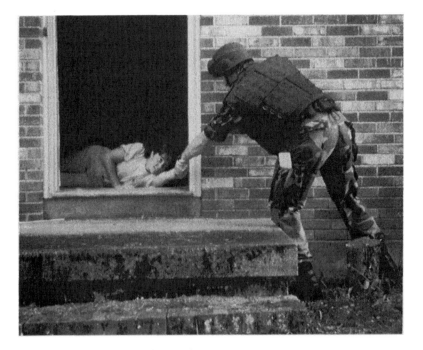

Figure 13-2 Rapid extraction from the hot zone.

possible exception of increased awareness of forensic considerations. Injured persons in the cold zone may be evaluated and treated without undue risk.

Warm Zone

The warm zone is the area in which TEMS decision making is most dramatically affected. It is defined as that area in which there is a potential hostile threat, but the threat is not immediate or direct. This is the same concept used in tactical field care (discussed in chapter 1, The Tactical Environment of Care). Here, the threat is often poorly defined and highly dynamic. For example, the grounds immediately surrounding a house where the suspect is believed to be contained would be considered a warm zone. If an armed subject were in the window, it would be a hot zone. If intelligence assets confirmed that the suspect had left the area, then it could be considered a cold zone. It is in the warm zone where the benefits of on-the-spot medical evaluation and treatment must be carefully weighed against the risk of remaining in the warm zone and delaying extraction. It is here that the difficult and defining decisions must be made. Should CPR be initiated? Should a backboard be applied? Should an endotracheal tube be inserted?

Threat Level

Multiple factors must be considered in only a very brief time. Among these factors is the relative threat level. Not all threats are equal. Some are more severe than others for a variety of reasons, including credibility, intelligence, type of weapon (if any), nature of injuries that could be inflicted, and consequences of being wrong in your threat assessment. Some warm zones are simply warmer than others.

Benefit of Interventions

The potential benefit of any medical intervention must also be considered (Figure 13-3). Spinal immobilization is of comparatively little value in patients with penetrating head or neck wounds. CPR probably has little role in the warm zone since the likelihood of successful outcome following cardiac arrest secondary to trauma is near zero. (The exceptions are arrest due to electrocution, hypothermia, near drowning, and toxic exposure, in which cases, the supportive therapy of artificial ventilation can be therapeutic; see chapter 1, Tactical Environment of Care.) On the other hand, hemorrhage control for an extremity wound might be lifesaving.

Transit Risk

The transit risk is another one of the multiple factors that must be considered in TEMS decision making. Transit risk consists of three components. The first is the amount of time it takes to move the casualty to a safer area. If it's a matter of a few seconds, then time is inconsequential. But if it's a matter of minutes or tens of minutes, then some treatment in the warm zone might be prudent. Route of travel is the second component of transit risk. It may be necessary to travel through a hotter part of the warm zone, or

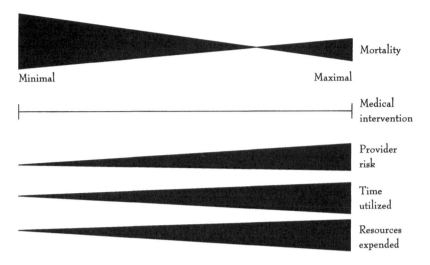

Figure 13-3 Relative risks and benefits of medical interventions in TEMS

even cross a hot zone, in order to extract the casualty to an area of greater safety. Under such circumstances, digging in and providing care may be more attractive than transporting immediately. Finally, the third component of transit risk is capability to deliver care during the move. Although short transit times can make this component less important, the inability to deliver care during the extraction may require that certain stabilizing measures be performed before heading for safer haven. For example, if the airway is being maintained by jaw thrust and the 4-minute extraction will be performed using an improvised litter on the run, then taking the time and risk to insert a nasopharyngeal airway might be indicated since it will not be possible to maintain a jaw thrust during transit. Table 13-1 outlines the components of transit risk.

Zone Shape

Resist the temptation to think of the TEMS treatment zones as contiguous, concentric circles surrounding a crisis site. Indeed, the zones may be discontinuous. In the Texas Tower

---

TABLE 13-1

COMPONENTS OF THE TRANSIT RISK

Duration of transit (time)
Route of travel
Ability to deliver care on the move

---

sniper incident, a germinal event for modern SWAT thinking, there were pockets of hot zone many blocks from the crisis site itself because the sniper had a clear line of fire from his high vantage point. On the other hand, owing to the cover afforded by some neighboring buildings, there were pockets of cold zone close to the tower. The TEMS treatment zones may assume irregular shapes and may change rapidly during an incident (Figure 13-1).

The advantage of thinking in terms of hot, warm, and cold treatment zones is that it provides a framework within which the tactical medic can prospectively and retrospectively analyze options available under highly fluid conditions, when opportunities to gather a consensus and make collective judgments are minimal. It also simplifies a very complex problem by essentially eliminating the cold zone as a region where modified practice might be appropriate and reducing the complexity of decisions made in the hot zone.

Zone Concept Summary

In summary, TEMS decisions can be made in the context of three echelons: the hot zone, warm zone, and cold zone. In the hot zone, there is a direct and immediate threat. Extraction is usually the only appropriate medical option. The warm zone is the area where a potential, but poorly defined and highly dynamic, threat exists. Some warm zones may be hotter than others. In this zone, the benefits of medical intervention must be carefully weighed against the risks of operating in this zone. Modified scope and practice are most appropriate here. The cold zone is an area of relative safety and security where normal EMS practices can usually be applied. The transit risk must be evaluated when deciding to move from a hotter zone to a cooler zone. It consists of transit time, transit route, and transit care or the capability to deliver essential care while transporting.

CARE IN THE WARM ZONE

As noted earlier, the principle difference between everyday EMS and TEMS is not the specific medical interventions, but the need to weigh constantly the costs of intervention in terms of increased risk against the benefits (Figure 13-3). However, some out-of-hospital practices should be routinely modified for those operating in the tactical environment. The discussion is similar to the concept outlined in chapter 1, The Tactical Environment of Care. It is reinforced here because of the special considerations involved in TEMS.

Airway

Some authors have argued that, in the warm zone, if the patient is sufficiently obtunded to require airway support secondary to trauma, then the liklihood of a good outcome is very small even with airway support. However, since there is not universal agreement regarding this premise, each case should be evaluated individually, again weighing the threat against the potential benefit of intervention. If the medic elects to provide airway support, then it should be aggressively pursued, with minimal reliance on manual techniques that require constant attention. Meticulous monitoring is not always possible, particularly during transit. If the patient will tolerate a nasopharyngeal airway, it should be inserted. Endotracheal intubation and cricothyrotomy should be considered if mechanical obstruction of the airway is the primary cause of respiratory insufficiency. If a bag-valve device is being used to ventilate these patients, it should have an extender between the bag and the exhalation valve. This allows for more movement of the hand-held bag during transport without dislodging the tube. It is critical that the device be capable of attaching the exhalation valve at the endotracheal tube side of the extender; otherwise, a column of expired air would accumulate in the extender tube, causing less optimal oxygenation (Figure 13-4).

Cardiopulmonary Resuscitation

CPR and artificial ventilation have limited utility in the hot and warm zones. The successful resuscitation rate from cardiac arrest secondary to trauma is sufficiently low, and the risk of performing CPR or ventilation in the tactical environment is sufficiently high, that it makes little sense to begin such procedures under the circumstances. If movement to the cold zone can be quickly achieved, then everyday EMS standards should prevail when the cold zone is reached. However, CPR cannot be justified in the hot zone and only occasionally makes sense in the warm zone.

The exceptions to this rule are those situations in which CPR or artificial ventilation are, in themselves, therapeutic and likely to make a difference in outcome. These situations include electrocution, hypothermia, near-drowning, and toxic exposure (see chapter 1, The Tactical Environment of Care). In each of these cases, if cardiorespiratory function can be maintained for a limited time, restoration to normal function is possible. For example, in lightning injury, death is often due to paralysis of the respiratory muscles, and there will be a spontaneous return to normal respiratory effort over time.

Cervical Spine Immobilization

Proper immobilization of the cervical spine requires significant time (approximately 5 minutes) and at least two personnel. This represents a serious exposure risk for rescuers when compared to immediate extraction from the warm zone. There is evidence that immobilization does not contribute significantly to an improved outcome in cases of penetrating injury to the neck. It is probably reasonable to extrapolate this evidence to all penetrating injuries, but not to blunt trauma. Therefore, it is inappropriate automatically

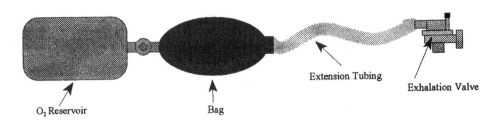

O₂ Reservoir   Bag   Extension Tubing   Exhalation Valve

Figure 13-4 Extender tube and BVM assembly.

to immobilize the c-spine in the warm zone following a gunshot wound. Rather, the decision to delay immobilization must consider the specific clinical findings and the tactical circumstances. Absent a compelling reason to the contrary, immobilization should be delayed until it can be done safely. Even though the same general decision paradigm applies to instances of blunt trauma resulting in potential c-spine injury, the medic must bear in mind that blunt trauma is more likely to result in occult injury in which immoblilization will be of value (see chapter 1, The Tactical Environment of Care).

Chest Wounds

Traditional teaching in prehospital care was to treat all chest wounds as if they were sucking chest wounds and to seal them with an occlusive dressing. However, in the TEMS environment, the medic is often unable to monitor the patient closely after initial treatment and might not have the opportunity to recognize a tension pneumothorax created by the seal (Figure 13-5). This is especially true when transit from the warm zone to the cold zone is required. Since most chest wounds are not truly sucking chest wounds, and since many patients will do well for a short time with a small, open pneumothorax, it is

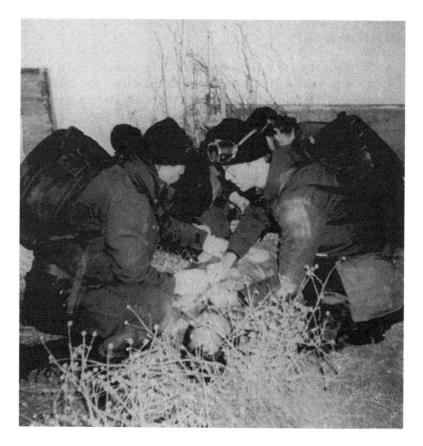

Figure 13-5 Treating a chest wound in the TEMS environment.

recommended that a chest wound not be sealed. If the wound is sealed, then the medic must exercise extreme diligence to ensure that a simple pneumothorax is not converted to a tension pneumothorax. The patient's respiratory status must be carefully monitored and the pressure released if increasing distress develops.

RAPID AND REMOTE ASSESSMENT METHODOLOGY

The Rapid and Remote Assessment Methodology (RAM) was developed by the Counter Narcotics Tactical Operations Medical Support (CONTOMS) program at the Department of Defense medical school, the Uniformed Services University of the Health Sciences. The goal of this assessment technique is to maximize the benefit to the patient while minimizing the risk to the provider. Consider the following military scenario:

> On patrol, one member of a squad is shot in the left elbow (patient A). He shouts that he has been hit and calls for medical aid.
>
> During a similar patrol situation, another squad member is hit in the head (patient B), and is lying quietly on the ground with a small amount of bleeding from the head wound.
>
> Which of these patients requires immediate treatment and transport? In fact, neither of them requires immediate treatment and transport. Patient A has a minor injury and could extract himself. Patient B is likely dead, and extraction will not alter outcome at all. These are actual cases drawn from Vietnam era archives. The real events occurred like this:
>
> Patient A-A medic came to the aid of the patient, and while evaluating his injuries, the medic was shot in the head and killed. A second rescuer came to the aid of both parties and was shot in the chest and killed. The patient subsequently crawled about 50 meters to a more secure area and was evacuated.
>
> Patient B-Another member of the squad was applying a dressing to the head, and he was shot in the right hand and left wrist. Another member came to their aid, and he was shot in the forearm. Another came to help and was shot in the left shoulder. When yet another platoon member came to their aid, he was shot in the right side of the chest and right hip. A sixth platoon member was shot in the left posterior thorax when he tried to help. Finally, a seventh member was wounded in the right thigh when he came to help. Patient B was dead due to massive head trauma from a gunshot wound.

Auto Extraction

Auto extraction, that is, having the casualty move to a position of safety under his or her own power, is an important concept that can save lives in the warm zone. Distinguishing between the recovery of the deceased and rescue of a viable patient is

TABLE 13-2

PRINCIPLE CONCEPTS OF RAM

1. Do not sacrifice personnel when the likely benefits are minimal (e.g., patient is dead or does not have a life-threatening injury).
2. Assess from a safe location initially, and expose the provider only if medically indicated.
3. Provide only critical treatment (e.g., airway support, hemorrhage control) until the cold zone has been reached. Normal stabilization and extrication procedures must be evaluated against the risk-benefit ratio.

equally important. The RAM methodology is directed at making these differentiations from a position of cover and concealment, minimizing the initial risk to the medic. The principles of RAM are listed in Table 13-2.

Principles of RAM

First, determine if the area is secured. Next, establish if the patient is one of the perpetrators and therefore likely to be a threat to providers. Under such circumstances, medical extraction is inappropriate until the threat has been controlled. Attempt to evaluate the current level of injury or stability of the victim. This can be accomplished in a number of ways. Observation is the first technique that should be employed. This allows the medic to gather a lot of information about the casualty without revealing his or her position or intent to the opposing force. *Using a good pair of binoculars or night-vision goggles can often help ascertain if the patient is breathing, the rate and quality of respirations, the presence of extensive hemorrhage, and the presence of obvious wounds incompatible with life, such as brain evisceration.* In cold weather, a respiratory condensation plume can often be seen from the patient's mouth. The medic should establish prearranged signals with team members that will allow them to give an "okay" sign that is not easily detected by others who don't know to look for it. For example, one might use a rhythmical flexing of the little finger on the side closest to friendly forces. Figure 13-6 shows the decision pathways for the RAM algorithm.

MEDICINE ACROSS THE BARRICADE

Medicine Across the Barricade (MAB) is another useful technique developed as part of the CONTOMS program at the Uniformed Services University of the Health Sciences. It has been successfully employed in numerous barricade situations and resulted in the saving of lives and perhaps even the early resolution of some situations.

MAB Concept

MAB was designed to provide a mechanism of addressing medical problems among hostages, hostage-takers, or barricaded subjects without placing caregivers at increased risk.

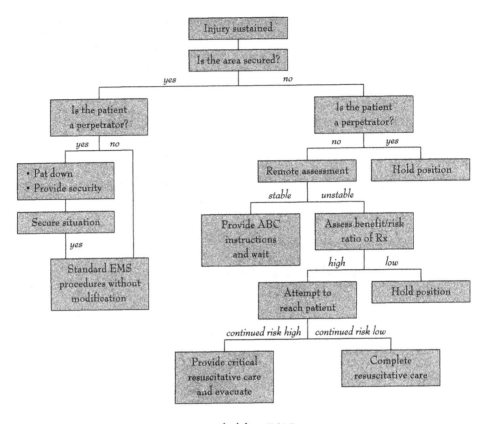

Figure 13-6 Rapid and Remote Assessment Methodology (RAM).

The concept is modeled, in part, after public access communications systems that provide prearrival instructions to citizens on the scene of a medical emergency. However, a tactical law enforcement scenario such as a hostage situation is much more complex than most EMS calls and involves concerns and objectives that may override the medical issues. Therefore, in order for MAB to be successful, it must be well integrated into the other aspects of the mission, such as negotiations, intelligence, tactics, and command (Figure 13-7).

Communications

Communication with the barricaded subject(s) is usually conducted via telephone (Figure 13-8), public address system, or direct speech. Generally, but not always, the situation on the far side of the barricade will not be visible to the medic. Therefore, it is important to paint a highly realistic picture of the far side situation. As information is acquired about the position of the patient, it may be useful to have another person role-play as the patient and position himself or herself exactly as described by the far side

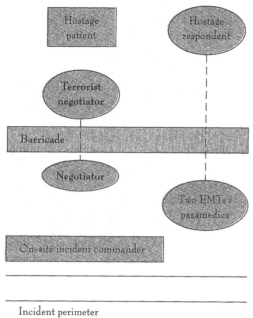

Incident perimeter

Figure 13-7 Medicine Across the Barricade (MAB)

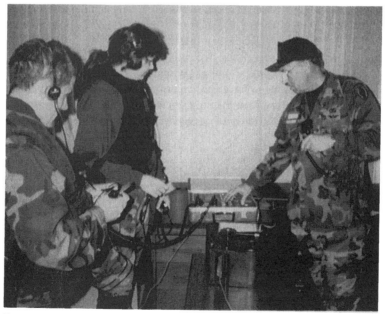

Figure 13-8 Communicating across the barricade.

respondent. This permits the medic to form a clear impression of the physical features of the scenario and facilitates the development of reasonable intervention options for relay.

Working with Negotiators

Although many negotiators initially respond negatively to the concept of MAB, it has been demonstrated that medical personnel sometimes have an instant credibility with subjects because they are perceived as "neutral" or "unbiased" parties. This can be used to the negotiators' advantage, resulting in early resolution. Furthermore, it is possible for the medic to act as the negotiator's medical expert, without ever talking to the subject himself or herself. Although the protocol shown in Table 13-3 is designed for clarity, this is not a technique that is easily learned from a book alone, and medics are cautioned to obtain plenty of practice under expert guidance before attempting this technique in an actual situation.

CLEARANCE FOR INCARCERATION

Once a tactical medical element is established as part of a SWAT team, the question of medically clearing subjects for incarceration will inevitably arise. Team commanders will often ask the medic to determine if the prisoner can go directly to a detention facility or if further medical care or evaluation is required. This is a difficult issue that is highly dependent on local laws, regulations, and circumstances. However, some general guidance can be useful.

Medical Clearance

Medically clearing subjects for incarceration from the scene can be extremely valuable to the tactical team. Relying on the judgment of a trained medical professional to determine whether the patient needs care at a fixed treatment facility can avoid the dangerous situation of delivering a seriously sick or injured prisoner to a lockup when he or she really needed to be in a hospital. Appropriate referral for evaluation and care can prevent some in-custody deaths. On-scene evaluation by a medical professional can also avoid unnecessary visits to the hospital emergency department, which represents a credible security risk and consumes time and manpower.

Clearance Versus Screening

In reality, the term medical clearance is a misnomer. *The subject is not being cleared of all medical problems, rather he or she is being screened for conditions likely to need urgent medical attention. This is a determination of whether an emergency medical condition exists.* If there is any suspicion of a potential problem, always err on the side of patient safety. That is the TEMS medic's top priority in this circumstance. In all cases, follow the protocols established by the medical director for medically screening subjects for incarceration.

Medical Capability

Before the medic can make any judgment about clearance for incarceration, he or she must know the medical capability at the detention facility. This capability can range from

TABLE 13-3

MEDICINE ACROSS THE BARRICADE PROTOCOL

1. Work with a partner.
2. Identify yourself, your partner, and your role—medical assistance. Calm and reassure.
3. Ask respondent what he or she would like to be called and whether or not he or she has had any prior medical training—regardless of how simple or rudimentary. Establish rapport.
4. Ask what happened—pertinent history.
5. Ask to describe the patient—what can respondent see. Visualize scene.
   a. Patient position and behavior
   b. Signs of injury or illness
6. Tell respondent not to move patient—control head and neck. Is there anyone to assist you?
7. Direct systematic assessment using specific simple instructions.
   a. A (airway). Visualize what you want done.
   b. B (breathing). What is the rate and quality?
   c. C (circulation). Have respondent count pulse while you time.
   d. D (disability). Determine neurologic status.
   e. E (expose)
   f. Secondary survey
8. Direct appropriate interventions, and evaluate responses using simple terms.
   a. Visualize what you want done.
   b. Use material at the scene.
   c. Use no more than two steps at a time.
9. If respondent loses confidence in you, have partner take over.
10. If patient removal is essential, tell the respondent.
11. Contact medical control for advice if appropriate.
12. Maintain contact with respondent.
13. Report findings and recommendations to on-site incident commander.

full-time staff physician and nurse coverage to no medical coverage at all. Most detention facilities in the United States probably fall at the lower end of this continuum, with little or no medical expertise available on site. Obviously, the availability of further medical observation and follow-up makes it more reasonable for the team medic to screen certain patients for incarceration. The medic should also be aware of his or her own capabilities and limitations. Evaluating an individual in the field is necessarily brief and limited to a few diagnostic instruments (for example, sphygmomanometer). Do not overextend your training or abilities in making important patient safety judgments. Seek online medical direction whenever appropriate, and always follow established medical protocols.

Screening for incarceration should not focus only on acute, minor trauma that may have occurred, but also needs to consider pertinent medical history. For example, patients with communicable diseases may need to be evaluated and have their illness controlled before being admitted to the general detention population. Medics can be helpful in sorting out a prisoner's medication and determining which legitimate pharmaceuticals should be taken to the lockup with the prisoner.

Though specific criteria for exclusion from out-of-hospital screening for incarceration will vary from one area to another, there are minimum exclusion criteria. If any of these findings are present, the patient should be evaluated at a medical treatment facility prior to incarceration. Table 13-4 outlines medical "clearance" or screening for incarceration.

The environment that exists during a law enforcement tactical operation in which a subject is taken into custody can be seen by some as intimidating and coercive. It is important that this not interfere with the rendering of sound medical judgment regarding the fitness of the subject to be incarcerated. If there are any doubts, it is usually best to err conservatively and have the subject evaluated again at a hospital. Furthermore, the ability to render such judgments will depend highly on the qualifications and scope of practice of the individual medic. Physicians acting in this role will be able to clear some patients whom a basic EMT would not be able to clear.

PATTERNS OF INJURY

Through the CONTOMS program, data are collected on a regular basis from more than 180 tactical law enforcement teams that have medical support programs. This information can be used to characterize the nature of the injuries that will present in this unique environment and to identify opportunities for aggressive injury control practices that will improve operations and outcome for all involved. It is useful to examine these data as a snapshot of what you might expect in supporting a SWAT team.

Agencies of different sizes and with different mission profiles, have contributed to this database. Some agencies run a large volume of missions each year, whereas others run very few. To help compare dissimilar agencies, casualty rates, rather than just the

---

TABLE 13-4

MEDICAL SCREENING FOR INCARCERATION

1. Airway compromise
2. Respiratory compromise—wheezing, lung congestion, excessive coughing
3. Perfusion compromise—pulse rate, blood pressure, or room air SaO_2 abnormal
4. Altered mentation
5. Compromised mental health
6. Skeletal compromise, including gross deformity and abnormalities affecting function
7. Integument compromise, including significant lacerations, deep lacerations to the hands, and burns
8. Septic compromise, including body temperature over 38.3°C (101°F), severe dental abscess or infection, significant cellulitis
9. Noncompliance with prescribed medications
10. Complaint of severe pain

TABLE 13-5

CASUALTY RATES PER 1000 PERSON-MISSIONS
(ACTIVITY TYPE BY PERSONNEL STATUS)

	TACTICAL TEAM	LAW ENFORCEMENT	PERPETRATORS	BYSTANDERS
High-risk warrant	4.6	1.9	18.2	3.6
Barricade	7.0	2.6	246.2	6.6
Hostage rescue	5.5	1.5	207.3	22.1
Dignitary protection	0.0	0.9	0.0	0.0
Crowd control/civil disorder	0.0	1.5	0.1	0.2
Training	8.8	2.4	0.0	13.8
Other	7.7	2.3	27.9	0.0

number of casualties, are examined. The primary variables that affect a team's overall risk of injury are the number of personnel placed at risk and the number of times they are at risk. The concept of a "person-mission" accounts for these two variables. One person present at one mission represents a person-mission. If you are a member of a tactical team that consists of 10 personnel, and your team runs 100 calls each year, the team would have 10 x 100 = 1000 person-missions per year. Use of the person-mission denominator-that is, x casualties per 1000 person-missions-helps account for differences in team size as well as team activity levels.

Table 13-5 shows the casualty rates per 1000 person-missions for various categories of participants and types of typical missions. Table 13-6 shows the distribution of mission types that produce casualties. It is clear from the tables that tactical officers are at higher risk of injury than other law enforcement officers, except in crowd control and dignitary protection operations. *Although high-risk warrant service accounts for most SWAT injuries (36.9% of all missions that result in casualties), barricades and hostage rescues are actually riskier situations.* They have a casualty rate of 7.0, and 5.5 casualties per 1000 person-missions, respectively, compared to the casualty rate for high-risk warrant service of 4.6 per 1000 person-missions. Barricades and hostage rescues produce fewer numbers of injuries (19% and 4% of all missions that produced casualties, respectively) for the SWAT officers because they occur less frequently.

Table 13-6 shows that training accounts for 23.9% of all missions that produce casualties. Those teams that do not include their medical element on training missions are probably making a mistake and missing an opportunity to reduce injury and its consequences. The overall high rate of bystander casualties (Table 13-5) is also noteworthy and adds to the rationale for having a tactical medical element for civilian law enforcement tactical operations.

Table 13-7 shows the outcome of injuries incurred during SWAT operations. The majority of injuries (89%) do not require admission to the hospital. However, about 6% of all casualties die, and another 5% suffer serious injuries as evidenced by their admis-

TABLE 13-6

DISTRIBUTION OF MISSIONS AND CASUALTIES BY OPERATION TYPE

	NUMBER OF INCIDENTS	PERCENT	INCIDENTS WITH CASUALTIES	PERCENT	TOTAL CASUALTIES	PERCENT
High-risk warrant service	2206	49.7	226	36.9	304	19.8
Barricade	384	8.7	114	18.6	197	12.8
Hostage rescue	77	1.7	25	4.1	50	3.2
Dignitary protection	64	1.4	2	0.3	2	0.1
Crowd control/riot	56	1.3	14	2.3	622	40.4
Training	1248	28.1	146	23.9	242	15.7
Other	400	9.0	85	13.9	122	7.9
Total	4435	99.9	612	100	1539	99.9

TABLE 13-7

OUTCOME BY PERSONNEL STATUS

	TACTICAL TEAM	LAW ENFORCEMENT	PERPETRATORS	BYSTANDERS	TOTAL	PERCENT (OF TOTAL)
Treated and released	322	65	193	44	624	88.9
Admitted to hospital	6	3	23	5	37	5.3
Died at hospital	0	0	6	0	6	0.9
Died en route to hospital	0	0	1	0	1	0.1
Died at scene	0	1	28	5	34	4.8

sion to the hospital. Table 13-8 shows that abrasions and contusions are the most common injuries, but gunshot wounds account for 13% of all injuries.

In this database, airway adjuncts, such as an oropharyngeal airway, endotracheal tube, or bag-valve-mask, were used in approximately 2% of all treatments rendered. Among these casualties, only one-third survived until arrival at the hospital. Seven and a half percent of the casualties received IV fluid administration. Nearly 90% of these casualties survived. The majority of the injuries were to the face, head, hand, and eye. Examination of the details of these injuries suggests that the use of protective equipment such as face shields, helmets, gloves, and ballistic eyewear could offer significant protection and reduction in the casualty rate.

SUMMARY

The development of tactical emergency medical support for law enforcement operations has achieved credibility and acceptance in recent years. It is a science that borrows heavily from military medicine and the lessons learned through centuries of

TABLE 13-8

DISTRIBUTION OF INJURIES BY INJURY TYPE

	TACTICAL TEAM	LAW ENFORCEMENT	PERPETRATORS	BYSTANDERS	TOTAL	PERCENT (OF TOTAL)
Fracture	10	4	1	2	17	2
Dislocation	5	3	0	0	8	1
Sprain/strain	45	9	21	5	80	8
Heat/dehydration	9	3	1	0	13	1
Cold injury	0	1	1	0	2	0
Electrical injury	6	0	9	0	15	2
Toxic exposure	21	3	7	2	33	3
Abrasion	62	15	78	2	157	15
Contusion	50	16	83	6	155	15
Laceration	43	9	44	4	100	10
Puncture	7	9	14	2	32	3
Amputation	0	0	2	0	2	0
Cut by sharp instrument	20	6	27	5	58	6
Gunshot	20	5	92	15	132	13
Blunt internal	0	0	7	3	10	1
Burn	18	0	4	2	24	2
Other	113	11	37	19	180	18
Total	429	94	428	67	1018	100

military medical support. However, there are important differences between the two fields, and lessons drawn from one environment must be cautiously modified and applied to the other. The essential difference between everyday EMS and TEMS is that in everyday EMS, the delivery of medical care is the mission, whereas in TEMS, medicine is a tool to help achieve the overall tactical mission. Certain specific techniques or modifications of existing techniques contribute to successful operation in this specialized environment.

FOR FURTHER READING

REESE K, Jones J, Kenepp G, Krohmer J: Into the Fray: Integration of Emergency Medical Services and Special Weapons and Tactics (SWAT) Teams. Prehospital and Disaster Medicine, 1996; Vol. 11(3): 202-206.

HEISKELL LE, Carlo P: Scoop and Run vs Stay and Treat: Some Tactical Considerations. The Tactical Edge, 1996; Vol. 14(3): 61-63.

CARMONA RH, Rasumoff D: Trends in Tactical Emergency Medical Support. The Tactical Edge, 1996; Vol. 14(2): 52.

Leibovich M, Speer CW: Physician Involvement in Police Tactical Teams. The Tactical Edge, 1995; Vol.13(4): 48-50.

Carmona RH, Rasumoff D: Use of TEMS on SWAT Operations. The Tactical Edge, 1995; Vol. 13(3): 69.

Carmona RH, Rasumoff D: The Integration of Tactics and Emergency Medical Support. The Tactical Edge, 1995; Vol. 13(1): 69-70.

Heiskell LE, Carmona RH: Tactical Emergency Medical Services: An Emerging Subspecialty of Emergency Medicine. Annals of Emergency Medicine, 1994; Vol. 23(4): 778-785.

Rasumoff D, Carmona RH: Position Paper: Use of Physicians in the Tactical Environment. The Tactical Edge, 1994; Vol. 12(2): 77-86.

McArdle DQ: Integration of Emergency Medical Services and Special Weapons and Tactics (SWAT) Teams: The Emergence of the Tactically Trained Medic. Prehospital and Disaster Medicine, 1992; July-September.

Burg M: Tactical EMS Emergency Medical Services, 1992; Vol. 21: 76-77.

Carmona RH, Rasumoff D: Tactical Emergency Medical Support (TEMS): An Emerging Specialized Area of Prehospital Care. Prehospital and Disaster Medicine, 1991; 394.

Rasumoff D, Carmona RH: Burns in the Tactical Environment. The Tactical Edge, 1990; Vol. 9(1): 54.

Appendix A

MEDICATIONS FOR THE TACTICAL ENVIRONMENT

Prescription Drugs Listed
1. Albuterol (Ventolin)
2. Amyl Nitrite
3. Atropine
4. Cefazolin (Ancef)
5. Diazepam (Valium)
6. Morphine
7. Pyridostigmine
8. Sodium Iodine
9. Sodium Nitrite
10. Sodium Thiosulfate
11. Pralidoxime (2-pam-chloride)

Nonprescription (Over-the-Counter) Drugs Listed
1. Acetaminophen (Tylenol)
2. Antacids (Tums, Mylanta, Maalox)
3. Attapulgite (Kao-Pectate)
4. Bacitracin
5. Diphenhydramine (Benadryl)
6. Calamine Lotion
7. Dextromethorphan
8. Oil of Clove (Eugenol)
9. Ibuprofen (Advil, Nuprin, Motrin IB)
10. Pseudoephedrine (Sudafed)

PRESCRIPTION MEDICATIONS

The prescription medications listed in this appendix are for use by properly trained medics (usually trained and certified at the advanced EMT level) under the close supervision of a medical director. Specific, written protocols are an important aspect of prehospital drug administration, and their use is strongly encouraged.

The medications listed were chosen because of their particular significance to tactical emergency care. Other important medications are needed to treat effectively many emergencies not peculiar to the tactical environment. Readers are encouraged to review one of the many fine paramedic-level EMT textbooks available for a complete review of emergency drugs used in general prehospital practice.

Albuterol (Ventolin, Proventil)
Class: Beta-2 agonist.
Description: Sympathomimetic that is selective for Beta-2 adrenergic receptors.
Mechanism of action: Stimulates smooth muscle of airway to cause bronchodilation

Indications: Relief of bronchoconstriction caused by pulmonary or riot control chemical agents. Also indicated for bronchoconstriction due to asthma, anaphylaxis, and chronic lung disease.

Contraindications: Known hypersensitivity to albuterol.

Precautions: Always monitor the patient's vital signs when administering albuterol. Use with caution in elderly persons or patients with known ischemic heart disease. Auscultate breath sounds before and after treatment.

Side effects: Anxiety, nervousness, tachycardia, palpitations, dizziness, headache, dysrhythmias, hypertension, nausea, and vomiting.

Interactions: Simultaneous use with other sympathomimetics may increase incidence of side effects. Beta-blockers may blunt or completely negate the effects of albuterol.

Dosage: 2.5 mg (0.5 ml of a 0.5% solution) mixed in 5-ml normal saline nebulized. A metered dose inhaler (MDI) delivers 90 g of albuterol in each puff. Administer 2 puffs per dose. Dosing can be repeated every 20 min up to 3 doses. For long evacuation, repeat this dosing protocol every 3-4 hours if needed.

Pediatric dosage: 0.15 mg (0.03 ml)/kg in 2.5-5 ml normal saline nebulized.

How supplied: Solution for nebulization is supplied in single-dose vials containing 2.5 mg (0.5 ml) albuterol. MDIs contain approximately 300 90 g puffs.

Amyl Nitrite

Class: Cyanide antidote; nitrite.

Description: Reducing agent that converts hemoglobin to methemoglobin. Methemoglobin preferentially binds cyanide.

Mechanism of action: Forms methemoglobin in blood by reducing hemoglobin.

Indications: Cyanide poisoning with severe symptoms.

Contraindications: IV established and able to give sodium nitrite.

Precautions: May cause life-threatening methemoglobinemia. A potential drug of abuse, therefore it must be properly secured.

Side effects: Hypotension, vasodilation, euphoria.

Interactions: May potentiate methemoglobin formation when used with sodium nitrite.

Dosage: 1 ampule crushed and inhaled.

Pediatric dosage: Same.

How supplied: A component of the Pasadena Cyanide antidote kit. However, not available in all kits supplied to the military.

Atropine

Class: Anticholinergic.

Description: Parasympatholytic (anticholinergic) that is derived from *Atropa belladonna* plant.

Mechanism of action: A potent anticholinergic that acts by blocking acetylcholine receptors, thus inhibiting parasympathetic stimulation. It is an important antidote for nerve agent and organophosphate insecticide poisoning.

Indications: Nerve agent poisoning. Also, cardiac arrest, hemodynamically significant bradycardia, and organophosphate poisoning.

Contraindications: None for emergencies.

Precautions: The traditional maximum dose of 0.04 mg/kg (approximately 3 mg for an adult) may need to be exceeded in nerve agent poisoning. Life-threatening heat stroke may result if given in very hot climates because atropine inhibits sweating.

Side effects: Blurred vision, dilated pupils, dry mouth, tachycardia, drowsiness and confusion.

Interactions: None in the tactical setting.

Dosage: For nerve agent poisoning and mild symptoms; 2 mg IV/IM. For severe symptoms, 6 mg IV/IM/ET. May be repeated in 2-mg increments for a total of 12 mg until secretions are dry. During prolonged evacuation, redose 2 mg every 5 min up to 20 mg total or until secretions dry.

Pediatric dosage: 0.02 mg/kg (0.1 mg minimum dose).

How supplied: Available in autoinjector form (Mark I) containing atropine 2 mg. Also available in prefilled syringes for IV/IM use containing 1 mg atropine in 10 ml solution.

Cefazolin (Ancef)

Class: Antibiotic.

Description: Cephalosporin antibiotic. It is chemically related to the penicillins, but is effective against a broader range of bacteria.

Mechanism of action: Prevents and fights bacterial infections. Inhibits the synthesis of bacterial cell walls, which kills the bacteria.

Indications: Prophylaxis against infection from serious gunshot, shrapnel, or other missile wound.

Contraindications: Allergy to penicillin or cephalosporin antibiotics.

Precautions: Should be given only for serious wounds when evacuation time exceeds 1 hour. Give only after all immediate life-threats have been addressed first.

Side effects: Usually well-tolerated.

Interactions: None in the tactical setting.

Dosage: 2 gm IV/IM given once.

Pediatric dosage: 50 mg/kg IV/IM given once.

Note: Cefoxitin, ceftriaxone, and other cephalosporin antibiotics have similar activity and profiles. Substitution (at the appropriate dose) is permissible if authorized by a physician.

Diazepam (Valium)

Class: Anticonvulsant, sedative.

Description: Benzodiazepine, which is used as an anticonvulsant and sedative.

Mechanism of action: Suppresses the spread of seizure activity across the brain. Does not appear to suppress the seizure focus, however. Induces sedation and muscle relaxation by directly stimulating specific brain receptors.

Indications: Convulsions associated with nerve agents. Also used to stop other seizures, and as a sedating and antianxiety agent for cardioversion and other painful or uncomfortable procedures.

Contraindications: Known hypersensitivity to diazepam.

Precautions: Diazepam is a relatively short-acting drug. During prolonged evacuation, seizures may recur. Injectable diazepam is irritating to veins, so use the largest IV catheter possible when administering by IV. A controlled substance and must be properly secured. Diazepam can be reversed with flumazenil (Romazicon).

Side effects: Hypotension, drowsiness, headache, amnesia, respiratory depression, blurred vision, nausea, and vomiting.

Interactions: Diazepam is incompatible with many medications. Any time diazepam is given intravenously, be sure to flush the line before and after administration. The effect of diazepam can be additive with other CNS depressants and alcohol.

Dosage: For convulsions associated with nerve agent poisoning 10 mg IV/IM/ET. May be repeated in 5-mg increments every 5 minute up to 20 mg or until convulsions stop.

For prolonged evacuation, dose up to 10 mg every 2-3 hours as needed to control seizures.

Pediatric dosage: 0.2 mg/kg IV/IM/ET up to 10 mg.

How supplied: Available as autoinjector containing diazepam 10 mg. Also available in ampules and prefilled syringes containing 10 mg in 2 ml solvent.

Note: Other benzodiazepines such as lorazepam (Ativan) are equally effective in controlling seizures. Substitution (at the appropriate dose) is permissible if authorized by a physician.

Sodium Iodine

Class: Essential trace element.

Description: Trace mineral required by the thyroid gland to produce thyroid hormone.

Mechanism of action: Blocks the uptake of radioactive iodine by the thyroid gland.

Indications: When radioactive iodine has been (or there is an imminent threat) released into the air or contaminates the food supply.

Contraindications: Known hypersensitivity to sodium iodide.

Precautions: None.

Side effects: Possible skin rashes, swelling of the salivary glands, a metallic taste in the mouth, and sore teeth, throat, and gums. More severe but very rare effects include fever, joint pain, facial or body swelling, and shortness of breath.

Interactions: None.

Dosage: One tablet (130 mg) per day. Preferably start the medication several days before or soon after exposure to radioactive iodine. However, the medication may be given at any time after exposure.

Pediatric dosage: One table (130 mg) per day for children 1 year and older. Half tablet (65 mg) per day for children under 1 year old. Crush tablet and mix with food or drink as needed.

How supplied: Multitablet vial of 130-mg tablets.

Morphine

Class: Narcotic analgesic.

Description: Naturally occurring CNS depressant and potent analgesic derived from opium.

Mechanism of action: Acts on opiate receptors in the brain and spinal cord, providing analgesia and sedation. Generally depresses CNS function. The potent analgesic properties of morphine make it an ideal pain reliever for serious wounds and injuries.

Indications: Severe pain and suffering associated with gunshot, blast, or burn injuries. Also used for relief of pain in extremity injuries and myocardial infarction.

Contraindications: Known hypersensitivity to morphine. Morphine is contraindicated in isolated serious head injury, isolated altered mental status, and hypotension.

Precautions: High potential for abuse. Requires secure storage and careful record keeping. At very high doses, can cause significant respiratory depression. Morphine can be reversed with naloxone (Narcan).

Side effects: Nausea, vomiting, abdominal cramps, blurred vision, constricted pupils, altered mental status, respiratory depression, headache, and hypotension.

Interactions: The CNS depressant properties of morphine can be increased when administered with other CNS depressants and alcohol.

Dosage: 2 mg IV/IM. May be repeated in 2-mg increments up to a total of 10 mg (0.25 mg/kg). Titrate to relieve suffering, not to induce sedation. Prolonged evacuation may require redosing at 2-10 mg every 4 hours as needed

Pediatric dosage: 0.05 mg/kg IV/IM. May be repeated in 0.05 mg/kg increments up to a total of 0.25 mg/kg. Prolonged evacuation may require redosing at 0.05-0.25 mg/kg every 4 hours as needed.

How supplied: 1-ml ampules/vials containing 5, 8, 10, and 15 mg, and tubex syringes containing 1 ml volume of 2, 4, 8, 10, and 15 mg.

Pyridostigmine

Class: Cholinergic-stimulating agent.

Description: Carbamate acetylcholinesterase (AChE) inhibitor.

Mechanism of action: Temporarily blocks the enzyme AChE. When taken as a pretreatment, pyridostigmine blocks some of the AChE receptors. These blocked receptors are then unavailable for binding with nerve agents. After a few hours, the pyridostigmine releases the AChE, restoring normal function.

Indications: Pretreatment when the risk of nerve agent exposure, particularly soman (GD) is high. May not be effective for sarin (GB) or VX nerve agents.

Contraindications: Known hypersensitivity to pyridostigmine. Not an antidote and may worsen nerve agent toxicity and so is contraindicated if exposure has already occurred. Also contraindicated in urinary and gastric obstruction.

Precautions: May precipitate severe respiratory distress in asthmatics.

Side effects: Nausea, vomiting, abdominal cramps, salivation, increased bronchial secretions, constricted (pinpoint) pupils, sweating, and skin rash. Can also cause weakness and fasciculations (localized muscle twitching).

Interactions: Effects can be additive if taken with similar medications such as neostigmine or physostigmine. Over time, tablets of pyridostigmine can become mottled from exposure to moisture. This does not affect the medication.

Dosage: 30 mg po every 8 hours.

Pediatric dosage: Not established for pretreatment. However, based on information on the use of pyridostigmine in children for other reasons, a dose of 0.5 mg/kg po every 8 hours may be effective.

How supplied: 30-mg tablets in a 7-day (21 tablets) blister-pack. Also available as 60-mg scored tablets (half tablet is 30 mg) and in syrup form, 60 mg per 5 ml.

Sodium Nitrite

Class: Cyanide antidote; nitrite.
Description: Reducing agent that converts hemoglobin to methemoglobin. Methemoglobin preferentially binds cyanide.
Mechanism of action: Forms methemoglobin in blood by reducing hemoglobin. Methemoglobin preferentially binds cyanide.
Indications: Cyanide poisoning with severe symptoms.
Contraindications: None in emergencies.
Precautions: May cause life-threatening methemoglobinemia.
Side effects: Hypotension, vasodilation, euphoria.
Interactions: May potentiate methemoglobin formation when used with amyl nitrite.
Dosage: 300 mg IV over 2-4 minutes.
Pediatric dosage: 6 mg/kg IV over 2-4 minutes.
How supplied: Available in Pasadena Cyanide antidote kit as a 10-ml ampule containing 3% sodium nitrite.

Sodium Thiosulfate

Class: Sulfate-forming compound.
Description: A sulfate-forming compound that reacts with cyanide-methemoglobin.
Mechanism of action: Reacts with cyanide-methemoglobin complex in blood to detoxify the cyanide and allow excretion by the kidneys.
Indications: Suspected cyanide poisoning with severe symptoms.
Contraindications: Do not administer until after sodium nitrite is administered.
Precautions: Does not detoxify cyanide unless a nitrite (amyl or sodium nitrite) is administered first.
Side effects: Hypotension is the chief side effect.
Interactions: Works together with nitrites to detoxify cyanide.
Dosage: 12.5 gm IV.
Pediatric dosage: 250 mg/kg IV.
How supplied: Available in Pasadena cyanide antidote kit as a 50-ml ampule of 25% sodium thiosulfate.

Pralidoxime (Protopam, 2-Pam-Chloride)

Class: Oxime.
Description: Regenerator of acetylcholinesterase (AChE) that has been inactivated by a nerve agent or organophosphate insecticide.
Mechanism of action: Breaks the bond between the nerve agent and AChE, thus restoring its function.
Indications: Nerve agent poisoning.
Contraindications: None in emergencies.
Precautions: Will variably regenerate AChE depending on the type of nerve agent and the time elapsed since exposure. Some nerve agents age with time (minutes to hours) and become resistant to pralidoxime effects.
Side effects: Inconsequential in the setting of nerve agent poisoning.
Interactions: Works synergistically with atropine, and the two should always be used together.
Dosage: For mild symptoms, 600 mg IV/IM. For severe symptoms, 1800 mg IV/IM. For prolonged evacuation, redosing may be required at 1000 mg IV/IM administered over 20 minutes every 60 min or until spontaneous respirations return.
Pediatric dosage: For mild symptoms, 10 mg/kg IV/IM. For severe symptoms, 30 mg/kg up to 1 gm IV/IM. For prolonged evacuation, redosing may be required at 15 mg/kg IV/IM administered over 20 minutes every 60 min or until spontaneous respirations return.

How supplied: Available in autoinjector (Mark I) containing pralidoxime 600 mg. Also available in vials containing 1 gm of powder for reconstitution with 20-ml sterile water.

NONPRESCRIPTION (OVER-THE-COUNTER) MEDICATIONS

The medications listed in this formulary are intended for use in otherwise healthy adults. Medics dispensing these medications must be properly trained and authorized in their use. Clear protocols and strong medical direction are essential for effective and safe use of these medications. Medics must be thoroughly familiar with the safe and effective use of any medication dispensed. Carefully read and follow the manufacturer's instructions before using any medication.

The dispensing of medications outlined in this formulary is intended for military medics treating active-duty service members. There is little experience to date with EMS or prehospital personnel (military or civilian) dispensing medications to civilians. Therefore, this latter approach cannot be recommended. Consultation and close coordination with medical control and local authorities is required before attempting to use these medications in any manner not consistent with traditional EMS or prehospital practice.

Allergies and Contraindications Some patients will experience serious adverse reactions to medications. Medics must carefully determine if a patient has any suspected allergy or contraindication to a medication prior to administering it. If in doubt, consult a physician prior to dispensing the medication.

Pregnant Women and Nursing Mothers Pregnant women or women in whom pregnancy is suspected, as well as nursing mothers, should avoid medications when possible. The medic should question every female patient of childbearing age (roughly 11-55 years) about the possibility of pregnancy and nursing prior to administering any medication. Also counsel the female patient to avoid getting pregnant while taking medications. If in doubt, consult a physician prior to dispensing the medication.

Acetaminophen (Tylenol)

Class: Nonnarcotic analgesic (pain reliever).
Description: Nonnarcotic analgesic and antipyretic unrelated to aspirin or NSAIDs.
Mechanism of action: Inhibits the formation of pain-producing substance at the cellular level.
Indications: Temporary relief of minor aches and pains associated with the common cold, toothache, and muscular aches.
Contraindications: Known hypersensitivity to acetaminophen. Avoid in patients with chronic alcoholism and liver failure.
Precautions: Avoid if the patient regularly consumes 3 or more alcoholic drinks per day or has liver problems. Serious overdosage produces little or no initial symptoms; however, death from liver failure may occur days later. All overdoses need physician attention, even if asymptomatic.
Side effects: Remarkably few side effects.
Interactions: Do not take with other acetaminophen-containing medications.
Dosage: 650-1000 mg po q 4 hours.
How supplied: Tablets 325 mg (regular strength), 500 mg (extra strength).

Antacids (Tums, Mylanta, Maalox)

Class: Antacids.
Description: Alkaline compounds of calcium, aluminum, and/or magnesium.
Mechanism of action: Reduces stomach acid by neutralizing acid.
Indications: Temporary relief of discomfort from acid indigestion (dyspepsia) or heartburn or upset stomach.
Contraindications: Known hypersensitivity to any of the antacid components.
Precautions: Persistent use may mask serious symptoms and delay seeking of a physician's care. Avoid in patients with kidney disease.
Side effects: Diarrhea and constipation are possible with continued use.
Interactions: Antacids can interfere with the absorption of many prescription medications, including tetracycline. Consult a physician or pharmacist if the patient is taking prescription medications.

Dosage: Calcium carbonate (Tums) 1000 mg po chewed; aluminum and magnesium hydroxide (Mylanta, Maalox) 3 tablets chewed or 15 ml po.
How supplied: Calcium carbonate: 500-mg tablets. Aluminum and magnesium hydroxide: tablets or liquid.

Attapulgite (Kao-Pectate)

Class: Antidiarrheal.
Description: Refined clay (kaolin).
Mechanism of action: Acts to bind loose stools.
Indications: Temporary relief of minor diarrheal symptoms.
Contraindications: Known hypersensitivity to the components of the drug.
Precautions: Serious or persistent diarrhea requires physician attention.
Side effects: Bloating, constipation.
Interactions: Few significant interactions. May bind some drugs in the gastrointestinal tract.
Dosage: 30 ml (2 tablespoons) po or 2 tablets (do not chew) after each bowel movement, up to 6 doses (180 ml or 12 tablets) in 24 hours.
How supplied: Liquid and tablets containing 750-ml attapulgite per tablet or 5 ml.

Bacitracin

Class: Antibiotic.
Description: Topical, broad-spectrum antibiotic in a white petrolatum base.
Mechanism of action: Antibiotic helps prevent infection in minor wounds, while the petrolatum helps speed healing.
Indications: Prevention of infection in minor, uncomplicated wounds.
Contraindications: Known hypersensitivity to bacitracin. Not for internal use.
Precautions: Not for routine use in deep or puncture wounds, animal bites, or serious burns except on the advice of physician. Will not treat established infection; refer all suspected infections to physician. Prolonged exposure of petrolatum will weaken latex gloves. Avoid contact with eyes and mucous membranes. Do not swallow or take internally.
Side effects: Possible skin irritation.
Interactions: None.
Dosage: Apply liberally to wound tid-qid.
How supplied: Tubes of ointment containing bacitracin 500 units per gm.

Calamine Lotion

Class: Topical desiccant.
Description: Suspension of tinted zinc oxide.
Mechanism of action: Soothes, coats, protects, and dries minor skin irritations.
Indications: Temporarily relief of minor discomfort from poison ivy, oak, or sumac, insect bites, and similar minor skin irritations.
Contraindications: Deep or serious wounds. Not for internal use.
Precautions: Avoid contact with eyes and mucous membranes. Do not swallow or take internally.
Side effects: Minor skin irritation.
Interactions: None.
Dosage: Apply liberally to affected area tid-qid and allow to dry.
How supplied: Liquid suspension of 8% calamine.

Dextromethorphan (Benylin, Maximum Strength Robitussin)

Class: Nonnarcotic antitussive.
Description: Nonaddicting opioid-related antitussive (cough suppressant).
Mechanism of action: Suppresses the cough reflex through opioid receptor complex.
Indications: Temporary relief of minor cough due to the common cold.
Contraindications: Known hypersensitivity to dextromethorphan.
Precautions: Excessive or prolonged use may cause altered mental status.
Side effects: May cause drowsiness or jitteriness.

Interactions: May cause additive effects (drowsiness) when taken with narcotics, alcohol, or other depressant drugs. Do not take with MAOI (monoamine oxidase inhibitor) drugs used for depression and Parkinson disease.
Dosage: 30 mg po q 6 hours.
How supplied: 15 mg per 5 ml liquid.

Diphenhydramine (Benadryl)

Class: H$_1$ blocker (antihistamine).
Description: H$_1$ specific antihistamine.
Mechanism of action: Blocks histamine (H$_1$) receptors on cells, blocking the effects of histamine. Histamine is a vasoactive substance that causes swelling, itching, vasodilation, and bronchoconstriction.
Indications: Temporary relief of minor itch caused by poison ivy, insect bites, and similar minor skin irritations. Also used intravenously in anaphylaxis.
Contraindications: Known hypersensitivity to diphenhydramine.
Precautions: Avoid use in high heat-stress environments (hot, humid weather) or while wearing a chemical protective ensemble. Avoid where high degree of alertness is required (driving, guard duty, etc.).
Side effects: Dry mouth, drowsiness, decreased sweating, urinary retention, and other anticholinergic symptoms.
Interactions: May cause excessive drowsiness or sedation when used with alcohol or other drugs that cause CNS depression.
Dosage: 25-50 mg po qid.
How supplied: Tablets 25 mg, liquid 12.5 mg/5 ml.

Oil of Clove (Eugenol)

Class: Topical anesthetic.
Description: Extract of clove.
Mechanism of action: Acts as a local anesthetic when applied to mucous membranes.
Indications: Temporary relief of minor dental or oral discomfort from toothache, chipped teeth, or oral mucosal sores.
Contraindications: Known sensitivity to clove oil.
Precautions: For topical use on oral mucous membranes only. Not for internal use.
Side effects: Minor gum irritation. May slow healing of infection.
Interactions: None.
Dosage: Apply 1-2 drops to affected area qid.
How supplied: Liquid.

Ibuprofen (Advil, Nuprin, Motrin IB)

Class: Nonsteroidal antiinflammatory drug (NSAID).
Description: Nonnarcotic, nonsteroidal, antiinflammatory, and analgesic.
Mechanism of action: Acts to inhibit the formation of inflammation and pain-producing substances.
Indications: Temporary relief of minor aches and pains associated with the common cold, headache, toothache, and muscular aches.
Contraindications: Known hypersensitivity to ibuprofen, other NSAIDs, and aspirin.
Precautions: Avoid if the patient regularly consumes 3 or more alcoholic drinks per day or has liver problems. Avoid in patients with history of peptic ulcer disease, kidney failure, or asthma, except under the advice of a physician. Take with meals, and avoid dehydration (drink plenty of liquids). Prolonged use may cause serious gastrointestinal bleeding.
Side effects: Mild gastrointestinal upset.
Interactions: Do not take with other ibuprofen or NSAID containing medications.
Dosage: 200-400 mg po q 6 hours.
How supplied: 200 mg tablets, liquid 100 mg/5ml.

Pseudoephedrine (Sudafed)

Class: Sympathomimetic.

Description: Adrenergic-agonist.

Mechanism of action: Causes vasoconstriction of blood vessels in mucous membranes, resulting in decreased edema and reduced secretions.

Indications: Temporary relief of runny nose and nasal congestion due to common cold or allergic rhinitis.

Contraindications: Known sensitivity to pseudoephedrine.

Precautions: May worsen preexisting hyperglycemia (diabetes), hypertension, or hyperthyroidism. May cause urinary retention in patients with enlarged prostate glands.

Side effects: Jitteriness, increased heart rate, anxiety, sleeplessness.

Interactions: Avoid in patients taking medication for hypertension, thyroid disease, diabetes mellitus, or difficulty urinating from enlarged prostate. Do not take with MAOI (monoamine oxidase inhibitor) drugs used for depression and Parkinson disease.

Dosage: 60 mg po q 6 hours.

How supplied: 30 mg tablets, or liquid 15 mg/5ml.

Appendix B

CHEMICAL AGENT PROTECTIVE MEASURES

Procedures Listed

I. Donning the M40 series mask and hood
II. Donning the M17 series mask and hood
III. Decontaminating using the M258 kit
IV. Decontaminating using the M291 kit
V. Donning the military chemical protective overgarment
VI. Decontamination procedure for litter patient
VII. Decontamination procedure for ambulatory patient

I. Donning the M40 series mask and hood (Figure B-1)

1. Don your mask within 9 seconds.
   a. Stop breathing.
   b. Close your eyes.
   c. Remove your headgear and place your headgear in a convenient location, avoiding contaminated surfaces, if possible.

WARNING
DO NOT WEAR CONTACT LENSES WITH PROTECTIVE MASK. REMOVE CONTACT LENSES WHEN THE USE OF CHEMICAL AGENTS IS IMMINENT.

   d. Take off your glasses, placing them in a safe place.
   e. Open the carrier with your left hand holding the carrier open.
   f. Remove the mask from the carrier by grasping the mask with your right hand.
   g. Put your chin in the chin pocket.
   h. Seal the mask.
      (1) Cover the openings at the bottom of the outlet valve with the palm of your hand.
      (2) Blow out hard so that air escapes around the edges of the mask.
      (3) Cover the inlet port of the canister with the palm of your hand.
      (4) Breathe in.
   Note: The facepiece should collapse against your face and remain so while you hold your breath. If it does, the facepiece is airtight. If the facepiece does not collapse, check for hair, clothing, or other matter between the facepiece and your face.
      (5) Remove anything preventing a seal from forming between your face and the mask.
   i. Don the head harness.
      (1) Pull the head harness over your head after grasping the tab.
      (2) Position the harness so that your ears are between the temple straps and the cheek straps.
   j. Tighten the face straps one at a time with one hand while holding the facepiece to your face with the other hand to maintain the seal.
   k. Center the headpad at the high point on the back of your head.
   Note: The straps should lie flat against your head.
   l. Clear your mask again.
   m. Recheck your facepiece for leaks.
   n. Resume breathing.
2. Don the hood so that it lies smoothly on your head.

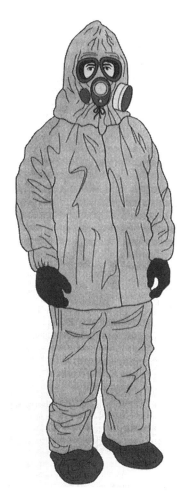

Figure B-1 M40 Mask and hood, worn properly.

CAUTION

BE VERY CAREFUL WHEN PULLING ON THE HOOD. THE HOOD COULD SNAG ON THE BUCKLES OF THE HEAD HARNESS AND TEAR.

    a. Grasp the back edge of the hood skirt.

    b. Pull the hood carefully over your head so that it covers the back of your neck, head, and shoulders.

    c. Zip the front of the hood closed by pulling the zipper slider downward.

    d. Tighten the draw cord.

    e. Secure the underarm straps by fastening and adjusting them.

    f. Put on your helmet.

    g. Close your mask carrier.

    h. Continue the mission.

3. Remove your protective mask with hood after the "all clear" order is given.

    a. Remove your helmet.

    b. Unfasten the underarm straps.

    c. Loosen the draw cord.

    d. Unzip the zipper on the hood.

4. Continue your mission.

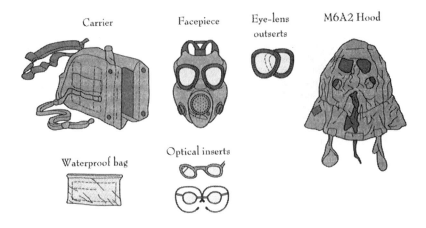

Carrier   Facepiece   Eye-lens outserts   M6A2 Hood

Waterproof bag   Optical inserts

Figure B-2 M17 mask and hood components.

II. Donning the M17 series mask and hood (Figure B-2)

1. Don your mask within 9 seconds.
   a. Stop breathing, holding your breath until the mask is sealed and cleared.
   b. Remove your headgear.
   c. Place your headgear in a convenient location, avoiding contaminated surfaces, if possible.
   d. Remove your glasses, placing them in a safe place (for example, the overgarment pocket), if appropriate.
   e. Open your mask carrier with your left hand holding the carrier open.
   f. Grasp your mask just below the eyepiece with your right hand.
   g. Pull the mask out of the carrier so that the hood hangs inside out in front of the facepiece.
   h. Grasp the facepiece with both hands. (Figure B-3)
   I. Slide your thumbs up and inside the mask, opening the head harness and facepiece as wide as you can.
   j. Put your chin in the chin pocket.
   k. Pull the head harness up over your head, making sure the head pad is centered at the back of your head and the mask is smooth against your face and forehead.
Note: Never put the head harness over your head first and then pull the mask down over your face.
   l. Adjust the mask by grasping the cheek straps with both hands and pulling them with moderate jerks.
   m. Clear the mask by the following steps:
      (1) Seal the outlet valve and voicemitter by cupping the heel of one hand over the outlet valve and placing the other hand over the voicemitter and applying pressure.
Note: You can put your hands either over or under the hood to do this.
      (2) Blow hard to force air out around the edges of the mask.
   n. Check the mask.
      (1) Place the palms of your hands over both inlet valve caps.
      (2) Seal the valves by applying pressure.
Note: You can either put your hands over or under the hood to do this.
      (3) Suck in and hold your breath.
   Note: If there are no leaks, your mask will collapse against your face and stay that way until you breathe out.
      (a) Go to step p, if you find your mask has no leaks.
      (b) Go to step o, if your mask does not collapse.
   o. Reseat a mask that leaks.

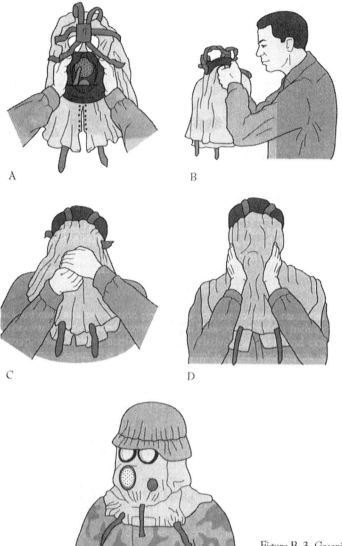

A   B

C   D

E

Figure B-3 Grasping facepiece of mask.

(1) Stop breathing.
(2) Check to see if there is anything, such as hair or clothing, between your face and the mask.
(3) Remove anything that would keep the mask from sealing against your face.
(4) Make sure the head straps and the head pad are not twisted.
(5) Tighten the head straps, if necessary.
(6) Clear your mask by repeating step m.
(7) Recheck your mask for leaks using step n.
p. Start breathing normally.
2. Don the hood within an additional 6 seconds.
   a. Pull the hood up and over your head and down onto your shoulders.

    b. Zip the front closed all the way, making sure the edge of the hood does not get caught in the collar of the overgarment.

3. Pull the draw cord slider snug, as the mission allows.
4. Fasten the underarm straps, adjusting them with buddy aid, if available as the mission allows.
5. Replace your headgear.
6. Close your mask carrier.
7. Continue your mission.

III.   **Decontaminating your skin and personal equipment using an M258A1 decontamination kit**

WARNING

THE M258A1 DECONTAMINATION KIT (OLIVE DRAB CASE AND WIPE PACKETS) WILL BE USED ONLY FOR ACTUAL CHEMICAL DECONTAMINATION. DO NOT USE WIPES ON YOUR EYES, MOUTH, OR OPEN WOUNDS. THESE AREAS SHOULD BE FLUSHED WITH WATER. FOR DECONTAMINATION OF BLISTERS, GIVE FIRST AID FOR BURNS.

1. Don your mask and hood without:
    a. Zipping the hood.
    b. Pulling the draw strings.
    c. Fastening the shoulder straps.
2. Seek overhead cover or use your poncho for protection against further contamination.
3. Decontaminate your hands with decontaminating wipe.
    a. Open the decontamination kit.
    b. Remove one decontaminating 1 packet.
    c. Fold the packet on the solid line marked BEND.
    d. Unfold the packet.
    e. Tear open the packet at the notch.
    f. Remove the wipe, fully unfolding it.
    g. Wipe your skin, starting with your hands.
4. Decontaminate your eyes, if necessary.
    a. Check your canteen for contamination.
      (1) Remove your canteen.
      (2) Unscrew the cap, avoiding possible contamination of the canteen cap by pushing up on the bottom of the canteen cover until you can grasp the canteen by its body.
      (3) Check the canteen mouth for contamination.
        (a) Obtain an uncontaminated canteen.
        (b) Decontaminate the canteen mouth with M258A1 decontamination kit.
    b. Unseal your mask as follows:
      (1) Hold your breath.
      (2) Close your eyes.
      (3) Lift the hood and mask from your chin.
    c. Flush your eyes with water from the canteen.
      (1) Look up, tilting your head to the side to be decontaminated.
      (2) Keep your eyes open.
      (3) Pour water slowly into your eye without letting the water run onto your clothing.
      (4) Flush the other eye, if necessary, using the same steps.
    d. Secure your mask by:
      (1) Resealing it.
      (2) Clearing it.
      (3) Checking it.
    e. Breathe.
5. Decontaminate your face, if necessary, with a decontaminating wipe 1.
    a. Unseal your mask as follows:
      (1) Hold your breath.

(2) Close your eyes.

(3) Lift the hood and mask from your chin.

b. Wipe up and down from ear to ear.

    (1) Start at your ear.

    (2) Wipe across your face to the corner of your nose.

    (3) Wipe across your face to the other ear.

c. Wipe up and down from your ear to the end of your jawbone.

    (1) Begin where step b ended.

    (2) Wipe across your cheek to the corner of your mouth.

    (3) Wipe across your closed mouth to the center of your upper lip.

    (4) Wipe across your closed mouth to the corner of your mouth.

    (5) Wipe across your cheek to the end of your jawbone.

d. Wipe up and down from one end of your jawbone to the other end of your jawbone.

    (1) Begin where you ended in step c.

    (2) Wipe across and under your jaw to your chin, cupping your chin.

    (3) Wipe across and under your jaw to the end of your jawbone.

e. Turn your hand out and quickly wipe the inside of the mask that touches your face.

Note: Do not wipe the mask lens. The decontaminating solution may leave a film on the lens.

f. Secure your mask by:

    (1) Resealing it.

    (2) Clearing it.

    (3) Checking it.

g. Breathe.

6. Decontaminate your neck and ears, if necessary, using the same decontamination 1 wipe.

7. Decontaminate your hands again with the same decontaminating 1 wipe.

8. Properly dispose of the contaminated wipe.

9. Prepare the decontaminating 2 wipe.

a. Pull out one decontaminating 2 wipe packet.

b. Crush the enclosed glass ampule between your thumb and fingers without kneading.

c. Fold the packet on the solid line marked CRUSH AND BEND.

d. Unfold it.

e. Tear the packet open quickly at the notch.

f. Remove the wipe.

g. Open the wipe fully.

h. Dispose of the crushed glass ampule by burying it.

10. Repeat steps 5 through 8 using the decontaminating 2 wipe.

11. Put on your protective gloves.

12. Fasten your hood.

13. Make sure all skin areas that you have decontaminated are covered.

14. Decontaminate your personal equipment.

Note: Do not use the decontaminating kit on protective overgarments.

a. Decontaminate weapons, gloves, helmet, and hand tools using decontaminating 1 wipe first, then decontaminating 2 wipe.

b. Decontaminate the exterior of the hood and mask.

    (1) Wipe eyelens outserts using a decontaminating 2 wipe.

    (2) Begin wiping the hood at the top working your way downward.

    (3) Repeat (1) and (2) above using decontaminating 1 wipe.

Note: Using the wipes in this order will prevent a residue from forming on the eyelens outserts.

15. Remove radiological contamination from your clothing, equipment, and exposed skin if necessary.

a. Shake or brush contaminated dust from your clothing, equipment, or exposed skin with a brush, broom, or your hands (if a brush or broom is not available).

b. Wash your body as soon as possible, giving special attention to the hairy areas and underneath your fingernails.

IV. **Decontaminating your skin using the M291 skin decontaminating kit (SDK)**
1. Inspect the M291 SDK for loose black powder.
   a. If no powder is detected, the kit is mission ready.
   b. If powder is detected, inspect each packet for leaks.
   c. Discard all leaking packets.
   d. Reinsert good packets into the carrying pouch.
2. Verify that there are at least four skin decontaminating packets in the kit.
Note: If there are fewer than four packets, request an additional kit, continuing to use your kit until all packets are gone.
CAUTION
FOR EXTERNAL USE ONLY. MAY BE SLIGHTLY IRRITATING TO THE SKIN OR EYES. KEEP DECONTAMINATING POWDER OUT OF YOUR EYES, CUTS, AND WOUNDS. USE WATER TO WASH TOXIC AGENT OUT OF YOUR EYES, CUTS, OR WOUNDS.
3. Decontaminate your skin with the M291 SDK within 1 minute of the suspected exposure.
   a. Put on your mask and hood without:
      (1) Zipping the hood.
      (2) Pulling the draw strings.
      (3) Fastening the shoulder straps.
   b. Seek overhead cover for protection against further contamination.
   c. Remove one skin decontaminating packet from the carrying pouch.
   d. Tear the packet open quickly at the notch.
   e. Remove the applicator pad from the packet.
   f. Properly dispose of the empty packet.
   g. Open the applicator pad.
      (1) Unfold the applicator pad.
      (2) Slip your finger(s) into the handle.
   h. Throughly scrub exposed skin on the back of your hand, palm, and fingers until completely covered with black powder from the applicator pad.
   I. Switch the applicator pad to the other hand, repeating the previous step on the other hand.
WARNING
DEATH OR INJURY MAY RESULT IF YOU BREATHE TOXIC AGENTS WHILE DECONT-AMINATING THE FACE. IF YOU NEED TO BREATHE BEFORE YOU FINISH, RESEAL YOUR MASK, CLEAR IT, AND CHECK IT. GET YOUR BREATH, THEN RESUME THE DECONTAMINATING PROCEDURE.
   j. Decontaminate your face and the inside of your mask.
      (1) Hold your breath.
      (2) Close your eyes.
      (3) Grasp the mask beneath your chin.
      (4) Pull the hood and mask away from your chin enough to allow one hand between the mask and your face.
      (5) Wipe up and down across your face, beginning at the front of one ear to your nose to other ear.
      (6) Wipe across your face to the corner of your nose.
      (7) Wipe extra strokes at the corner of your nose.
      (8) Wipe across your nose and the tip of your nose to the other corner of your nose.
      (9) Wipe extra strokes at the corner of your nose.
      (10) Wipe across your face to the other ear.
      (11) Wipe up and down across your face, beginning from the ear to your mouth to other end of the jawbone.
      (12) Wipe across your cheek to the corner of your mouth.
      (13) Wipe extra strokes at the corner of your mouth.
      (14) Wipe across your closed mouth to the center of your upper lip.
      (15) Wipe extra strokes above your upper lip.
      (16) Wipe across your closed mouth to the other corner of your mouth.

(17) Wipe extra strokes at the corner of your mouth.

(18) Wipe across your cheek to the end of your jawbone.

(19) Wipe up and down across your face, beginning from your jawbone, to your chin and to the other end of your jawbone.

(20) Wipe across and under your jaw to your chin, cupping your chin.

(21) Wipe extra strokes at the center of your chin.

(22) Wipe across and under your jaw to end of your jawbone.

(23) Decontaminate the inside of your mask by turning your hand out and quickly wiping the inside of the mask that touches your face.

(24) Properly dispose of the applicator pad.

(25) Seal your mask.

(26) Clear your mask.

(27) Check your mask.

(28) Breathe.

k. Remove the second packet from the carrying pouch.

l. Tear open the packet quickly at the notch.

m. Remove the applicator pad from the packet.

n. Discard the empty packet, employing litter discipline.

o. Open the applicator pad.

(1) Unfold the applicator pad.

(2) Slip your finger(s) into the handle.

p. Scrub throughly the skin of your neck and ears without breaking the seal between your face and the mask until they are completely covered with black powder.

q. Redo your hands until they are completely covered with black powder.

r. Properly dispose of the applicator pad.

s. Put on your protective gloves.

t. Fasten the hood.

u. Remove the powder with soap and water when operational conditions permit.

Note: It does not matter how long the powder stays on your skin.

V. Donning the military chemical protective overgarment

1. Put on an uncontaminated overgarment.

   a. Have your buddy open a package containing a new overgarment without touching the garment itself. (Figure B-4)

   b. Pull out the overgarment one piece at a time without touching the outside of the package.

      (1) Put on the new trousers, leaving the cuffs open.

      (2) Put on the jacket.

2. Put on the overboots. (Figure B-5)

   a. Have your buddy pick up a new package of overboots.

   b. Have your buddy open it without touching the overboots inside.

   c. Reach into the package.

   d. Remove the overboots.

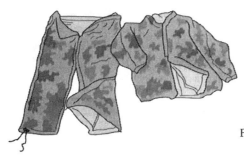

Figure B-4 Chemical overgarment.

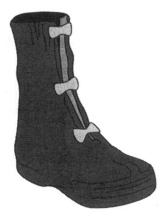

Figure B-5 Overboots.

    e. Put the overboots on.

3. Put on the green vinyl overboots (GVOs). (Figure B-5)
    a. Have your buddy pick up a new package of GVOs, opening it without touching the GVOs inside.
    b. Reach into the package, removing the GVOs.
    c. Put on the GVOs.

Note: GVO donning procedures are very basic; donning is done just like a regular wet weather boot.

4. Put on the gloves. (Figure B-6)
    a. Have your buddy pick up a package of new chemical protective gloves, opening it without touching the gloves inside.
    b. Remove the gloves from the package.

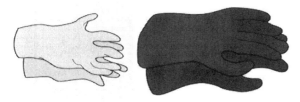

Figure B-6 Gloves.

    c. Put the gloves on.

5. Secure the hood.
    a. Have your buddy decontaminate his or her chemical protective gloves with the personal decontamination kit.
    b. Have your buddy reposition the hood as follows:

Note: The buddy's gloves must be decontaminated before proceeding with this step.

      (1) Unroll your hood.
      (2) Reattach the straps.
    c. Check all the zippers and ties on your hood and overgarment to ensure they are closed.

6. Repeat steps 3 through 5, taking the role of the buddy.

7. Secure your gear.
    a. Place the new chemical protective cover on your helmet.
    b. Put your individual gear back on.
    c. Check the fit of the secured gear of your buddy.
    d. Have him or her check your gear.

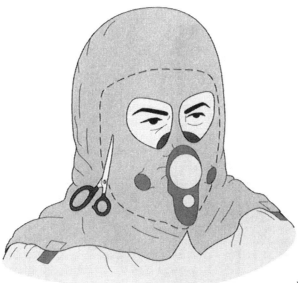

Figure B-7 Cutting off hood.

VI. Decontamination procedure for litter patient

1. Decontaminate the mask and hood: sponge down front, sides, and top of hood with 5.0% calcium hypochlorite solution, or wipe off with the M258A1 or the M291 Decon Kit.
2. Remove hood.
   a. Dip scissors in 5% hypochlorite (HTH) solution.
   b. Cut off hood. (Figure B-7)
      (1) Release or cut hood shoulder straps.
      (2) Cut/untie neck cord.
      (3) Cut/remove zipper cord.
      (4) Cut/remove drawstring under the voicemitter.
      (5) Unzip the hood zipper.
      (6) Cut the cord away from the mask.
      (7) Cut the zipper below voicemitter.
      (8) Proceed cutting upward, close to the inlet valve covers and eye lens outserts.
      (9) Cut upward to top of eye lens outsert.
      (10) Cut across forehead to the outer edge of the next eye lens outsert.
      (11) Cut downward toward patient's shoulder staying close to the eye lens outsert inlet valve cover.
      (12) Cut across the lower part of the voicemitter to the zipper.
      (13 Dip scissors in hypochlorite solution.
      (14) Cut from center of forehead over the top of the head.
      (15) Fold left and right sides of the hood to the side of the patient's head, laying sides on the litter.
   c. The Quick Doff Hood is loosened and removed.
3. Decontaminate protective mask/face.
   a. Use M258A1, M291, or 0.5% hypochlorite solution.
   b. Cover both inlet valve covers with gauze or hands.
   c. Wipe external parts of mask.
   d. Uncover inlet valve covers.
   e. Wipe exposed areas of patient's face.

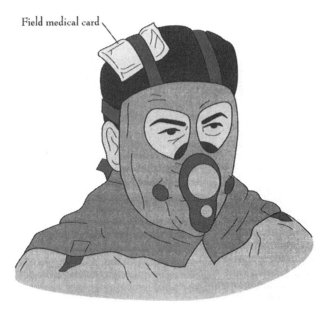

Field medical card

Figure B-8 Place field medical card (in plastic bag) in mask head straps.

      (1) Chin.
      (2) Neck.
      (3) Back of ears.
  4. Remove field medical care (FMC) or triage tag.
      a. Cut FMC tie wire.
      b. Allow FMC to fall into a plastic bag.
      c. Seal plastic bag and wash with 0.5% hypochlorite.
      d. Place plastic bag under back of mask head straps. (Figure B-8)
  5. Remove all gross contamination from patient's overgarment.
      a. Wipe all evident contamination spots with M258A1 Decon Kit, M291, or 5% hypochlorite.
      b. Wipe external parts of mask with M258A1 Decon Kit, or M291.
      c. Use wipe 1 then wipe 2, to clean exterior of mask; use wipe 2 then wipe 1 to clean interior.
  6. Cut and remove overgarments. Cut clothing around tourniquets, bandages, and splints. Two persons will be cutting clothing at the same time. Dip scissors in 5% hypochlorite solution before doing each complete cut to avoid contaminating inner clothing.
      a. Cut overgarment jacket. (Figure B-9)
         (1) Unzip protective overgarment.
         (2) Cut from wrist area of sleeves, up to armpits, and then to neck area.
         (3) Roll chest sections to respective sides with inner surface outward.
         (4) Tuck clothing between arm and chest.
         (5) Repeat procedure for other side of jacket.
      b. Cut overgarment trousers. (Figure B-10)
         (1) Cut from cuff along inseam to waist on left leg.
         (2) On right overgarment leg, cut from cuff to just below zipper and then go sideways into the first cut.
         (3) Allow trouser halves to drop to litter with contamination away from patient.
         (4) Tuck trouser halves to sides of body and roll the camouflage sides under between the legs.

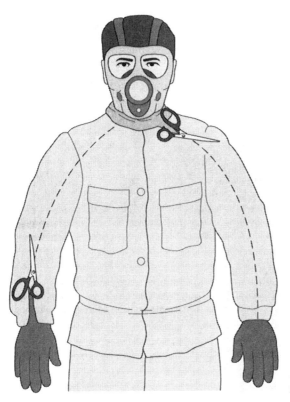

Figure B-9 Cut overgarment jacket.

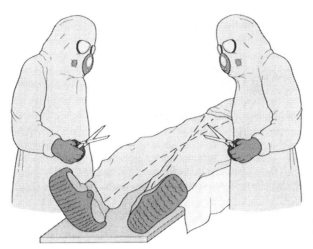

Figure B-10 Cut overgarment trousers.

7. Remove outer gloves. This procedure can be done with one medic on each side of the patient working simultaneously. Do not remove inner gloves. (Figure B-11)
   a. Lift the patient's arms by grasping his or her gloves.
   b. Fold the glove away from the patient over the sides of the litter.

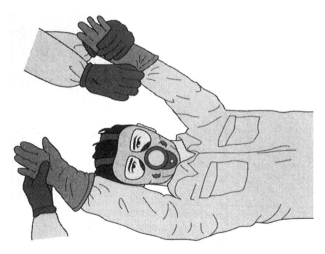

Figure B-11 Remove outer gloves.

c. Grasp the fingers of the glove.
d. Roll the cuff over the finger, turning the glove inside out.
e. Carefully lower the arm(s) across the chest when the glove(s) is removed. (Do not allow the arms to contact the exterior—camouflage side—of the overgarment.)
f. Dispose of contaminated gloves.
   (1) Place in plastic bag.
   (2) Deposit in contaminated dump.
g. Dip your own gloves in hypochlorite solution.

8. Remove overboots.
   a. Hold heels with one hand.
   b. Pull overboots downwards over the heels with other hand.
   c. Pull toward you until removed.
   d. Place overboots in contaminated disposal bag.

9. Remove personal articles from pockets.
   a. Place in plastic bags.
   b. Seal bags.
   c. Place in contaminated holding area.

10. Remove combat boots without touching body surfaces.
    a. Cut boot laces along the tongue.
    b. Pull boots downward and toward you until removed.
    c. Place boots in contaminated dump.

11. Remove inner clothing.
    a. Unbuckle belt.
    b. Cut BDU pants following same procedures as for overgarment trousers.
    c. Cut fatigue jacket following same procedures as for overgarment jacket.

12. Remove undergarments following same procedure as for fatigues. If patient is wearing a brassiere, it is cut between cups. Both shoulder straps are cut where they attach to cups and laid back off shoulders.

13. Clothing removal and skin decontamination: Transfer the patient to a decontamination litter. After the patient's clothing has been cut away, he or she is transferred to a decontamination litter or a canvas litter with a plastic sheeting cover. Three decontamination team members decontaminate their gloves and apron with the 5% hypochlorite solution. One member places his or her hands under the small of the patient's legs and thigh; a second member places his or her arms under the patient's back and buttocks; and the third member places his or her arms under the patient's shoulders and supports the head and neck. They carefully lift the patient using their knees, not their backs to minimize back strain. While

the patient is elevated, another decon team member removes the litter from the litter stands, and another member replaces it with a decontamination (clean) litter. The patient is carefully lowered onto the clean litter. Two decon members carry the litter to the skin decontamination station. The contaminated clothing and overgarments are placed in bags and moved to the decontaminated waste dump. The dirty litter is rinsed with the 5% decontamination solution and placed in a litter storage area. Decontaminated litters are returned to the ambulances.

14. Skin decontamination: The areas of potential contamination should be spot decontaminated using the M258A1 kit, the M291 kit, or 0.5% hypochlorite. These areas include the neck, wrists, lower face, and skin under tears or holes in the protective ensemble. After the patient is decontaminated his or her dressings and tourniquet are changed. Superficial (not body cavities, eyes, or nervous tissue) wounds are flushed with the 0.5% hypochlorite solution, and new dressings applied as needed. Cover massive wounds with plastic or plastic bags. New tourniquets are placed 0.5" to 1" proximal to the original tourniquet, then the old tourniquets are removed. Splints are not removed but saturated to the skin with 0.5% hypochlorite solution. If the splint cannot be saturated (air-splint or canvas splint), it must be removed sufficiently so that everything below the splint can be saturated with the 0.5% CI solution. The patient, his or her wounds, and the decontaminable stretcher have now been completely decontaminated.

15. Final monitoring and movement to treatment area: The patient is monitored for contamination using chemical agent detection equipment. The contents of the M258A1 kit (pad 1 and pad 2 when used separately or together) and hypochlorite on the skin do not affect most detection devices. Once the casualty is confirmed clean of chemical agent he or she is transferred via a shuffle pit over the hot line. The shuffle pit is composed of two parts Super Tropical Bleach (STB) and 3 parts earth or sand. The shuffle pit should be deep enough to cover the bottom of the protective overboots. The buddy system wash of the TAP apron and gloves in 5.0% hypochlorite solution precedes the transfer of the patient to a new clean canvas litter if the decontaminable stretchers are in limited supply. A three-person patient lift is again used as the litter is switched. If the litter, as well as the patient, was checked, both patient and the same litter can be placed over the hot line.

VII. Decontamination procedure for ambulatory patient

Decontamination of ambulatory patients follow the same principles as for litter patients. The major difference is the sequence of clothing removal to lessen the chance of patient contaminating himself or herself and others.

The first five steps are the same as in litter patient decontamination and are not described in detail.

1. Remove casualty's equipment.
2. Decontaminate mask and hood and remove hood.
3. Decontaminate skin around mask.
4. Remove field medical card (triage tag), and put it into a plastic bag.
5. Remove gross contamination from the outergarment
   a. Removal and bag personal effects from overgarment.
6. Overgarment jacket removal.
   a. Instruct patient to:
      (1) Clench his or her fist.
      (2) Stand with arms held straight down.
      (3) Extend arms backward at about a 30-degree angle.
      (4) Place feet shoulder width apart.
   b. Stand in front of patient.
      (1) Untie drawstring.
      (2) Unsnap jacket front flap.
      (3) Unzip jacket front.
   c. Move to the rear of the patient.
      (1) Grasp jacket collar at sides of the neck.
      (2) Peel jacket off shoulders at a 30-degree angle down and away from the patient.

(3) pull the inside of sleeves over the patient's wrists and hands.
   d. Cut to aid removal if necessary.
7. Removal of butyl rubber gloves.
   a. Patient's arms are still extended backward at a 30-degree angle.
      (1) Dip your gloved hands in 5% hypochlorite solution.
      (2) Use thumbs and forefingers of both hands.
      (a) Grasp the heel of patient's glove at top and bottom of forearm.
      (b) Peel gloves off with a smooth downward motion. This procedure can easily be done with one person or with one person on each side of the patient working simultaneously.
      (c) Place gloves in contaminated disposal bag.
   b. Tell the patient to reposition his or her arms, but not to touch trousers.
8. Remove patient's overboots.
   a. Cut overboot laces with scissors dipped in 5% hypochlorite.
   b. Fold lacing eyelets flat on ground.
   c. Step on the toe and heel eyelet to hold eyelets on the ground.
   d. Instruct the patient to step out of the overboot onto clean area. If in good condition, the overboot can be decontaminated and reissued.
9. Remove overgarment trousers.
   a. Unfasten or cut all ties, buttons, or zippers.
   b. Grasp trousers at waist.
   c. Peel trousers down over the patient's boots.
   d. Cut trousers to aid removal if necessary.
      (1) Cut around all bandages and tourniquets.
      (2) Cut from inside pant leg ankle to groin.
      (3) Cut up both sides of the zipper to the waist.
      (4) Allow the narrow strip with zipper to drop between the legs.
      (5) Peel or allow trouser halves to drop to the ground.
   e. Tell patient to step out of trouser legs one at a time.
   f. Place trousers into contaminated disposal bag.
10. Remove glove inner liners. Patient should remove the liners since this will reduce the possibility of spreading contamination.
   a. Tell patient to remove white glove liners.
      (1) Grasp heel of glove without touching exposed skin.
      (2) Peel liner downward and off.
      (3) Drop in contaminated disposal.
      (4) Remove the remaining liner in the same manner.
      (5) Place liners into contaminated disposal bag.
11. Final monitoring and decontamination.
   a. Monitor/test with M8 Detection Paper or CAM.
   b. Check all areas of patient's clothing.
   c. Give particular attention to:
      (1) Discolored areas.
      (2) Damp spots.
      (3) Tears in clothing.
      (4) Neck.
      (5) Wrist.
      (6) Around dressings.
   d. Decontaminate all contamination on clothing or skin by cutting away areas of clothing or using 5% hypochlorite solution, the M291, or the M258A1 for clothing or 0.5% hypochlorite and the M291, or the M258A1 for skin.
12. The medic should remove bandages and tourniquets and decontaminate splints, using the procedures described in the decontamination of a litter patient, during overgarment removal.

13. The patient is decontaminated and ready to be moved inside the hot line. Instruct patient to shuffle his or her feet to dust boots thoroughly as he or she walks through the shuffle pit.

In the clean treatment area, the patient can now be retriaged, treated, evacuated, and so forth. In a hot climate, the patient will probably be significantly dehydrated, and the rehydration process should start.

The clean area is the resupply point for the patient decontamination site. Water is needed for rehydration of persons working in the decon area. The resupply section should have an adequate stock of canteens with the chemical cap.

A location is needed in each decon area (75 meters from the working decon site) to allow workers, after they have deconned their TAP aprons, to remove their masks and rehydrate. There are generally not enough BDOs available to allow workers to remove them during the rest cycle and don new gear before going back to work. If these clean/shaded rest areas are not provided, the workers must remain fully dressed in protective ensembles even during rest periods, and water must be drunk through the mask via the drinking port. If all water consumption is by mask, there must be a canteen refill area adjacent to the vapor/clean line in which empty canteens can be deconned and placed for refill and clean full canteens are present for rehydration.

Appendix adapted from Soldier training Publication STP-21-1-SMCT Soldier's Manual of Common Tasks, Department of the Army, Washington, DC, 1994, and Medical Management of Chemical Casualties, Medical Research Institute of Chemical Defense, Aberdeen Proving grounds, MD, 1995.

Appendix C

FLUID AND MEDICATION PROCEDURES

The administration of medications and fluids to the combat casualty can be life saving. Field medications can counteract the effects of chemical warfare, relieve pain, and help the body combat infection. Fluid administration can replace, at least temporarily, the fluid volume lost through bleeding or burns. However, to introduce these agents into the body effectively and safely, you must establish a route. A direct route into the blood stream, and specifically a vein, is described as intravenous therapy. It is the quickest and most predictable method of drug and fluid administration. Medications may also be administered into the large muscles of the body, called intramuscular therapy. This route is easy to obtain, though distribution to the blood stream and body is slower and less predictable than the intravenous route.

Procedures Listed
I. Intravenous Catheter Introduction
II. Saline Lock Preparation
III. Intravenous Drip Administration
IV. Preparing a Solution for Administration
V. Intravenous Medication Administration
VI. Intramuscular Medication Administration

I. Intravenous Catheter Introduction
One of the most rapid and effective routes for administering fluids to a casualty is through an intravenous (IV) route. This method of administration delivers fluid through a catheter advanced into the vein, thereby giving you direct access to the casualty's blood stream. The fluid is carried to the heart, mixed with the blood supply, and distributed throughout the body in a matter of seconds.

The process of initiating an IV involves locating a larger superficial vein and introducing a flexible hollow tube into it. Because the process intrudes through the skin, there is the danger of introducing infection at the puncture site. When fluids or medications are administered to the patient, there is an associated danger that those fluids might not be compatible with the patient's blood stream and system. Fluids and medications must be sterile and carefully chemically balanced to be compatible with the human system.

The process of initiating an intravenous fluid line involves the following steps (see Figures C-1 to C-5):
1. Determine the patient's need for fluids or medication.
2. Don sterile gloves, and observe body substance isolation procedures.
3. Select a suitable vein for cannulation. Such a vein should be easily accessed and large enough to introduce a needle and associated catheter. Veins commonly used for IVs are those of the back of the hand, forearm, elbow, leg, thigh, or neck. The vein can be located by examining for slight bluish color, slight elevation above the skin, and spongy hollow feel. When selecting a suitable vein, choose one that is straight, does not roll about underneath the skin, and is free of valves in the region where the catheter will reside. Valves are small enlargements of the vein that have a firmer feel than the rest of the vein. They may resist catheter advancement or may slow fluid flow.
4. Place a venous tourniquet (an elastic constricting band) around the limb a few inches above the site you have chosen. In normotensive patients, this may cause the veins to engorge and stand out. In hypotensive patients, they may remain collapsed and difficult to find.

334

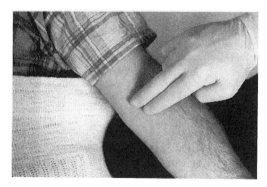

Figure C-1 Select suitable vein.

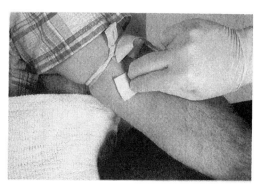

Figure C-2 Apply venous tourniquet and cleanse site.

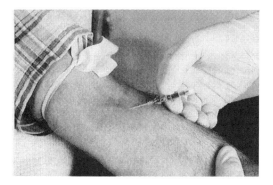

Figure C-3 Advance needle into vein at 30 degrees, obtain flashback, and thread catheter.

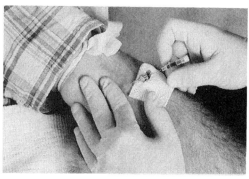

Figure C-4 Finger on vein at catheter tip, withdraw needle.

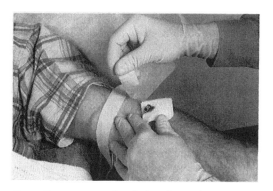

Figure C-5 Connect saline lock and securely tape.

5. Cleanse the site chosen for venipuncture with alcohol or Betadine, briskly cleaning the area in concentric circles moving outward from the site.
6. Select a large (18 to 14 gauge) needle in trauma patients because they may require rapid fluid resuscitation. Remove the protective cover from the needle and catheter, and draw the skin tightly over the intended venipuncture site with finger traction, drawn away from the selected site.

7. Place the needle against the skin at a 30- to 45-degree angle, bevel up. Penetrate the skin until you feel the needle gently "pop" as it enters the vein. Blood should move up the view port of the needle handle. This is called flashback.
8. Lower the needle to about 15 degrees, and thread the needle and catheter about a centimeter into the vein.
9. While holding the needle hub, advance the catheter hub to within a centimeter of the venipuncture site. Twist the catheter slightly during the advance to help it move off the needle and smoothly into the vein.
10. Place a finger just above the tip of the catheter, and apply gentle pressure on the vein to assure blood does not flow through the catheter. While holding the catheter hub in place, withdraw the needle.
11. Place the needle where there is no danger of an accidental needle stick. Select a biohazard puncture-proof needle box (sharps container) or other secure location.
12. Connect the fluid administration set or saline lock with a twisting motion while holding the catheter hub firmly in place.
13. Release the venous tourniquet.
14. Open the administration set or flush the saline lock to assure there is free fluid flow through the tubing, catheter, and into the vein. (See the procedure on IV administration set or saline lock setup.)
15. Observe the venipuncture site to assure there is no infiltration (fluid flowing into the skin) or developing hematoma (a swelling and discoloration reflective of bleeding from the vein).
16. Carefully tape the catheter in place. Do this by placing a long thin piece of tape underneath the catheter, sticky side up, and then fold both ends across the catheter hub. Place a small amount of bacteriostatic ointment over the venipuncture site and cover the entire site with a sterile gauze pad held in place with tape.
17. Loop the patient end of the IV administration tubing or saline lock, and tape it so, if pulled, it won't tug on the venipuncture site.
18. Consider splinting the limb to limit movement at the venipuncture site, especially if you have used a vein close to the elbow or one of the veins of the back of the hand.

II. Saline Lock Preparation

The saline lock is an easy and convenient way to maintain IV access while not having the cumbersome IV bag and administration set associated with fluid administration. The saline lock is a small length of IV tubing with adapters at one end to fit the IV catheter and at the other to fit a syringe or standard IV administration set. The saline lock may also have injection ports where medications may be administered using a syringe and needle.

You will fill the saline lock with normal saline fluid and then attach it to the venous catheter. Push a small amount of fluid through the lock and catheter to assure flow into the vein is accomplished. Then cap the lock for later use as an intravenous fluid or medication administration site.

When selecting a saline lock, assure you use a nonflow restrictive one. This is a saline lock with a large internal diameter. It will not impede the rapid administration of fluids for the shock or serious burn patient.

1. Assemble the needed equipment, including the saline lock, a multidose vial of normal saline, a 5- or 10-ml syringe, a 1 1/2" 21-gauge needle, and an alcohol swab (Figure C-6).
2. Don sterile gloves, and observe body substance isolation procedures.
3. Inspect the vial to assure it is sterile, has no particulate matter within it, and is not expired.
4. Expose and cleanse the needle port of the vial with the alcohol swab.
5. Attach the needle to the syringe, remove the needle cap, and inspire about 5 ml of air.
6. Invert the vial, and insert the needle through the port and just into the vial.
7. Expel about 5 ml of air, and then draw slightly more than 5-ml solution into the syringe, and withdraw the needle from the vial.
8. While holding the syringe and needle pointing upward, tap the syringe to move any air bubbles upward, and expel any excess fluid, leaving the syringe with just 5 ml of solution (Figure C-7).
9. Remove the needle from the syringe, and connect the syringe to the saline lock.
10. Inject saline into the lock until it begins to flow through the other end of the tubing.

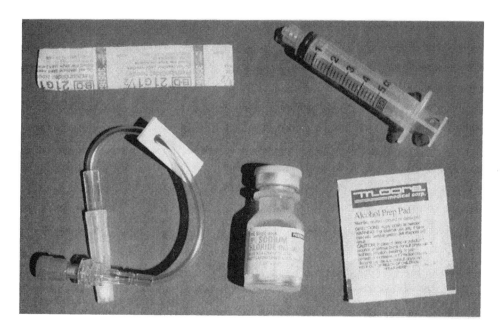

Figure C-6 Equipment (saline lock, multidose vial NS, 5- or 10-ml syringe, a 1 1/2 21-gauge needle, alcohol swab).

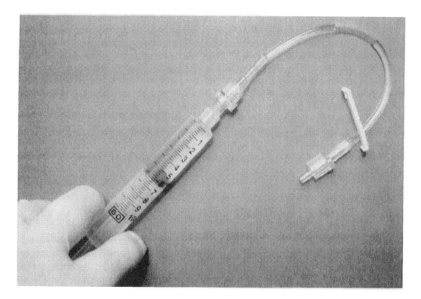

Figure C-7 Syringe connected to lock and fill.

At this time, you would set the saline lock aside and place an IV catheter.
11. Remove the protective cap and connect the saline lock to the IV catheter.
12. Inject the remaining saline fluid to assure the catheter is patent.
13. Remove the syringe, cap the saline lock, and then tape it firmly in place (Figure C-8).

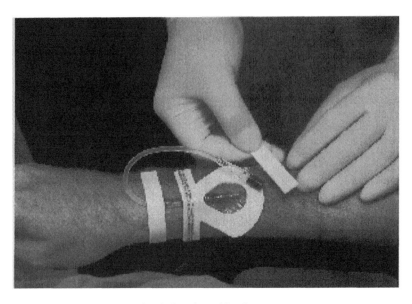

Figure C-8 Syringe connected to lock and taped firmly in position.

III. Intravenous Drip Administration

Intravenous fluids are used in trauma to help replace some of the fluid volume lost because of internal or external hemorrhage, and for fluids lost because of serious burn injury. An intravenous fluid line may also be used to maintain an open vein so that drugs can be administered in other medical emergencies. Normal saline (a 0.9% solution of sodium chloride and water) is the fluid of choice and is usually available in 1000-ml plastic bags.

The plastic fluid bag has two ports. One is covered with a removable tab and is designed to accept an administration set. The other is provided to accommodate the addition of medications to the solution, if so needed. The solution and bag are contained in a plastic disposable outer liner to protect the solution's sterility. The bag clearly identifies its contents and an expiration date.

The administration set consists of a long tube for fluid travel with a clear chamber for fluid flow measurement (a drip chamber). There is a plastic spike for insertion into the fluid bag at the end near the drip chamber. The other end has a connector for insertion into the catheter hub, covered to maintain sterility. Along the tubing will be a flow regulator, operated by turning a rolling cylinder (or other mechanism), and one or more ports for medication or additional fluid administration.

The procedure for fluid administration setup is as follows:
1. Inspect the fluid bag to assure the container is sealed and its contents are clear and free of particulate matter. Check the solution to assure it is the correct solution and concentration for the patient, and is not expired (Figure C-9).
2. Remove the plastic solution wrapper, and remove the bag's administration set port cover. Open the administration set container and locate the solution bag spike. Remove the spike cover and insert it, with a twisting motion, into the bag port (Figure C-10).
3. Open the flow regulator and, while holding the bag up, squeeze it so the fluid flows through the drip chamber, tubing, and out the catheter-connector end.
4. The drip chamber should be one-third to one-half full of fluid. If it contains no or little fluid, squeeze the chamber while the bag and administration set are upright. If it is filled with fluid, invert the bag and drip chamber, and squeeze the drip chamber. Release the pressure, and the chamber should fill partially with air. Return the drip chamber and bag to their normal orientation, and adjust the flow regulator to halt the fluid flow.

At this time, you would set the administration set aside and place the intravenous catheter.

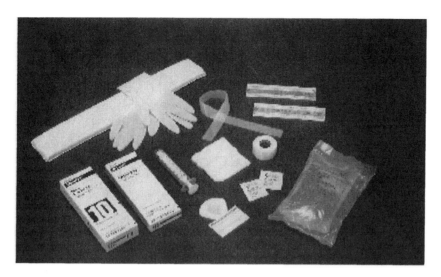

Figure C-9 Inspect fluid bag, and set out solutions, administration set, and IV equipment.

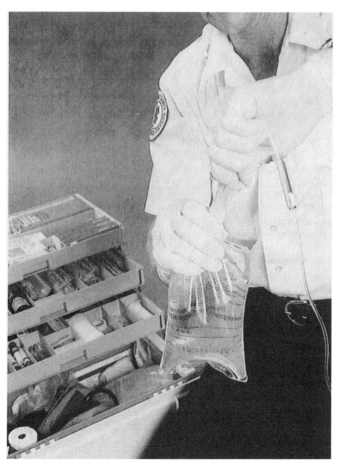

Figure C-10 Spike the bag.

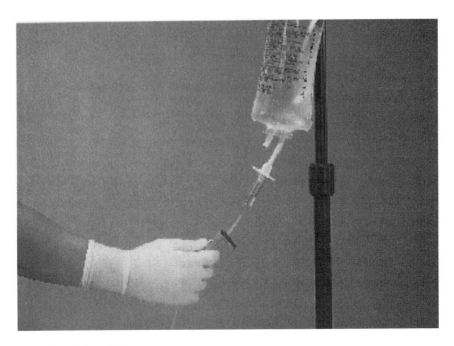

Figure C-11 Adjust the flow rate.

5. Remove the catheter connector cover, and connect the administration set directly to the catheter or saline lock.
6. Regulate the fluid flow by adjusting the flow regulator and counting the drips in the drip chamber (Figure C-11). For trauma, use either trauma tubing or a macro drip set (10 drips per ml). Calculate the fluid administration rate by counting the drips for 15 seconds, and multiply the result by 4. For every 10 drops you administer 1 ml of fluid (with the 10-drop per ml set). For a 60-drop per ml set (a microdrop set), the number of drops per minute equals the milliliters per hour you administer.
7. Monitor the administration set for fluid flow. If the rate slows or stops, raise the IV bag, check for kinked or trapped tubing, and examine the catheter site for infiltration or hematoma. Adjust the flow regulator as needed.
8. In the tactical situation, it may not be appropriate to elevate the fluid bag to administer fluid. You may use a pressure bag or a blood pressure cuff, pressurized to maintain the desired fluid flow. However, in shock and serious burns, you may administer fluid as a bolus. Here the fluid is administered rapidly, in a few minutes, under your direct observation.

IV. Preparing a Solution for Administration

Medications come packaged in many ways. Some drugs come in their own prefilled syringe or auto-injector, whereas others come in multidose vials. To administer a drug when packaged in a multi-dose vial, you must first preload the syringe. This procedure is described as follows:
1. Assemble the needed equipment, including a vial of the solution (medication), a 5- or 10-ml syringe, a 1 1/2" 21-gauge needle, and an alcohol swab.
2. Don sterile gloves and observe body substance isolation procedures.
3. Inspect the vial to assure it is sterile, the correct drug, in the correct concentration, has no particulate matter within it, and is not expired.
4. Attach the needle to the syringe, and draw the plunger back to the volume of drug you will draw (Inspiring air).

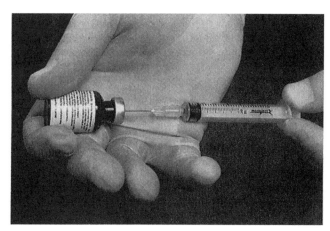

Figure C-12 Insert needle in vial, introduce air.

5. Expose and cleanse the injection port of the multidose vial with a clean alcohol swab, and allow it to dry.
6. Remove the needle cover, and insert the needle into the medication vial. Push the air in the syringe into the vial (Figure C-12).
7. Invert the vial with the needle passing only millimeters past the inside surface of the injection port (this assures you will draw in only the medication).
8. Withdraw the plunger slowly, drawing up just slightly more medication than you desire.
9. Withdraw the needle from the vial, hold the syringe and needle facing upward, tap the syringe to move any air bubbles upward, and expel any air and excess fluid from the syringe.
10. Recap the prefilled syringe and set it down, in preparation for administration.

V. Intravenous Medication Administration

Intravenous medication administration is one of the fastest and most effective routes for the administration of emergency drugs. It assures rapid mixing within the blood stream and distribution to all parts of the human system. The drugs administered by this route include morphine sulfate for pain, antibiotics to combat infection, and atropine to counteract the effects of chemical weapons.

Although it is possible to administer a drug from a syringe, through a needle, and directly into the vein, field medication administration should be through a saline lock or into an IV drip administration set. This assures the drug enters the blood stream and is less likely to be administered into the tissue surrounding the vein. The procedure for intravenous medication administration is as follows:

1. Assemble the needed equipment, including the prefilled syringe and an alcohol swab.
2. Don sterile gloves, and observe body substance isolation procedures.
3. Inspect the syringe to assure it is sterile, contains the correct drug, is in the correct concentration, has no particulate matter within it, and is not expired.
4. Cleanse the drug administration port of the administration set or saline lock with an alcohol swab, let it dry, and gently insert the needle (Figure C-13). With the saline lock, you may connect the syringe directly to the lock.
5. Depress the syringe plunger to inject the desired amount of the drug, at the rate prescribed for the drug (slowly, rapidly, or in increments, titrated to patient effect) (Figure C-14).
6. Remove the syringe. Do not attempt to recap the needle; dispose of it in a biohazard sharps container.
7. Run a small amount of fluid through the administration set or saline lock to assure all the drug was delivered to the patient's blood stream.

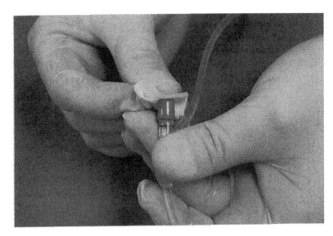

Figure C-13 IV administration set—medication port cleansing.

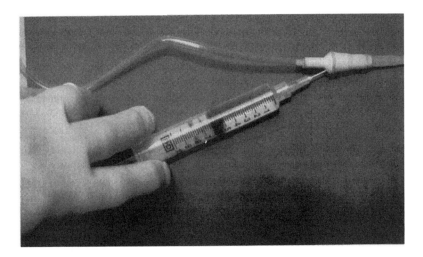

Figure C-14 Insert needle, introduce medication.

VI. Intramuscular Medication Administration

Intramuscular injection is a quick and easy method to administer a drug. The technique delivers the drug to the blood stream over time and does not necessitate starting an IV. It is, however, difficult to predict the rate of absorption by the body, and the rate may be very slow for patients with serious injuries or medical problems.

You may carry out intramuscular medication administration by using a commercially prepared prefilled syringe, an auto-injector, or by using a 5-ml or smaller syringe with a 1 1/2" 21-gauge needle. Administer no more than 5 ml of solution at one site by this method. The procedure for intramuscular administration (IM) is as follows:

1. Check the indications and contraindications for the drug you are about to administer, and assure it is appropriate for your patient.
2. Don sterile gloves, and observe body substance isolation procedures.
3. Assemble the necessary equipment, including the prefilled syringe, an alcohol swab, a small gauze dressing, and a small piece of adhesive tape (Figure C-15).

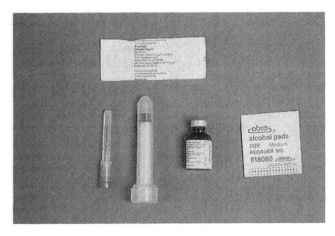

Figure C-15 Equipment, syringe, needle, and fluid; alcohol swab; tape; and small gauze dressing.

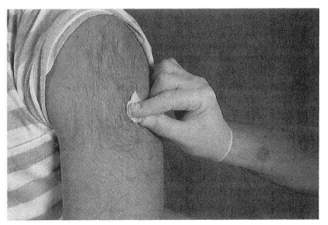

Figure C-16 Swabbing deltoid muscle.

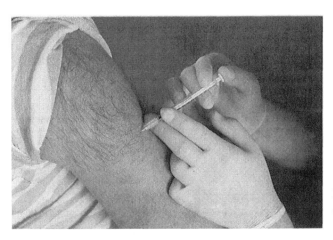

Figure C-17 Insert the needle at 90 degrees.

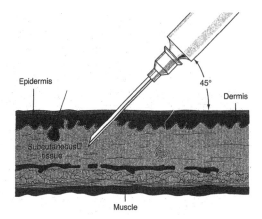

Figure C-18 Aspirating for blood.

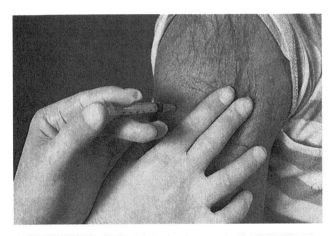

Figure C-19 Injecting medication.

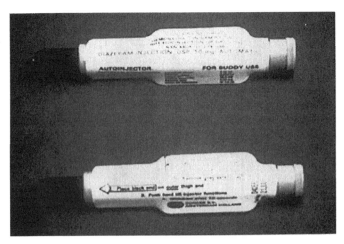

Figure C-20 Mark I autoinjector syringe.

4. Inspect the syringe to assure it is sterile, contains the correct drug, is in the correct concentration, has no particulate matter within it, and is not expired.
5. Select any large muscle mass, though the deltoid muscle of the shoulder is most convenient and accessible.
6. Briskly swab the intended site with the alcohol pad to remove any contaminants. Allow the alcohol to dry, killing most infectious agents that remain (Figure C-16).
7. Draw the skin down across the site with gentle thumb pressure. This makes the skin easier to penetrate and will cause it to obscure the needle's track after it is withdrawn and the finger tension is released (called Z-tracking).
8. Quickly push the needle deep (1 to 1 1/2 cm) into the muscle at a 90-degree angle (Figure C-17).
9. Pull back on the syringe to assure you are not in a vein or artery. If you aspirate blood, withdraw the needle and reinsert it nearby, and then repeat this step (Figure C-18).
10. Inject the required amount of medication over 1-2 seconds (Figure C-19).
11. Withdraw the needle quickly, and release your finger pressure.
12. Place the gauze dressing over the needle entry site, and hold it firmly in place with your finger for 1 minute. Then hold it in place with the small piece of tape.
13. Dispose of the needle in a proper biohazard container, do not attempt to recap the needle.

Nerve agent antidote Mark I kit

A special circumstance occurs when you are called to administer the nerve agent antidote (from the Mark I kit; Figure C-20) or other autoinjector via the intramuscular route. Administer the medication by firmly striking the barrel of the injector directly against a large muscle of the lateral thigh. Do not remove the soldier's protective NBC ensemble since this would risk chemical contamination. Inject the antidote directly through the suit and clothing, and do not attempt to clean the site. The risk of injury from the chemical agent far outweighs the risk of infection from the needle stick. Once the antidote is delivered (be sure to keep the autoinjector firmly pressed against the skin until all the medication is injected, usually 10-15 seconds), attach the syringe to the visible outer clothing of the casualty. This will help track the dosage of antidote the soldier has received.

Appendix D

ADVANCED AIRWAY PROCEDURES

Introduction

The airway is a tube passing from the openings of the mouth and nose to the individual air sacs of the lungs, the alveoli. The portion above the opening of the trachea is referred to as the upper airway. The upper airway and upper end of the digestive system intermingle. This leads to a dangerous situation when a patient becomes deeply unconscious and no longer controls the structures of this important passage. Although head positioning, suctioning, and oral and nasal airways help maintain the patency of the upper airway, only by placing a tube from the outside to the opening of the trachea can you definitively protect this vital passageway. The introduction of this tube is called endotracheal intubation.

In cases of severe trauma to the facial region, the structures of the upper airway may be destroyed such that it is impossible to open and maintain an airway, even with an endotracheal tube. In these circumstances, an emergency surgical airway, a cricothyrotomy, or a needle airway, a cricothyrostomy, may be the only way to secure the airway. These procedures open the membrane between the thyroid (Adam's apple) and cricoid cartilages, and permit air flow through an otherwise obstructed airway.

Relevant Anatomy

It is essential to understand the relevant anatomy and physiology to be successful at endotracheal intubation and the cricothyrotomy. Understanding how the airway functions and recognizing important landmarks during the procedures will better assure your success when employing these life-saving procedures.

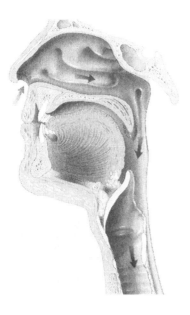

Figure D-1 Cross-sectional drawing of the airway.

The airway begins with the external openings of the nasal cavity, the nostrils or nares, and the mouth procedures (Figure D-1). The nasal cavity is divided into left and right sides by the nasal septum and is supplied by a rather rich supply of blood. The nasal cavity is separated from the oral cavity by a boney (or hard) and then cartilaginous (or soft) plate, called the palate. The oral cavity contains the large muscle of the tongue that guides food for chewing and also propels fluid and well-chewed food through the initial stages of swallowing. As the tongue moves backward, its upward pressure against the soft palate pushes it upward against the posterior and anterior wall of the nasal cavity. This prevents fluid and food from entering the nasal cavity during the swallowing process.

At the back of the throat, the tongue continues to propel food downward toward the opening of the esophagus. In the region just below the tongue's base is the opening of the trachea, called the larynx. The larynx has an upward cartilaginous and muscular cover called the epiglottis. This flap-shaped structure moves downward with swallowing and closes off the opening of the larynx. The space between the base of the tongue and the epiglottis is called the vallecula. The larynx is formed by a large, hollow, and cylindrical structure called the thyroid cartilage. It contains the vocal cords: two connective tissue bands that vibrate to produce a tone when we speak. These cords will spasm and close off the airway to prevent aspiration of food or other foreign materials.

Beneath the larynx is the trachea, a narrow tube about the size of a patient's little finger. It can be felt below the Adam's apple in the anterior neck. It is made up of cartilaginous Cs and shares its posterior surface with the esophagus. Just below the top of the sternum, the trachea divides into two tubes, the mainstem bronchi, supplying each lung with air exchange. The right mainstem bronchus is slightly larger, and at an angle less severe, than the left. This is because the heart displaces more of the left lower lung. This reduced angle and larger diameter results in objects breathed in (aspirated) or an endotracheal tube placed too deeply, to more likely lodge in the right mainstem bronchus.

Endotracheal intubation utilizes these landmarks to secure the airway by placing a tube from the outside into the trachea. Two intubation techniques are of great value to the field medic. They are oral endotracheal intubation and digital endotracheal intubation.

You must also recognize special structures to perform properly the cricothyrotomy or cricothyrostomy. The thyroid cartilage is located in the upper anterior neck (Figure D-2). In males, the thyroid cartilage is usually visible and easily palpable as a firm ridge in the upper anterior neck. In females, it is less visible but is usually palpable. In children, it can be challenging to

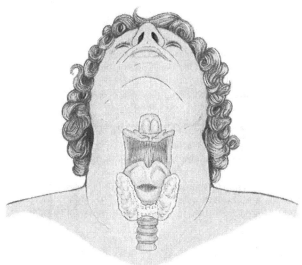

Figure D-2 Anterior neck showing landmarks.

locate the thyroid cartilage because it is smaller and softer than in adults. However, with careful palpation, it too can be located. Accurate identification of the thyroid cartilage is crucial to successful cricothyrotomy (surgical) and cricothyrostomy (needle).

Directly beneath the thyroid cartilage is a small membrane, called the cricothyroid membrane, and then the firm, ringlike, cricoid cartilage. This small membrane is best located by palpating the trachea in the middle anterior neck, then moving your fingers upward to the first firm ring. Above this ring, the cricoid cartilage, is the small indentation of the cricothyroid membrane. This is the location where the needle is inserted or the surgical incision is performed.

Procedures Listed
I.   Oral Endotracheal Intubation
II. Digital Endotracheal Intubation
III. Cricothyrotomy/Cricothyrostomy
IV. Pulse Oximetry
V.   Automatic Ventilators

I. Oral Endotracheal Intubation

Oral tracheal intubation provides the greatest advantages to protecting the airway in a casualty. Through the process, you see the endotracheal tube pass between the vocal cords and into the trachea. Though this procedure is relatively simple, you must use great care to protect the patient from further harm and assure that you place the tube in the trachea. If the tube is misplaced and ventilation occurs through it only, the patient is in great danger of apnea, anoxia, and death. For this reason, carry out this procedure with great care, and monitor the patient's respiratory status immediately and then frequently after tube placement.

Proper and rapid placement of the endotracheal tube requires you to be familiar with the anatomy of the oral cavity, pharynx, and larynx. Important landmarks include the base of the tongue, the epiglottis (the cover of the larynx), the vallecula (the space between the epiglottis and the base of the tongue), the larynx opening, and the vocal folds. The procedure of endotracheal intubation interrupts casualty ventilation, so it must be done very quickly, in around 15 to 30 seconds. Assure that all of your equipment is ready and easily at hand when you start the procedure, and hold your breath from the time ventilation stops to remind you that the time you take is taking breath from the patient (Figures D-3 to D-7).

1. Don sterile gloves, and observe body substance isolation throughout the procedure. Consider the use of a mask and eye protection since the patient's breath or ventilation attempts may propel blood or other fluids toward your face during the procedure.
2. Assure the patient is being ventilated adequately by another care provider. Watch for chest rise and a ventilation rate of about 24 breaths per minute. Have the patient hyperventilated for a few minutes just prior to the intubation attempt.
3. Set out the endotracheal tubes, tape, malleable stylet, laryngoscope, and 10-ml syringe.
4. Select an endotracheal tube about the same outside diameter as the patient's little finger.
5. Fill the syringe with 10 ml of air, attach it to the port on the endotracheal tube, and inflate the distal cuff. Assure air fills the cuff evenly and does not leak out. Then withdraw the air and collapse the cuff.

If the endotracheal tube is too pliable (as with warm temperatures), you may wish to stiffen it with a malleable stylet. Introduce the stylet to 1 cm from the tip of the endotracheal tube (if it protrudes, it may cause physical damage to the larynx or tracheal during insertion), and shape the tube and stylet into a large J.

6. Assemble the laryngoscope with a blade matched to the patient. Large adults may need a #4 blade, whereas small adults and children need a #2. Assure the light glows with a bright, nonflickering, white light. If not, replace the batteries, clean the handle and blade contacts, or replace the bulb.
7. Halt ventilation, and assume a position at the top of the patient's head. If neck trauma is not suspected, gently tilt the head back and move it forward to align the airway. This "sniffing position" permits the easiest visualization of the vocal cords, essential to successful intubation.

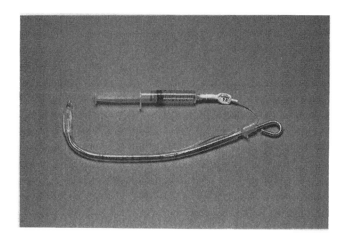

Figure D-3 Stylet in tube and preformed.

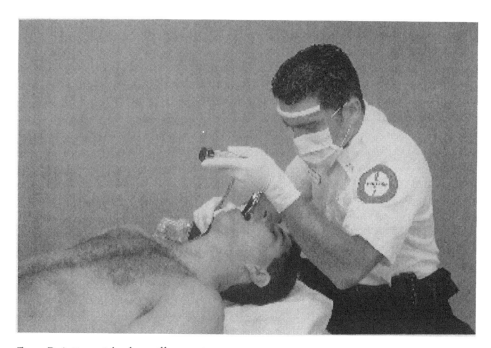

Figure D-4 Patient's head in sniffing position.

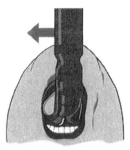

Figure D-5 Laryngoscope inserted and cords in view.

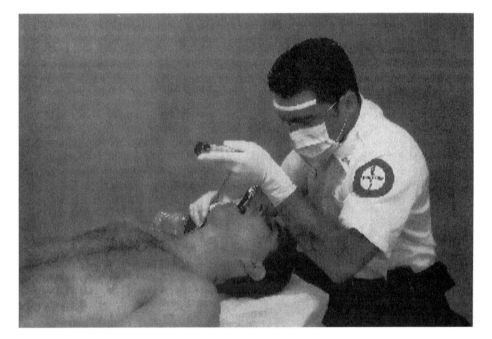

Figure D-6 Tube going through cords.

8. Grasp the laryngoscope in the left hand, and insert it into the mouth along the right side to the back of the tongue. Then move it and the tongue to the left, and look for landmarks. As you move the laryngoscope deeper into the pharynx, you will see the vallecula, then the two narrow white slits of the vocal cords, and the dark opening of the trachea. The curved laryngoscope (McIntosh) blade is designed to fit into the vallecula, whereas the straight (Miller) blade physically lifts the epiglottis out of the way.

It takes a great deal of effort to lift the tongue and jaw to visualize the tracheal opening clearly. Be careful to lift these tissues, and not pry them by rotating the laryngoscope handle. Keep the blade off the teeth since pressure may easily brake the teeth and cause other soft tissue damage.

9. Once you visualize the opening of the trachea, grasp the endotracheal tube with your right hand and guide its tip through the vocal cords and into the trachea. The tip should travel about 2-3 cm beyond the vocal cords.

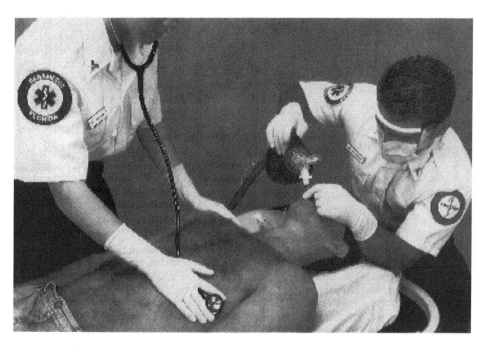

Figure D-7 Checking breath sounds.

10. Carefully hold the endotracheal tube in place and withdraw the laryngoscope. With a bag-valve-mask, ventilate the patient, watch for chest rise, and listen for breath sounds over both lung fields and the epigastric region (just below the sternum).
11. If you hear good breath sounds and no gurgling sounds over the epigastric region, secure the tube firmly with tape and note its location (the number on the tube where the tube exits the corner of the mouth). Then inflate the cuff with 5 to 10 ml of air.

If breath sounds are heard on the right side only or they are much stronger than the left, withdraw the tube 1 cm and recheck. The tube may have passed too deeply and entered the right mainstem bronchus. Withdrawing the tube slightly should restore bilateral ventilation.

If breath sounds are weak and there are sounds of gurgling over the epigastric area, the endotracheal tube may not have entered the trachea. Withdraw the tube and reattempt intubation.

12. Hyperventilate the patient, then continue ventilation, and monitor breath sounds, chest rise, skin color, and other signs of respiratory effectiveness.

II. Digital Endotracheal Intubation

Digital intubation differs from oral intubation in that the laryngoscope is not used and the patient's head need not be tilted for placement. It does not have the surety of placement as does the oral route but may be beneficial under hostile fire since it does not require illumination or head movement and may be attempted while you are at the patient's side, not above his or her head.

This procedure requires that your fingers extend deep into the throat. If the patient is allowed to bite down during your intubation attempt, you may be seriously injured. Therefore, only completely unresponsive patients are candidates for this procedure. As an additional precaution, carefully assure that the jaw is held open by using a bite block or portion of an oral airway. The procedure is best attempted by persons with long narrow fingers and may be unsuccessful in patients with large heads, simply because of the depth of finger insertion needed for proper tube placement.

Because you do not observe the endotracheal tube pass between the vocal cords, you must be extra careful in assuring the tube has been placed properly. This includes carefully monitoring the breath sounds, epigastric sounds, chest rise, and skin color immediately after the procedure and frequently thereafter. Use of an end-tidal CO_2 detector can also confirm proper placement.

1. Don sterile gloves, and observe body substance isolation throughout the procedure. Consider the use of a mask and eye protection since the patient's breath or ventilation attempts may propel fluid toward your face during the procedure.
2. Assure the patient is being ventilated adequately by another care provider. Watch for chest rise and a rate of about 24 breaths per minute. Have the patient hyperventilated for a few minutes just prior to the intubation attempt.
3. Set out the endotracheal tubes, tape, malleable stylet, and 10-ml syringe.
4. Select an endotracheal tube about the same outside diameter as the patient's little finger.
5. Fill the syringe with 10 ml of air, attach it to the port on the endotracheal tube, and inflate the distal cuff. Assure air fills the cuff evenly and does not leak out. Then withdraw the air and collapse the cuff.
6. Stiffen the endotracheal tube with a malleable stylet. Introduce the stylet to 1 cm from the tip of the endotracheal tube (if it protrudes, it may cause physical damage to the larynx or trachea during insertion), and shape the tube and stylet into a large J.
7. Assure the patient is unresponsive, halt ventilation, and place a bite block or oral airway partially into the patient's mouth. This prevents the patient from biting down and severely injuring your fingers.
8. Using just the first and second fingers of the hand closest to the patient, walk your fingers along the back of the tongue until you feel the flap covering the larynx (the epiglottis). Hold the epiglottis against the anterior of the pharynx with the first finger (Figure D-8).
9. Insert the endotracheal tube along the curve of the back of your hand. Guide it along the anterior surface of the larynx, past the epiglottis, and beyond. Advance the tube about 3 to 4 centimeters beyond the tip of your finger. If it travels along the anterior surface of the throat and epiglottis, it should enter the trachea.
10. Carefully hold the tube in place and withdraw the stylet. With a bag-valve-mask, ventilate the patient, watch for chest rise, and listen for breath sounds over both lung fields and the epigastric region (just below the sternum).
11. If you hear good breath sounds and no gurgling over the epigastric region, secure the tube firmly with tape and note its location (the number on the tube where the tube exits the corner of the mouth). Then inflate the cuff with 5 to 10 ml of air.

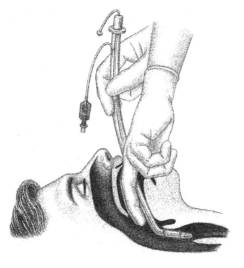

Figure D-8 Drawing of digital intubation process.

If breath sounds are heard on the right side only or they are much stronger than the left, withdraw the tube 1 cm and recheck. The tube may have passed too deep and entered the right mainstem bronchus. Withdrawing the tube slightly should restore bilateral ventilation.

If breath sounds are weak and there are sounds of gurgling over the epigastric area, the endotracheal tube may not have entered the trachea. Withdraw the tube and reattempt intubation.

12. Hyperventilate the patient and then continue ventilation, monitoring breath sounds, chest rise, skin color, and other signs of respiratory effectiveness.

III. Cricothyrotomy/Cricothyrostomy

The surgical or needle airway is a procedure employed only when there is a dire need for an immediate airway and all other methods have failed to obtain one. It is usually indicated in severe facial or upper airway trauma where the patient is unable to maintain the airway and endotracheal intubation has not been successful. It should be attempted only as permitted by your protocols.

1. Identify the need for an emergency surgical or needle airway and that attempts to secure the airway by endotracheal intubation have been unsuccessful.
2. Don sterile gloves, and observe body substance isolation procedures. Consider the use of a mask and eye protection since the patient's breath or ventilation attempts may propel fluid toward your face during the procedure.
3. Briskly cleanse the upper anterior neck with an alcohol swab in concentric circles outward from the base of the thyroid cartilage.
4. Set out the needed equipment, including an alcohol or betadine swab and:
   Cricothyrostomy-a large-bore needle (14 gauge or larger)
   Cricothyrotomy-a scalpel or sharp knife and a small oral airway
5. Palpate the trachea, cricoid cartilage, thyroid cartilage, and the membrane in between, the cricothyroid membrane (Figure D-9) .
6. Perforate the cricothyroid membrane.

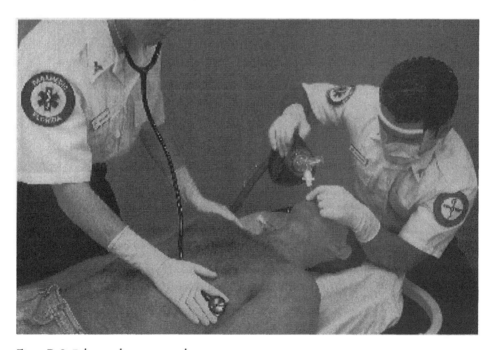

Figure D-9 Palpating the anterior neck.

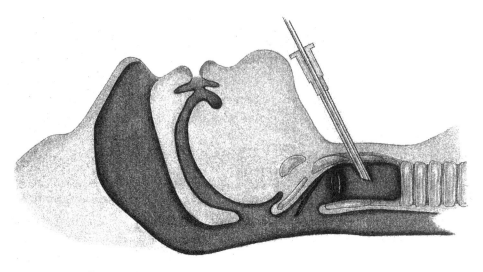

Figure D-10 Needle in cricothyroid membrane.

Cricothyrostomy

Insert the needle into the skin and membrane until you feel a "pop," advance it a few centimeters over the needle and then withdraw the needle (Figure D-10).

Cricothyrotomy

Insert the blade of a sterile scalpel into the skin and membrane until you feel a "pop." Enlarge the opening to accept a small (7 mm) shortened endotracheal tube (cut the tube to about 4" in length, bend it to an abrupt curve), and introduce it through the surgical opening.

    7. Ventilate the patient.

Cricothyrostomy

Remove the adapter from a pediatric 6.0 endotracheal tube, and connect it to the hub of the catheter. Attach it to the bag-valve-mask (without the mask) and ventilate. Ventilations will have to be quick since it takes a great deal of time for the patient to exhale through the very narrow lumen of the catheter.

Cricothyrotomy

Place a child mask on the bag-valve-mask, and seal it around or attach it directly to the endotracheal tube. Ventilate normally.

    Although the surgical approach to an airway provides a much larger route for ventilation, much less tissue damage and bleeding is associated with needle insertion. Needle insertion also leaves less of a scar, if any at all. However, a patient without an adequate airway will not survive. The needle approach is a short-term interim procedure that is marginally effective. The needle lumen and length seriously restrict the volume of air you can introduce, and even more severely restricts the air that the casualty can exhale. The resulting exchange will not sustain a patient but may lengthen the time before anoxic or hypoxic death. If you need to ventilate a patient for more than a few minutes before you arrive at a higher echelon of care, consider the surgical procedure.

IV. Pulse Oximetry

Pulse oximetry, in a noninvasive way, monitors oxygenated blood delivery to the body's most distal organ, the skin. The device-a sensor, an electrical black box, and a digital readout-evaluates pulsing

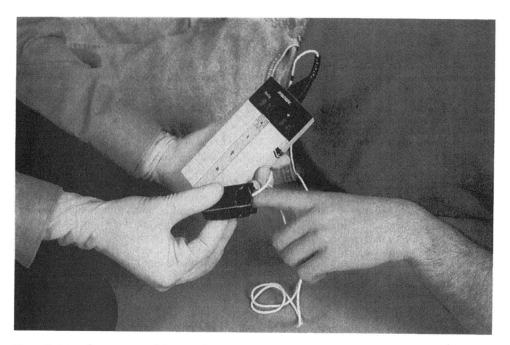

Figure D-11 Pulse oximeter and finger probe.

blood in the skin and determines how well it is oxygenated. This tells you how well the respiratory and cardiovascular systems are delivering oxygen to the body tissues on a real-time (second-to-second) basis. This information can be useful in guiding your care, including oxygen administration, ventilation, and overall shock therapy (Figure D-11).

How the Oximeter Works

The pulse oximeter probe sends light from two light-emitting diodes through the skin. On the other side of the probe, sensors pick up light that is not absorbed as it passes through the skin. The light is of different wavelengths (colors) and is filtered by oxygen-rich hemoglobin or by hemoglobin without oxygen. The electrical black box examines only the changing portion of the signal, the pulsing arterial blood. It also mathematically determines the ratio of oxygen-rich hemoglobin (bright red) to hemoglobin without oxygen (dark red or bluish), and then determines the percentage of oxygen-saturated hemoglobin. This saturation value is displayed digitally by the pulse oximeter.

Oxygen saturation is not directly associated with the oxygen carrying power of the blood. As the saturation drops from 100%, the amount of oxygen carried by the blood drops very quickly. Saturations at 100% carry about 120 mm hg partial pressure of oxygen. As the saturation drops to 95%, that figure plummets to about 75 mm hg, and as the saturation falls to 90%, the oxygen carried is about 60 mm hg. As the saturation drops from 90% to 80% the blood's carrying capacity drops another 12% to 15%, and more slowly thereafter. This large initial drop in carrying capacity with the first 10% drop in saturation demonstrates why it is so important to keep oxygen saturations upwards from 95% in any seriously injured casualty.

Oximeter Probes

The most common form of oximetry probe is a spring-loaded finger probe. This device simply and gently clamps to a finger or toe to sense oxygen saturation. Other probes may be an ear clip or self-adhering tape probe. All need to shine the light from the light-emitting diodes through a well-perfusing bed of tissue, not so thick as to obscure all the light nor so thin as not to allow good absorption.

Proper sensing requires some small arteries delivering blood to the area to be sensed. You can apply the probes to fingers, toes, earlobes, the bridge of the nose, or any well perfused fold of skin.

Once you apply the probe and turn the oximeter on, it reads in a matter of seconds. Blood takes about 15 seconds to reach the finger or 4 seconds to reach the ear lobe from the heart. Hence, pulse oximetry gives you a rapid and real-time evaluation of the cardiovascular system's ability to perfuse the body organs. Since the skin is not a critical organ, like the brain, heart, and kidneys, it is one of the first organs to receive reduced blood flow as the body begins to compensate for shock. This makes pulse oximetry a very valuable assessment tool for you as the medic.

Using the Pulse Oximeter

The pulse oximeter has value in both immediate and ongoing assessment. The oximeter reads the saturation quickly and gives you immediate information about the state of the respiratory and cardiovascular systems. If the reading is between 96% and 100%, the casualty is moving oxygen well. If the oximeter reads between 90% and 95%, the casualty needs supplemental, high-flow oxygen and careful respiratory monitoring. Any saturation level below 90% reflects serious respiratory compromise and the need for aggressive oxygen administration and possibly artificial ventilation.

Guide oxygen therapy, especially in austere tactical conditions, to a saturation of greater than 95%. If a casualty is oxygenated above that level on ambient air, do not apply oxygen unless there is more than an ample supply. Guide the oxygen administration for those who need it to obtain a saturation greater than 95% and administer no more. In those with saturations that do not respond to oxygen alone, consider overdrive ventilation. Monitor the oximetry reading carefully over time. Any change in saturation likely means a change in the casualty's condition and calls for your investigation.

The process for the use of the pulse oximeter:
1. Apply the finger probe to an exposed and warm finger.
2. Turn on the pulse oximeter
3. Assure the oximeter displays a saturation reading, and it stabilizes after a few seconds.
4. If the oximeter is equipped with a pulse rate read out, assure it agrees with any pulses you palpate.
5. If the oximeter reading is erratic or the unit fails to display, try another location or warm the finger. If the oximeter still is erratic, try it on another patient or yourself. If it fails to read, have the unit serviced.
6. Leave the pulse oximeter in place during patient care, include its readings with vital sign reports, and watch the effect interventions have on the saturation.

Erratic, False, or Misleading Readings

There are some conditions where the pulse oximeter may have some trouble sensing or may give erratic, falsely high, or misleading readings. These are important concerns, but with the proper caution, pulse oximetry readings can be reliable and invaluable in guiding your patient care. The conditions that adversely effect oxygen saturation readings are carbon monoxide, low flow states (like shock, cold exposure, and hypovolemia), anemia, and high-intensity lighting.

Carbon Monoxide

Carbon monoxide behaves like oxygen. It attaches to the hemoglobin in the blood and turns the blood bright red just as oxygen does. The oximeter reads as though the blood is well saturated when the carbon monoxide prevents it from transporting oxygen to the cells. Carbon monoxide is the greatest threat to the use of oximetry because it provides a false high reading and may lead you to a false sense of security. Hence, any time you employ oximetry to monitor a casualty's cardiorespiratory status, you must rule out carbon monoxide poisoning.

Carbon monoxide is the product of incomplete combustion either from an internal combustion engine (like that of an auto) or a burning fire without adequate ventilation. The condition occurs in a confined space and usually anyone in the area for an appreciable time will complain of a general ill feeling (malaise), rushing in the ears, and headache. The cherry red discoloration reported with carbon monoxide poisoning is a late finding and may not be present with life-endangering doses. If there is any question of carbon monoxide poisoning, treat as though it exists.

Smokers, by the nature of their habit, inhale significant amounts of carbon monoxide. This gives them a chronic carbon monoxide level to which their body has adjusted. The oximeter displays a falsely high reading though, since it is chronic and well compensated for, it gives a reasonable reflection of their cardiorespiratory function. Because they have a portion of their hemoglobin saturated with carbon monoxide, they experience dyspnea and respiratory problems sooner than healthy, nonsmoking patients.

Certain other agents cause false oximetry readings. These are medications, generally given in the hospital, and over long periods. These drugs color the blood and cause the oximeter to display a lower reading than the true oxygen saturation. However, since these readings are only slightly lower than normal, they raise your concern about the casualty's cardiorespiratory condition and do not lead you falsely to believe the casualty is doing well. Because these conditions are rare, suspect them only in patients with extensive past medical history.

Low Flow States

Low flow states result in poor perfusion to the distal regions of the body. This limits the strength of pulsing in areas the probe senses and results in erratic signals displayed by the oximeter. Whether the reason for this condition is chronic or acute, it is of concern. Whenever the heart is not able to drive pulsing blood into the peripheral circulation, the body is cardiovascularly compromised. Conditions that may cause this are cold exposure, shock, and hypovolemia.

Cold exposure causes the peripheral blood vessels to constrict and limit blood flow through the cold tissue. This conserves body temperature but results in limited distal circulation. This poor circulation makes it very hard for the oximeter to identify which blood is pulsing and results in an erratic reading, if it reads at all. To correct the problem, warm the region where you locate the oximeter probe, and consider being more aggressive in helping the patient maintain body temperature (more blankets or turn up the vehicle heat). If the oximeter still reads erratically, consider other possible causes of the problem.

Hypovolemia and shock begin the body's compensatory response. The body directs circulation to critical organs like the heart, brain, and kidneys while it limits circulation to the skin. This decrease in circulation reduces the oximeter's ability to recognize arterial blood. The saturation reading becomes erratic, or the device does not read at all. Whenever you have difficulty obtaining a pulse oximetry reading in a patient, suspect shock and consider aggressively treating for it.

Anemia

Anemia is a condition of reduced and inadequate amounts of red blood cells and their oxygen-carrying component, hemoglobin. It can be either chronic or acute, as in sudden blood loss and rapid fluid resuscitation. Anemia does not lead to abnormal oxygen saturation readings though they may not be as strong because the bright red color of the blood is diluted. The oximeter registers an accurate oxygen saturation reading; however, the amount of hemoglobin available to carry oxygen is inadequate. Even if the saturation reads 95% to 100%, there may not be enough oxygen in the blood to support body functions. If a casualty you are treating is receiving aggressive IV fluid resuscitation, be wary of an acute anemia and assure high-flow oxygen and adequate ventilations.

High-Intensity Lighting

High-intensity lighting and bright sunlight overload the oximeter sensor and cause it to provide a reading closer to 100% than the actual saturation. Whenever you are in bright sunlight or under high-intensity lighting as in surgery or the emergency department, cover the oximeter probe with a towel or blanket. If the reading drops slightly, the lower reading is more accurate.

High Altitude

In high elevations, air exerts substantially less pressure than it does at sea level. This is the pressure that drives oxygen into the hemoglobin and gives the oxygen saturation value. At high altitudes, the oximeter reads correctly, but the saturation values are somewhat lower than at sea level. Persons living at altitude adjust by increasing the number of red blood cells and hence the available hemoglobin. If personnel are new to the altitude and unaccustomed to the reduced pressure, expect them to experience altitude sickness, a general fatigue that increases with exertion. Over time, the body creates additional red blood cells, and stamina will increase. When a person travels to a higher altitude in an aircraft without pressurization, this same reduced pressure reduces the efficiency of oxygen-carrying capacity of the blood. If the person is seriously injured, this phenomenon may make the patient worse. For this reason, apply pulse oximetry to any seriously injured casualties flying at altitudes greater than 1000 feet above ground, and use supplemental oxygen to keep the saturation above 95%.

Summary

The oximeter is a rapid, noninvasive device that tells you of the respiration and circulation efficiency. When part of a complete patient assessment, it tells you a great deal of critical information about your patient. You can use it to evaluate the casualty or to monitor care activities and interventions or to provide a continuing assessment of oxygenated circulation to the end organs. It can also guide care such as the administration of oxygen or the need and benefit of endotracheal intubation or artificial ventilation. However, as with any piece of electronic or mechanical equipment in support of your care, consider the information it provides with the results of your assessments when determining the overall patient condition and the care you offer.

V. Automatic Ventilators

Automatic ventilators are oxygen or electrically powered mechanical devices administering a predetermined volume of oxygen to a patient at a predetermined rate. You will find them useful and effective in ventilating nonbreathing casualties over moderate to long periods. They can be a great advantage when transporting patients needing overdrive or positive pressure ventilation over long distances or prolonged transport times. They do, however, have some important limitations. Automatic ventilators are often in limited supply in the tactical setting, do not permit you directly to sense respiratory compliance, and consume rather large volumes of oxygen during their operation.

Ventilator Operation

Automatic ventilators use pressurized oxygen from a cylinder to deliver a timed flow to either a mask or endotracheal tube. This flow is about 30 liters per minute for adults. Settings on the control module permit you to adjust the length of oxygen delivery and, hence, the volume of oxygen, usually between 200 and 1200 ml per breath (Figure D-12). You also may adjust the rate of ventilation between 8 and 28 breaths per minute. The settings should normally deliver a volume of between 10 and 15 ml/kg for each breath at a rate of about 12 breaths per minute. The normal adult should receive at least 8 liters per minute (minute volume) with that volume adjusted up or down depending on the casualty's size. Note that greater numbers of breaths per minute and greater volumes of each breath (longer inspiration times) limit the remaining time for exhalation. Since exhalation is passive, this may not permit a full exhalation and may result in a residual back pressure.

If your ventilator has adjustments for children, it will deliver about 15 liters per minute of ventilatory flow with breath per minute rates slightly faster than for the adult (20 breaths per minute for small children and infants). Weight adjust tidal volumes in the 10 to 12 ml/kg range (see chapter 9, Evacuation Care).

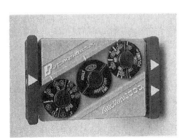

Figure D-12 Autovent control unit.

Oxygen-powered ventilators have safeguards to protect against increasing or high resistance to ventilation. If the airway is blocked or the ventilatory volume is too high for adequate exhalation, an audible alarm sounds. Upon hearing this, assure the airway is patent and the ventilatory volume or rate is not too high. If the alarm sounds early in the respiratory cycle, suspect airway obstruction. If it sounds late in the cycle, suspect the respiratory volume is too high and/or the rate is too fast. Lower the volume, and slightly increase the rate (or vice versa) to maintain an adequate minute volume without a residual back pressure.

You may use the oxygen-powered ventilator on patients with a mask or an endotracheal tube in place. Employ the ventilator with an endotracheal tube when possible because the ventilator works less efficiently as the dead air space increases. Without the direct access to the airway that the endotracheal tube provides, the ventilator must pressurize the oral, nasal, and laryngeal pharynx with each inspiration. This pressurization increases the oxygen volume necessary to ventilate the casualty adequately and increases the resistance to air flow into the lungs. It also endangers the airway since the ventilator does not recognize when the patient vomits or has other fluids in the airway. Continued ventilation may drive emesis into the trachea and lungs. Even when you attach the automatic ventilator to an endotracheal tube, you must monitor ventilation carefully to assure the patient remains adequately oxygenated.

If you chose to ventilate a casualty with a mask in place, assure you maintain a tight mask seal throughout care. This means one care provider continues to hold the mask position at all times while the ventilator is operating.

Some oxygen-powered ventilators operate as a demand ventilator when the ventilation rate is set to zero or off. A breathing casualty generates a negative pressure during inhalation. This opens the patient valve head to a flow of oxygen. This flow provides supplemental oxygen rather inefficiently, so you should switch to a nonrebreather oxygen mask as soon as possible. It also requires a tight mask seal, maintained by one caregiver.

Oxygen-powered ventilators consume a large supply of oxygen during their operation. They should be supplied from a vehicle mounted G or H cylinder though smaller cylinders will work for short times. An oxygen-generating device is ideal for ventilator use. A full E cylinder will operate a ventilator on an adult casualty for about 45 minutes.

Ventilator Operation

Assure the casualty is ventilated by bag-valve-mask while you set up the ventilator. Check the oxygen supply to assure it will be adequate for the transport, and then assemble the ventilator components. Introduce an endotracheal tube, confirm its position, and secure it well to the border of the mouth. Continue ventilating the casualty with the bag-valve-mask, and adjust the ventilator for your patient.

Secure the oxygen hose to a good supply of oxygen, either a large vehicle-mounted or a full E cylinder. Set the volume between 500 and 1000 ml for normal ventilation, with 800 ml being a good starting valve for adults. Initially turn the ventilation rate to 12 times per minute, and listen for proper ventilator operation (a cycling on and off of the oxygen flow). Cover the ventilation port with your hand and stop the oxygen flow. The audible alarm should sound. If it does not, do not use the machine. (Ventilators are not practical during time of noise discipline.)

Attach the patient valve head securely to the endotracheal tube and monitor ventilation. Watch chest excursion, and listen to lung sounds. The lungs should be bilaterally equal and clear on both sides. Carefully monitor the patient for color, capillary refill, and oxygen saturation readings. Guide ventilation to achieve oxygen saturations of 95% or higher in serious casualties. If the alarm sounds, reduce either the ventilation rate or volume. If there is no alarm and the casualty's condition does not stabilize or improve, increase the volume or rate slightly, and again assess the casualty.

Monitor the lung sounds and other patient signs and symptoms frequently to assure continuing and proper endotracheal tube placement, chest excursion, and ventilation. Also auscultate the epigastric region to assure there is not gastric insufflation, either from a misplaced tube or from air moving around the tube's cuff.

Appendix E

MANUAL CARRY AND LIFT PROCEDURES

The skills necessary to position, lift, drag, and carry casualties are essential to your function in the tactical setting, during extraction from the fire zone, evacuation rearward, and during transport to definitive care. Positioning the casualty shifts the casualty to a position where you can employ assessment, care, a lift, a drag, or a carry. Lifts elevate the patients to a position where you can place them on a spine board, litter, or other movement device or position them for a carry. You employ a drag to move the casualty along the ground and away from danger. A carry is a technique you use rapidly to transport a casualty higher above the ground than with a drag. Carries may be emergent and move the casualty from danger, or elective, where you move the patient to a casualty collection point or higher care location. Select the various positioning, lifting, dragging, and carrying techniques to afford the greatest safety to you, other caregivers, and the patient.

Procedures Listed

I. Positioning Techniques
    Positioning techniques are procedures you use to move the casualty to a position appropriate to begin assessment, emergency care, or to drag, lift, or carry the casualty.

II. Lifts
    Lifts are movement techniques you use to place a casualty on a litter or elevate the casualty so that you can then carry him or her.

III. Drags
    Drags are one-rescuer techniques you use for rapid casualty movement out of an area of immediate danger to safe cover or concealment.

IV. Carries
    Carries are techniques you use to move a casualty away from the combat zone and to an area of more formal evacuation and transport. Carries include one-person and two-person carries.

V. Stretcher Carries
    Stretcher carries are two-, four-, or more-person carries using a rigid or semirigid device to support the casualty during the move. They are very versatile and are the mainstay of casualty transport (once out of danger) to the transport vehicle, aid station, or hospital.

I. Positioning Techniques

In many cases, the casualty is not found in a position that facilitates immediate lifting or carrying. In these cases, you roll the patient to the supine or prone position. Here assessment; casualty care; or lifting to a horizontal, semistanding, or standing (vertical) position occurs. You will use the log roll, and several of its variations, to accomplish most patient positioning in the tactical operation.

Log Roll

Use the log roll to rotate the casualty along his or her body's long axis to arrive at either a full supine or prone position. You can accomplish this move with anywhere from one to four rescuers; however, spinal alignment is easier to obtain with more assisting rescuers. It is best to move casualties with suspected spinal injury using three or four rescuers when possible.

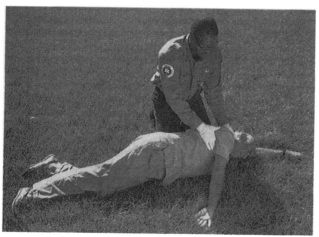

Figure E-1 One-person log roll.

Whenever you employ the log roll, attempt to maintain alignment of the nose, sternum, navel, and toes. When you use multiple rescuers, instruct each one in his or her particular responsibilities and in the cadence you will be using; for example, "we will roll the patient on the count of four." (Note, a four count allows the rescuers a better opportunity to anticipate the move.)

You may also use the log rolls to move casualties on their side so that you can negotiate a stretcher or spine board under them, then roll them back to the supine position and onto the stretcher or spine board.

One-Person Log Roll (Figure E-1).

1. Position the casualty by taking his or her leg farthest from you and crossing it over the closer leg. This applies to either the supine or prone patient.
2. Position the casualty's arms straight above his or her head (not crossed).
3. Place your hand closest to the casualty's head under the arm on the upper, lateral chest, and the other on his or her hip.
4. Gently and gradually roll the casualty toward you until he or she assumes the desired position.
5. You may use the one-person log roll to insert a stretcher or spine board. Roll the casualty halfway through the log roll, steady him or her with one hand, insert the movement device, then roll him or her back onto the device.

Two-Person Log Roll

1. Position the casualty by taking his or her leg farthest from you and crossing it over the closer leg. This applies to either the supine or prone patient.
2. Position the casualty's arms straight above his or her head (not crossed).
3. The rescuer at the head inserts his or her arm closest to the head under the casualty's head and cradles both the head and neck.
4. The rescuer at the head places his or her other hand on the casualty's lateral chest just below the arm pit.
5. The second rescuer places one hand just above the hip and the other on the lower thigh.
6. Using a cadence determined by the rescuer at the head, the rescuers gently and gradually roll the casualty to the desired position.
7. The rescuers may use the two-person log roll to insert a stretcher or spine board. They roll the casualty halfway through the log roll (the casualty on his or her side), insert the movement device, then roll him or her back onto the device.

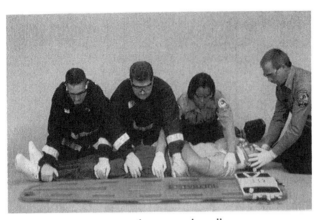

Figure E-2 Supine-to-supine four-person log roll.

Four-Person Log Roll (Spinal Injury)

Your log roll for the spinal injury casualty places him or her supine on the long spine board. Accomplish this by rotating the casualty to his or her side then back down when found supine or to his or her side, then continue the roll to supine when you find the casualty in a prone position.

Supine-to-Supine Log Roll (Figure E-2)

1. The rescuer at the head assumes stabilization of the head in a neutral position.
2. Position the casualty for the log roll, with his or her arm (on the side of the roll) above the head and the feet crossed.
3. A second rescuer applies a properly sized cervical collar.
4. The second rescuer then kneels with his or her knees directly against the casualties rib cage.
5. The second rescuer then places one hand on the casualty's opposite shoulder and the other on the lower lateral chest with the casualty's arm across the chest.
6. The third rescuer kneels with his or her knees directly against the casualty's pelvis and thigh.
7. The third rescuer places one hand on the opposite hip and the other on the opposite thigh.
8. The fourth rescuer readies the spine board for insertion.
9. Using a cadence determined by the rescuer at the head, gently and gradually roll the casualty to his or her side.
10. Insert the spine board to where the casualty meets the ground, tilting it as necessary to assure the edge of the board meets the edge of the casualty.
11. Using a cadence determined by the rescuer at the head, gently and gradually roll the casualty back to the full supine position and on the spine board or stretcher.
12. If the casualty is not centered on the spine board, the team gently and gradually shifts him or her to a centered position using a cadence determined by the rescuer at the head.

Prone-to-Supine Log Roll

The prone-to-supine log roll rolls the patient 90 degrees, allows for repositioning of the rescuers, and then concludes with a second motion (roll) to bring the patient to the full supine (or prone) position.

1. The rescuer at the head assumes stabilization of the head in a neutral position.
2. Position the casualty for the log roll, with his or her arm (on the side of the roll) above the head and the feet crossed.
3. A second rescuer applies a properly sized cervical collar.

4. The second rescuer then kneels with his or her knees directly against the casualty's rib cage.
5. The second rescuer then places one hand on the casualty's opposite shoulder and the other on the lower lateral chest with the casualty's arm across the chest.
6. The third rescuer kneels with his or her knees directly against the casualty's pelvis and thigh.
7. The third rescuer places one hand on the opposite hip and the other on the opposite thigh.
8. Using a cadence determined by the rescuer at the head, gently and gradually roll the casualty to his or her side.
9. Rescuers carefully move back from the casualty while maintaining the casualty's position on his or her side.
10. The fourth rescuer gently and carefully negotiates the spine board between the casualty and rescuers.
11. Using a cadence determined by the rescuer at the head, gently and gradually continue the roll to the full supine position.
12. The rescuer at the head has to reposition his or her hands due to the 180-degree rotation of the casualty. Another rescuer assumes the head support grasping the occiput and the jaw. The rescuer at the head then releases support and moves his or her hands back to the normal head support position.
13. If the casualty is not centered on the spine board, the team gently and gradually shifts him or her to a centered position using a cadence determined by the rescuer at the head.

II. Lifts

You will often find it necessary to elevate a casualty to place a spine board, stretcher, or other movement device beneath him or her. You may also need to position a casualty in an upright position to then move him or her off the battlefield or over rough terrain, using a carry. Such techniques, called lifts, use body mechanics and the casualty's momentum to move the casualty's center of gravity upwards. Ultimately, lifts result in the casualty elevated to a vertical or horizontal position.

Horizontal Lifts

Four-Person Lift

The four-person lift elevates a casualty for insertion of a stretcher, spine board, or other movement device.
1. Place the first rescuer at the casualty's shoulders on one knee with one hand passing under the neck supporting the neck and head while the other passes under the casualty's back and supports the lower chest.
2. Place the second rescuer at the casualty's hip on one knee with one hand passing under the small of the back supporting the pelvis and the other under the thigh.
3. Place a third rescuer at the casualty's knee on one knee with one hand passing under the lower thigh and the other under the lower calf.
4. Place the fourth rescuer opposite the other rescuers with his or her hands under the shoulder and hip.
5. Using a cadence determined by the rescuer at the head, have the rescuers lift the casualty and rotate the casualty toward the three rescuers.
6. Have the fourth rescuer place the movement device under the casualty.
7. Have the three rescuers, guided by the fourth rescuer and using a cadence determined by the rescuer at the head, lower the casualty to the movement device.

Two-Person Lift

The two-person lift accomplishes what the four-person lift does, though it is more awkward, and there is greater danger in injuring the casualty and rescuers (Figure E-3).
1. Place the first rescuer at the casualty's shoulders on one knee with one hand passing under the neck supporting the neck and head while the other passes under the casualty's back and supports the lower chest.
2. Place the second rescuer at the casualty's hip on one knee with one hand passing under the small of the back supporting the pelvis and the other under the upper leg, just above the calf.

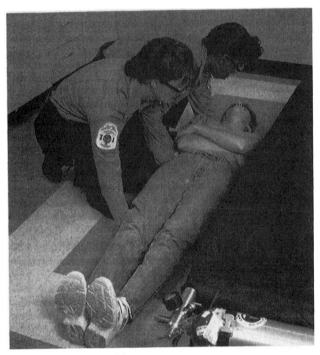

Figure E-3 Two-person lift.

3. Using a cadence determined by the rescuer at the head, have the rescuers lift the casualty and rotate him or her toward the rescuers.
4. Have the rescuers move to a standing position and walk with the casualty to an awaiting movement device.
5. Using a cadence determined by the rescuer at the head, have the rescuers lower the casualty to the awaiting movement device.

Straddle Lift

The straddle lift uses several rescuers, straddling the casualty and gently lifting him or her a few inches off the ground. Insert the movement device beneath the casualty from the head or feet. With four rescuers, the straddle slide accommodates spinally injured casualties. It is also effective in moving casualties into and out of devices like the Stoke's basket and SKED.

1. Position the casualty in the supine position.
2. Place the first rescuer above the casualty's head straddling the casualty with his or her legs spread just wider than the spine board or stretcher. Facing the casualty's feet, he or she supports the casualty's head.
3. Place a second rescuer straddling the casualty at the casualty's waist with his or her legs spread just wider than the spine board or stretcher. Facing the casualty's head, he or she supports the casualty's shoulder.
4. Place a third rescuer straddling the casualty at the casualty's thighs with his or her legs spread just wider than the spine board or stretcher. Facing the casualty's head, he or she supports the casualty's hip.
5. Place a fourth rescuer at the casualty's head facing the other rescuers with his or her feet spread just wider than the spine board or stretcher. He or she carefully inserts the movement device after the lift.
6. Using a cadence determined by the rescuer holding the head, have the rescuers lift the casualty a few inches higher than the clearance needed for the movement device.

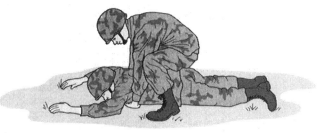

A

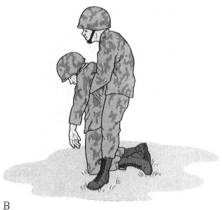

B

Figure E-4 Vertical lift—torso approach—to knees.

7. The fourth rescuer gently inserts the movement device, pushing the feet up as it is inserted fully.
8. Using a cadence determined by the rescuer at the head, the rescuers lower the casualty to the movement device.

Vertical Lift

The vertical lift moves the casualty from a supine or prone position to a full upright position. There you can get under the casualty or bring his or her arms over your shoulders to effect one of the carries listed later in this appendix.

Torso Approach
1. Place the patient in the prone position with his or her arms above their head.
2. Stoop at about the casualty's midback, straddling him or her.
3. Lock your hands under the casualty's arms and in front of his or her chest.
4. Using your legs, and keeping your weight back, pull the casualty backward to his or her knees (Figure E-4).
5. Rocking, then moving back one step, lift the casualty to his or her feet.
6. To turn the casualty, lift one arm above your head, tuck your head under his or her arm, and step around the casualty.

Head Approach
1. Place the casualty in the prone position with his or her arms to the side.
2. Position yourself squatting at the casualty's head.
3. Place your hands under the casualty's arms, and lift him or her toward the kneeling position Figure E-5).

4. Lock your arms behind the casualty's back, and draw him or her to a full kneeling position.
5. Gradually move to a standing position (Figure E-6).
6. Move your hands to under the casualty's upper rib cage.
7. Lift the casualty to his or her feet and walk forward one step. This will lock the casualty's legs.

III. Drags

Drags are movement techniques intended to extract a casualty from danger. Although you can effect drags without assistance, they may aggravate the casualty's injuries. Select such a technique when you need to limit casualty and rescuer exposure to enemy fire and when concern for causing further injury is less than potential injury by leaving them where they lie. Use drags to move the casualty from danger to safe cover or concealment where further, more extensive care and stabilization can be offered. Then use carries to more safely evacuate the casualty.

Cradle Drop (or Cloths) Drag

During the cradle drop drag, you grasp the cloth of the casualty's shirt or jacket at the shoulders and upper back. The pull exerts a force on the shoulders while you cradle the neck and head with your hands and forearms. This drag minimizes the danger of aggravating any spinal injury and moves the casualty along the long axis of the body. The procedure is somewhat awkward since you

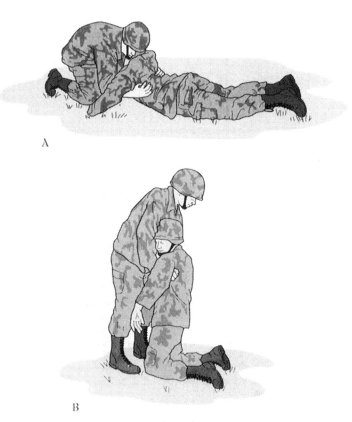

A

B

Figure E-5 Vertical lift—head approach—to knees.

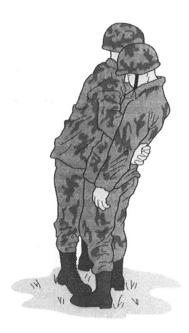

Figure E-6 Vertical lift—head approach—to standing.

move backward to move the casualty. It is most often successful when you are larger than the casualty (Figure E-7).

1. Position the casualty in the supine position with his or her arms and legs aligned along the axis of the body.
2. Position yourself squatting at the casualty's head.
3. Grasp the cloth of the casualty's shirt at the shoulder and upper back on each side of the head and neck.
4. Cradle the head and neck between your hands and forearms.
5. Pull strongly and smoothly along the axis of the body while backing away from the casualty. Assure the clothing does not place pressure on the casualty's neck during the move.

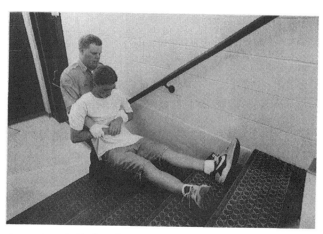

Figure E-7 Cradle drop drag.

6. Keep the casualty's head and neck as close to the ground as you can while still maintaining your balance and ability to move the casualty.

Sling Drag

The sling drag uses a short (6-8', continuous loop) length of wide diameter rope, two pistol belts connected together, or a fabric loop to move the casualty. Place the loop across the casualty's chest and under the arms, and behind the back. Then you either pull along the long axis of the body or loop the other end of the belt or rope over your head and shoulder to pull as you crawl. When you pull along the long axis of the body, this technique limits movement of the head and neck (Figure E-8).

1. Place the casualty in the supine position with his or her hands tied together over the upper abdomen.
2. Place the loop across the casualty's chest, under his or her arms, and coming out under the head. If you tie the rope, belt, or fabric behind the casualty's neck, it will provide a more direct pull on the shoulders.
3. Grasp the rope at its end and pull along the long axis of the casualty's body, or place your head and arm through the loop and crawl, dragging the casualty. With the crawl method, the casualty's head and neck remain unsupported.

Neck Drag

The neck drag moves the casualty along the axis of the body while you remain stable on all fours. The technique is not a quick move and does not protect the casualty's head and neck. However, the procedure is one that uses good body mechanics to move the casualty and allows a small rescuer to move a rather heavy casualty (Figure E-9).

1. Position the casualty in the supine position and align the arms and legs along the axis of the body.
2. Tie the casualty's hands together with a cravat or short length of webbing or rope.

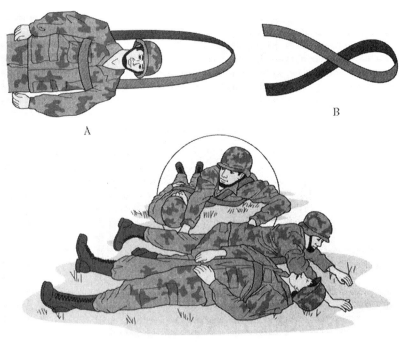

A

B

C

Figure E-8 Sling drag.

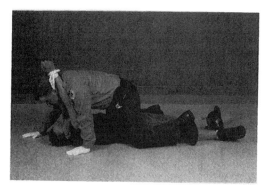

Figure E-9 Neck drag.

3. Position yourself straddling the patient with your head at the casualty's head.
4. Place your head through the casualty's tied hands and arms.
5. Crawl on all fours using your neck and shoulders to pull the casualty along.
6. If possible, crawl on your knees and one hand while using the other hand to cradle the casualty's head and neck.

IV. Carries

Carries are one- and two-person procedures you use to move casualties rapidly from the field of battle or over rough or debris strewn terrain. One-person carries include the support, saddle back, pack-strap, and fireman's carries. They are relatively unstable and expose both the rescuer and casualty to more enemy fire than the lower profile drags. Two-person carries include the support, fore and aft, and two-hand seat carries.

One-Person Carries

Support Carry

The support carry is a one person technique that supports a semicooperative casualty rather than lifting his or her entire weight. Although the casualty must be able to move somewhat on his or her own, the rescuer can guide and stabilize the casualty's movement to safe cover or concealment (Figure E-10).
1. Help the casualty up to the standing position, possibly using one of the lifting techniques addressed earlier.
2. Place the casualty's arm over your shoulder, grasp the wrist tightly, and pull down with your hand.
3. Wrap your opposite hand around the casualty's back and help stabilize him or her as he or she walks.

Saddleback Carry

The saddleback carry requires a conscious or semiconscious casualty that can at least hold on to your shoulders and neck during the carry. It also carries the casualty very high, resulting in your instability when traveling over rough terrain (Figure E-11).
1. Squat down while the casualty straddles your hips.
2. Grasp each of the casualty's legs, just above the knees, from around the outside and lock your hands in front of the abdomen.
3. Have the casualty lean forward and wrap his or her arms around your neck and shoulders.
4. Rise to a full standing position and walk.

Pack-Strap Carry

The pack-strap carry accommodates an unconscious casualty and keeps his or her weight slightly lower than the saddleback carry. It employs good mechanical advantage to lift the casualty but can move the casualty only for a moderate distance (Figure E-12).

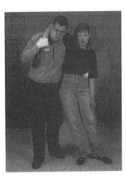

Figure E-10 Support
carry—one person.

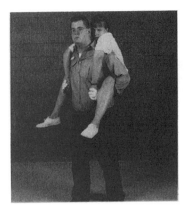

Figure E-11 Saddleback carry.

1. Using a lift, bring the casualty to an upright position. Then, position the casualty standing behind you.
2. Bring the each of the casualty's arms over your respective shoulder.
3. Pull the casualty's arms downward by placing your forearm across his or her arms.
4. Lean forward, lifting the casualty's weight with your shoulders and legs.
5. Walk, carrying the casualty.

Fireman's Carry

The fireman's carry permits you to easily carry a casualty and for a reasonable distance. However, it is difficult to get the casualty up and on your shoulders. Once there, your center of gravity is very high, leading to instability (Figure E-13).

1. Using a lift, bring the casualty to an upright position. Then, position yourself face to face with the casualty.
2. Grasp the casualty's left arm, and place your head under his or her arms and chest.
3. Quickly drop to one knee and allow the casualty to bend at the waist and come to rest across your shoulders while bringing the casualty's left hand down to your waist.
4. Reach around the casualty's left leg and grasp the casualty's left wrist.
5. Rise to a full standing position.
6. Walk, carrying the casualty.

This carry may be reversed, using the casualty's right arm and wrist.

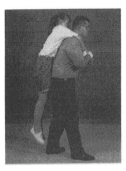

Figure E-12 Packstrap
carry.

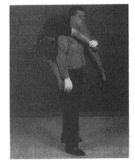

Figure E-13 Fireman's
carry.

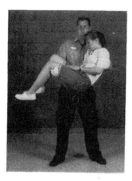

Figure E-14 Arm's carry.

Arms Carry

The arms carry uses one rescuer to carry the casualty in his or her arms. It is only useful for short distances, like transferring a casualty from one stretcher or bed to another or for short moves. It is awkward and does not support the casualty well. It also places the weight of the full casualty on one rescuer during movement to the standing position (Figure E-14).

1. Place the casualty in the supine position.
2. Kneel next to the casualty and place your hands under the upper back and the casualty's knees.
3. Rotate 90 degrees and hold the casualty against your body.
4. Rise to a standing position, then walk with the casualty.

Two-Person Carries

Two-Person Support Carry

The two-person support carry supports a casualty without carrying his or her full weight. The casualty need not be conscious because you may use the technique to drag him or her to safe cover or concealment (Figure E-15).

1. Bring the casualty up to the standing position, using one of the lifting techniques addressed earlier.
2. You and an assisting rescuer place the casualty's arms over your shoulders, then each of you grasp the casualty's wrist tightly and pull down.
3. Both of rescuers then wrap your free hands around the casualty's back and help stabilize him or her as he or she walks.

This carry may be modified by the rescuers supporting and lifting the casualty's thighs instead of placing their hands behind the casualty's back. This permits you to carry the casualty over rough ground. It is, however, useful only for short distances.

Fore and Aft Carry

The fore and aft carry is a simple and effective technique to move a casualty short distances over smooth to moderately rough terrain. It does not provide spinal support or accommodate casualty injuries very well. It does permit movement through narrow trails or hallways (Figure E-16).

1. Position the casualty supinely, then have one rescuer approach from the head, squat, move the casualty to a semiseated position, place his or her hands under the casualty's arms, and lock them across the chest. *In an alternative technique, the rescuer places the casualty's arms crossed over the chest and hands under their opposite arm pits. The rescuer then grasps the casualty's wrists.*
2. Direct the second rescuer to stand between the casualty's feet, facing away. He or she then squats down and grasps the casualty's legs from the outside and just above the knees.
3. Using a cadence determined by the rescuer at the head and chest, have both rescuers move from the squatting to full standing position.
4. The casualty moves as both rescuers walk with direction provided by the rescuer at the casualty's feet.

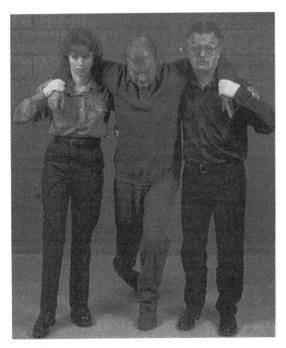

Figure E-15 Two-person support carry.

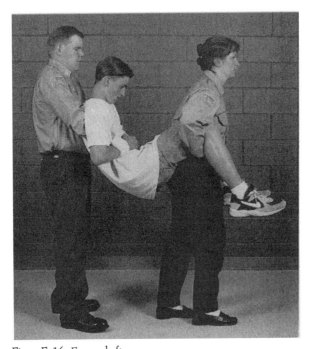

Figure E-16 Fore and aft carry.

372 *Tactical Emergency Care*

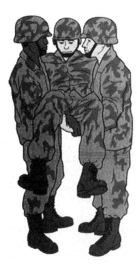

Figure E-17 Two-hand seat carry.

5. You may alter this procedure by directing the rescuer at the feet to face the casualty before the lift. Then the team can move sideways with the casualty.

Two-Hand Seat Carry

The two-hand seat carry is a efficient carry when you have easy access to both sides of the casualty and your evacuation route is relatively wide. The carry is difficult for long distances since rescuers stand and move sideways to the direction of travel (Figure E-17).

1. Position the casualty supine on the ground.
2. You and another rescuer approach the casualty from opposite sides.
3. Squat at the casualty's side, bring the casualty to a seated position, and lock your hands under his or her midback and upper thighs.
4. Using a cadence determined by you, you and the other rescuer rise to a standing position.

V. Stretcher Carries

The stretcher is a movement device popular and effective for moving casualties since their transport and care became important, early in warfare. It remains a very important and useful movement and evacuation device during the modern tactical operation. Stretcher carries use the stretcher, spine board, or other devices as a platform supporting the casualty while two, four, or more bearers move the casualty.

Traditionally, military medics spent a great deal of time learning and practicing litter bearer team drills. The goal was to achieve a coordinated, flowing execution of litter commands, much akin to military drill and ceremony. Although coordinated movement is important, overemphasis on crisp commands and flawless execution detract from the primary goal: safe and effective casualty movement. The modern approach keeps the principles of fluid, coordinated movement, but deemphasizes repetitive drill.

The "prepare to lift" and "prepare to lower" commands are the most important because they prepare and direct your team to raise up and set down the litter. These actions place the most risk on the bearers and patient because of the changing loads and direction. Other commands, such as "prepare to move, move" and "prepare to stop, stop" are likewise useful. Other commands like "prepare to rotate, rotate" may be useful; however, the emphasis should be on smooth and safe casualty movement.

Two-Person Stretcher Carry

1. Load the casualty on the stretcher using one of the lifts or carries previously mentioned.
2. Place one bearer at the head and one at the foot end facing to move the casualty feet first.
3. Both bearers squat and grasp the pole ends.
4. Using a cadence determined by the bearer at the head, they, together, lift the stretcher as they move to the full standing position.

Four-Person Stretcher Carry (Figure E-18)

1. Load the casualty on the stretcher using one of the lifts or carries previously mentioned.
2. Place one bearer on either side of the stretcher at the foot and head end.
3. They squat, facing to move the casualty feet first, and grasp the stretcher pole end with the inside hand.
4. Using a cadence determined by one of the bearers at the head, they move to the standing position, lifting the stretcher and casualty with them.

When moving up a steep hill, move the casualty with a head first direction of travel. This will prevent the apprehension from being moved head down. Otherwise, the direction the casualty faces with respect to travel is secondary to a smooth and safe transport. When approaching a sharp drop or rise in terrain or a barrier, have two litter bearers go ahead and accept the stretcher as it is raised or lowered.

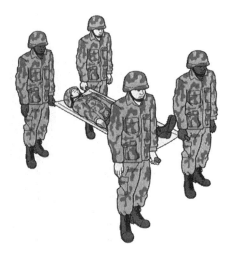

Figure E-18 Four-person stretcher carry.

Glossary

Acetylcholine is a critical neurotransmitter in neuromuscular and glandular control. Nerve agents disrupt the orderly degradation of acetylcholine.

Ambulatory is able to walk, as in ambulatory patient.

Angle of Louis is a palpable notch on the anterior surface of the sternum 1 1/2 to 2 inches from its superior edge, used to locate the second and third intercostal space.

Auto Extraction is having a patient move himself out of a hazardous zone.

Ballistics is the study of projectile motion and the interaction among the gun, air, and target.

Biological Agent is a natural substance which causes serious effects on man at low concentrations and is often lethal.

Blast is an extremely high pressure caused by explosives.

Body Surface Area is the amount (in percent) affected by burns.

Caliber is the diameter of a bullet expressed in 100ths of an inch (22 caliber = .22 inches).

Capnometer is a device to measure expired carbon dioxide level.

Care Under Fire is the first stage of tactical care, occurs while the casualty is still threatened by enemy fire.

Carry is a rapid movement technique where the carrier remains standing and the casualty is lifted above the carrier's waist.

Casualty Evacuation Care is the third stage of tactical care, occurs only once the casualty is being moved to definitive care.

Catheter is a hollow plastic tube covering a metal tube, inserted into a vein to provide venous access for administering fluids and medications.

Cavitation is the energy wave creating pressure, stretching, and a temporary cavity during bullet passage through a semi-fluid medium.

Chemical Agent is a man-made substance which causes serious effects on man at low concentrations and is often lethal.

Concealment is an object that hides your presence from the enemy, e.g., bushes or camouflage netting.

Cover is an object or terrain that provides protection against small arms fire, e.g., boulder or large tree.

Cricothrotomy is a surgical incision through the cricothyroid membrane to establish an emergency airway.

Cricothyrostomy is an emergency airway established by inserting one or several large-bore needles through the cricothyroid membrane.

Cyanide is a prototypical chemical agent that causes cellular hypoxia by disrupting key respiratory and metabolic enzymes.

Cytochrome a3 is a critical enzyme of cellular respiration. Inactivated by cyanide.

Delayed is the second highest triage category.

DNA (Deoxyribonucleic Acid) is a major building block of the body's cell and contains genetic information needed to synthesize proteins.

Dosimeter is a personnel monitoring device that measures the amount of ionizing radiation absorbed by the wearer.

Drag is a rapid movement technique that moves the casualty along the ground.

End expiratory CO_2 detector is a colormetric (different colors reflect different concentrations) device used to detect expired CO_2 and thereby identify proper endotracheal tube placement.

Endotracheal Tube is a cuffed hollow plastic tube placed into the trachea to provide a protected airway for ventilation and suctioning.

Echelon is a level.

Expectant is the lowest priority triage category.

Extraction is the rapid movement of a casualty from the risk of enemy fire to cover or concealment.

Firestorm is an intense area of combustion caused as debris ignited by the heat of a nuclear blast, and is fanned by the air drawn as the mushroom cloud rises.

Fission is the breaking apart of a large nucleus into smaller ones to release nuclear energy.

Fusion is the combining of two smaller nuclei into a larger one to release nuclear energy.

Geneva Conventions—see "Laws of War."

Gray is a standard unit of absorbed nuclear radiation energy.

Hemoglobin is the primary oxygen-carrying protein in red blood cells.

HMMWV is a wide track four wheel drive military utility vehicle that can be configured as an ambulance.

Humvee—see HMMWV.

Immediate is the highest priority triage category.

Irrigation is the application of sterile fluid to rinse away contamination from a wound.

Isotope is a molecular variation of an element that may be unstable and give off radioactive particles and rays.

Kinetic Energy is the energy of an object in motion related to its mass and velocity.

Laryngoscope is a lighted metal tongue blade and handle used to visualize the oral pharynx, vocal folds, and trachea to guide proper placement of the endotracheal tube.

Lateral Recumbent is a body position where the patient is placed on the side (recovery position).

Laws of War are a set of laws that guide the conduct of combatants and noncombatants alike during war. Also called the "Geneva Conventions."

Lift is a technique that moves the casualty in preparation for drag or carry.

Litter Patient is a patient who is unable to walk.

M-113 is a tracked armored personnel carrier that may be configured to carry casualties.

Mass is the quantity of matter as measured by its inertia. Weight is an object's mass as attracted to the earth by gravity.

Medevac refers to the medical evacuation of casualties, usually by helicopter.

Medical Direction is the physician oversight of all medical care.

Methemoglobin is hemoglobin chemically reduced by nitrites or other medications.

Minimal is the third highest triage category.

Nerve Agent is a type of chemical agent that inhibits the critical enzyme Acetylcholinesterase. This causes widespread cholinergic crisis, paralysis, and death.

Nucleus is the massive center of the atom. It contains neutrons and protons.

Portal of Entry is a route by which a chemical or biological agent enters the body (e.g., skin, respiratory tract).

Precedence is the priority for transport of the wounded casualty in a multi- or mass casualty circumstance.

Profile is the bullet surface area exposed to the target. It is the energy exchange surface.

Prognosis is the anticipated outcome for a casualty based on the known mechanism of injury, signs and symptoms determined by the field of evaluation.

Projectile is an object traveling in flight. It has kinetic energy and the potential to cause damage.

Pulmonary Agent is a group of chemical agents that cause direct damage to the respiratory tract leading to pulmonary edema, hypoxia, and death.

Pulse Oximetry is a device that measures oxygen levels in the arterial hemoglobin of distal tissues such as the skin. It gives a real-time evaluation of the effectiveness of the cardiorespiratory system.

REM (Roentgen Equivalent Man) is a standardized dosage of nuclear radiation based on the effects it has on man. Some radiation is more damaging than other of equal energy. Living at sea level results in a radiation exposure of about 30 milliREM per year.

Resiliency is the ability of tissue to return to its original position after the stretching due to a projectile's cavitational wave passage.

Riot Control Agents are a group of chemical agents that are not normally lethal but cause temporary incapacitation (e.g., eye pain and tearing).

Rules of Engagement are a set of rules that guide tactical personnel in interacting with perpetrators or the enemy.

Saline Lock is a short length of intravenous tubing attached to a catheter to serve as an intravenous access port.

Shrapnel are fragments of metal and other debris propelled at high speed by an explosion.

Spall is the spray of fragments from the inside of an object struck by a projectile.

Stylet is a malleable metal rod inserted into an endotracheal tube to stiffen and prebend it for endotracheal intubation.

Tactical Field Care is the second stage of care, occurs once the casualty is no longer under imminent threat of hostile fire. Includes many of the emergency care principles traditionally found in prehospital care, but tailored for the tactical environment.

Tactical Medic is a medical personnel, usually trained to the EMT or paramedic level, who supports military or civilian tactical operations.

Trajectory is the path traveled by a projectile.

Vector is an animal (usually an insect) that transmits disease.

Velocity is the movement of an object over time, its speed.

Vesicant Agent is a type of chemical agent that causes direct skin and mucous membrane damage leading to serious chemical burns.

Yaw is the cyclic sideways movement or rotation (wobble) of a projectile during flight.

Abbreviations

ABC   Airway, Breathing, and Circulation
AC   Hydrogen Cyanide
ACH   Acetylcholine
ACHE   Acetylcholinesterase
AVPU   Alert, Verbal, Painful Stimuli, and Unresponsive

BEM   Blast Effect Munition
bid   Twice Daily
BP   Blood Pressure
BSA   Body Surface Area

CG   Phosgene
CK   Cyanogen Chloride
CN   Mace
CNS   Central Nervous System
CONTOMS   Counter Narcotic Tactical Operations Medical Support
CO_2 Carbon Dioxide
CPR   Cardiopulmonary Resuscitation
CS   "Tear Gas"

D5W   5% Dextrose in water solution

ECG   Electrocardiograph
ED   Emergency Department
EMS   Emergency Medical Services
EMT   Emergency Medical Technician
ET   Endotracheal
$ETCO_2$ End-Tidal Carbon Dioxide

FMC   Field Medical Card

GA   Tabun
GB   Sarin
GD   Soman

HC   Smoke
HMMWV   High Mobility Multipurpose Wheeled Vehicle

ICS   Incident Command System
IM   Intramuscular
IR   Infrared
IV   Intravenous

KVO   Keep Vein Open

MAB   Medicine Across the Barricade
MASCAL   Mass Casualty (incident)
MAST   Medical Antishock Trousers
MCI   Mass Casualty Incident
MRE   Meal Ready to Eat

NATO   North Atlantic Treaty Organization
NBC   Nuclear, Biologic, and Chemical

OC   Oleoresin Capsicum (pepper spray)
OP ORDER   Operations Order
OSHA   Occupational Safety and Health Administration
OTC   Over the Counter

PA   Physician Assistant
PASG   Pneumatic Antishock Garment
po   By Mouth

qd   Once Daily
qid   Four Times Daily

RAM   Remote Assessment Methodology
RF   Radio Frequency

SEB   Staphylococcal Enterotoxin B
SLUDGE   Salivation, Lacrimation, Urination, Diarrhea, Gastric Emptying
SOP   Standard Operating Procedure
SQ   Subcutaneous
START   Simple Triage and Rapid Treatment

TEMS   Tactical Emergency Medical Support
tid   Three Times Daily
TKO   To Keep Open
TNT   Trinitrotoluene

SWAT   Special Weapons and Tactics

UV   Ultraviolet

WBGT   Wet Bulb Globe Temperature (index)
WP   White Phosphorous

Index

intra-abdominal and thoracic, 23

Blisters, 276, 281–82

Blood cells, radiation exposure injury and, 159

Blood pressure (BP)
in projectile injury casualties, 59–60
sphygmomanometer for measuring, 218

Blunt trauma, from nuclear detonation, 174

Body armor, for laser protection, 87

Body surface area (BSA), in burn injuries, 76

Bolus administration, 22

Bone, projectile injuries in, 42–43

Bone marrow, radiation exposure injury and, 159

Botulinum, 138–39

Bowel injuries
in blast casualties, 70–71
radiation exposure injury and, 159

Breathing (ventilation), 17. See also Airway
assessment of projectile injury casualties and, 54–55
evacuation and assessment of, 212–14
evacuation of casualties and, 220

Brucellosis, 135, 137

Bruises, 276

Bug bites. See Insect bites

Bullets. See also Projectile injuries
travel (trajectory) of, 31–36

Bumps and bruises, 276, 282–83

Burn injuries, 66, 73–90. See also Laser injuries
body surface area (BSA) affected by, 76
from flame and incendiary weapons, 79–81
from laser beam devices, 81–86
management of, 76
from masers and microwave devices, 87–89
mechanism of, 74
medical effects of, 74–75
thermal, from nuclear detonation, 157–58

Calamine lotion, 317

Caliber, 34

Cancer, radiation exposure injury and, 160

Cannon, 38

Capnometer, 219–20

Carbamate insecticides and medications, 97

Carbon monoxide
pulse oximeter and, 359
poisoning, 277

Cardiac arrest
evaluating, 25
nontraumatic, 24–25

Cardiac dysrhythmias, 218

Cardiopulmonary resuscitation (CPR), 24
tactical exceptions to use of, 25
in the warm zone, 298

Cardiovascular system, radiation exposure injury and, 160

Care. See Medical care

Carries, 192, 372–77
one-person, 372–74
stretcher, 376–77
two-person, 374–76

Casualties, evacuation of. See Evacuation

Casualty assessment. See Assessment of casualties

Catheter
bladder, 228
intravenous, 336–38

Cavitation, 39

Cefazolin (Ancef), 62, 313

Cefoxitin (Mefoxin), 62–63

Cervical spine, immobilization of, 16–17, 298–99

Chain of command, 7

Chain reaction, in nuclear explosions, 152–53

Chemical agents (chemical weapons). See also Nerve agents
current threat of, 94
cyanide poisoning, 105–9
decontamination of casualties, 122–25
history of, 94
nature of, 94–95
portal of entry of, 95
protection from, 115–22, 320–36
individual decontamination, 119
litter patients, decontamination procedure for, 328–33
M17 series mask and hood, 322–24
M40 series mask and hood, 320–22
M258A1 decontamination kit, 324–25

M291 skin decontaminating kit (SDK), 326–27
overgarments, 327–28
physical removal, 119–22
prophylaxis, 118–19
pulmonary agents, 109–13
treaty banning, 94
types of, 95
vesicants, 103–5

Chemical injuries, 93–125

Chest wounds
sucking, 18, 20
in TEMS environment, 299–300

Children, maintenance fluids for, 226

Chipped teeth, 276, 286, 287

Chlorine levels of water, 259–60

Choking agents. See Pulmonary agents

Cholera, 135–36

Circulation, 20
assessment of projectile injury casualties and, 55–56
evacuation and assessment of, 214–15
evacuation of casualties and, 224

Clearance for incarceration, 303–5

Cold environment, 4

Cold injuries, 255–58

Cold zone, 294–95

Comfort of patients, evacuation and, 228–29

Communication with barricaded subject(s), 302

Concealment, 10

Connective tissue, projectile injuries in, 42

Consciousness, level of, 52

Convenient casualties, 187

Cornea, laser injuries to, 85

Cough, 276, 277–78

Counter Narcotics Tactical Operations Medical Support (CONTOMS), 300, 301, 306

Cover, 10

CPR. See Cardiopulmonary resuscitation

Cradle drop (or cloths) drag, 370–71

Cricothyrostomy, 54

Cricothyrotomy, 16, 54

Cricothyrotomy (cricothyrostomy), 355–57

Cuts and scratches, 276, 283–85

Cyanide (cyanide poisoning), 105–9

Cytochrome a3, 106

thermal burn injuries from nuclear detonation, 158
Fallout, nuclear, 154–56
Feet, cold injuries to, 257
Fever, 276
    ambulatory care of, 279
    Argentine hemorrhagic, 137
    dengue, 135, 137
    Q, 134
    Rift Valley, 137
    viral hemorrhagic, 135, 137–38
    yellow, 135, 137, 138
Field sanitation, 262–66
Firestorm, 158
Fission, nuclear, 151
Flail chest, 55
Flame and incendiary weapons, 79–81
Fluid resuscitation, 21–22
    in burn injuries, 76–78
    in projectile injury casualties, 59–60
    in shock, 23
Fluids, maintenance, evacuation of casualties and, 225
Focused physical assessment of projectile injury casualties, 57
Foodborne illness, 258–60
Food preparation and handling, 260–62
Fragmentation of bullets, 35
Frostbite, 255
Fusion, nuclear, 153

Gamma radiation, 154–55
Garments, protective, 115–18, 327–28
    removal of, 123
Geneva Conventions (Laws of War), 10
Gloves, 51

Handguns, 36–37
Handwashing, 261–62
Hantavirus, 137
Hazmat (hazardous materials) teams, 115
Head, projectile injuries in, 44, 56
Headache, 276, 277
Hearing loss, blast injuries and, 70, 71, 72
HEAT (high-energy antitank) rounds, 38
Heat injuries, 253–55
Helicopters, evacuation by, 5–6, 202–5
Hemoglobin, 107

Hemorrhage (hemorrhage control)
    assessment of projectile injury casualties and, 55–56
    control of, 12
Hemorrhagic fevers
    Argentine, 137
    viral, 137
High-energy antitank (HEAT) rounds, 38
HMMWV (humvee) vehicles, 199–201
Hollow organs
    in blast casualties, 71, 72
    projectile injuries in, 42
Hot zone, 294
"Huey" helicopters, 202
Hygiene, personal, 262–63
Hypothermia, 255
Hypoxia, endotracheal tube suctioning and, 222

Ibuprofen (Advil, Nuprin, Motrin IB), 318
Immediate category, 239, 240
Immediate category of triage, 234–35, 239, 240
Immersion foot, 255
Immobilization, cervical spine, 298
Immunization. See also Vaccine
    against biological weapons, 146–47
Incarceration, clearance for, 303–5
Incendiary devices, 79–81
Incident command system (ICS), 244
Infection, wound, 286–87
Initial assessment, 52
    and care, 11
    and management, 15–16
Inner perimeter, 293
Insect bites, 276, 280–81
Insects, disease-carrying, 266–67
Intramuscular medication administration, 344–47
Intravenous
    catheter introduction, 336–38
    drip administration, 340
    fluids (intravenous fluid therapy), 21, 27
    (IV) access, 20–22
    medication administration, 343–44
Irrigation, 59
    of cuts and scratches, 285–86
    for vesicant-exposed casualties, 104–5

Jungle environment, 3–4
Kao-Pectate (attapulgite), 317
"Keep vein open" drip rate, 22
Kinetic energy, projectile, 32
Knives, 39

Landing zone for helicopters, 203–4
Laryngoscope, 53
Laser beams
    attenuation of, 83
    characteristics of, 82
    reflection of, 82
Laser injuries, 81–87
    assessment of, 85
    beam characteristics, 82
    burns, 85
    definitive care for, 86–87
    management of, 85
    medical effects of, 83
    protection from, 87
    supportive care, 85–86
Lassa fever, 137
Latrines, 263–66
Law enforcement, medical support for. See Tactical Emergency Medical Support (TEMS)
Laws of War (Geneva Conventions), 10
Lens, laser injuries to, 84
Level of consciousness, 52
Lewisite, 103–5
Lifting and movement of casualties, 184, 191–95, 363–77
    carries, 192, 194, 372–77
    drags, 192, 193, 368–72
    four-person log roll (spinal injury), 364
    horizontal lifts, 366–67
    lifts, 192–93
    log roll, 363–64
    one-person log roll, 364
    positioning of casualties, 192
    prone-to-supine log roll, 365–66
    stretcher carries, 194–95
    supine-to-supine log roll, 365
    two-person log roll, 364
    vertical lifts, 367–68
Lifts, 192–93, 366–68
Log roll, 363–64
    four-person (spinal injury), 364
    one-person, 364
    prone-to-supine, 365–66
    supine-to-supine, 365
    two-person, 364
Low flow states, 360

Lungs
blast injuries and, 69–70, 71
nerve agents and, 97
projectile injuries in, 42

**M17 series mask and hood,
322–24**
M40 series mask and hood,
320–22
M-113 armored and tracked vehi-
cles, 199–201
M258A1 decontamination kit,
324–25
M291 skin decontaminating kit
(SDK), 326–27
Maalox, 316–17
MAB (Medicine Across the
Barricade), 301–3
Mace, 113
Machine gun, 37
Magnesium burns, 79
Maintenance fluids, evacuation of
casualties and, 225
Marburg virus, 137
Masers, 87–89
Masks
for biological agents, 145–46
for chemical agents, 115
M40 series, 320–22
Mass, projectile kinetic energy
and, 32–34
Mass casualty incidents (MCI or
MASCAL), 243–46
MAST (medical antishock
trousers), 23, 209–10
Meal, ready to eat (MRE), 261
Medical care
under fire, 9
principles of, 8
stages of, 9
Medical clearance for incarcera-
tion, 304
Medical direction, 8
Medical evacuation (medevac),
180
helicopters, 202–5
Medical intelligence, 253
Medical threat assessment,
251–53
Medications (drugs), 24, 311–19
evacuation of casualties and,
227
preparing a solution for administration, 342–43
redosing of, during evacuation,
27
Medicine Across the Barricade
(MAB), 301–3
Medics. See also specific topics
definition of, 3
mission of, 6–8

role of, 8
Mefoxin (Cefoxitin), 62–63
Mental status, evacuation and
assessment of, 216
Methemoglobin, 108
METTAGs, 244–46
Microwave devices, 87–89
Military overgarment, 116–17
Minimal category, 241
of triage, 235
Mission of tactical medic, 6–8
Mobility, 4–6
Moisture, cold injuries and,
255–56
Monitoring of patients, during
evacuation, 27, 216–20
Morphine, 314
for projectile injury casualties,
62
Motrin IB, 318
Mountainous environment, 3
Mouth sores, 276, 288
Movement of casualties. See
Lifting and movement of casu-
alties
Moving casualties, 11
Mustards, 103–5
Mycotoxins, trichothecene, 142
Mylanta, 316–17

Napalm, 79
NATO standard method of triage,
234
Nausea, 276, 278
Neck drags, 372
Negotiators, working with, 303
Nerve agents (nerve agent poisoning), 95–103
antidote Mark I kit, 347
antidotes to, 99–100
assessment of, 97–98
autoinjectors for, 100
emergency care, 98–99
identification of an attack, 98
initial resuscitation, 99
overview of, 95–96
signs and symptoms of, 98
toxicity of, 96
triage and decision making,
102–3
Nervous system, radiation exposure injury and, 160
Neutron radiation, 155
Nuclear accidents, 164–65
triage and, 167
Nuclear casualties, 150–76. See
also Nuclear explosions
(nuclear detonation)
assessment of, 160–61, 165
care of, 169
supportive care, 173–75

decontamination of, 172–73
evacuation and sheltering of,
171–72
search and rescue of, 169–71
Nuclear explosions (nuclear detonation), 151
injury mechanisms, 154–58
radiation exposure injury from,
158–60
strategic detonation, 161–62
tactical detonation, 163–64
terrorist detonation, 162–63
thermal burns from, 157–58
triage and, 165
Nuclear fission, 151
Nuclear fusion, 151
Nuprin, 318

Oil of clove (Eugenol), 318
Ongoing assessment of projectile
injury casualties, 58
Organophosphate, 97
Outer perimeter, 293
Overgarments, protective. See
Garments, protective
Oxygen, supplemental (oxygen
therapy), 26–27
Oxygenation, evacuation of casu-
alties and, 223–24

**Pain medication, for projectile
injury casualties, 62**
Paradoxical respiration, 55
Paramedics. See Medics
Particle beam weapons, 89–90
Penetrating torso trauma, 18
Pepper spray (oleoresin capsicum,
OC), 113
Pericardial tamponade, 55
Permanent cavity, 41
Personal safety, mission and, 6
Phosgene, 109–13
Physician assistants (PAs), 8
Plague, 133
Pleural decompression, in projec-
tile injury casualties, 60–61
Pneumatic Anti-Shock Garment
(PASG), 209–10
Pneumonia-like biological agents,
132
Pneumonic plague, 133
Pneumothorax
blast injuries and, 71–72
tension, 18, 19, 55. See also
Pleural decompression
in blast casualties, 71–72
signs and symptoms of, 61
Poisoning. See also Chemical
agents
with biological toxins, 138–42
carbon monoxide, 277